THE OFFICIAL PATIENT'S SOURCEBOOK

on

MUSCULAR DYSTROPHY

JAMES N. PARKER, M.D.
AND PHILIP M. PARKER, PH.D., EDITORS

ii

ICON Health Publications
ICON Group International, Inc.
4370 La Jolla Village Drive, 4th Floor
San Diego, CA 92122 USA

Printed in the United States of America.

Last digit indicates print number: 10 9 8 7 6 4 5 3 2 1

Publisher, Health Care: Philip Parker, Ph.D.
Editor(s): James Parker, M.D., Philip Parker, Ph.D.

Publisher's note: The ideas, procedures, and suggestions contained in this book are not intended as a substitute for consultation with your physician. All matters regarding your health require medical supervision. As new medical or scientific information becomes available from academic and clinical research, recommended treatments and drug therapies may undergo changes. The authors, editors, and publisher have attempted to make the information in this book up to date and accurate in accord with accepted standards at the time of publication. The authors, editors, and publisher are not responsible for errors or omissions or for consequences from application of the book, and make no warranty, expressed or implied, in regard to the contents of this book. Any practice described in this book should be applied by the reader in accordance with professional standards of care used in regard to the unique circumstances that may apply in each situation, in close consultation with a qualified physician. The reader is advised to always check product information (package inserts) for changes and new information regarding dose and contraindications before taking any drug or pharmacological product. Caution is especially urged when using new or infrequently ordered drugs, herbal remedies, vitamins and supplements, alternative therapies, complementary therapies and medicines, and integrative medical treatments.

Cataloging-in-Publication Data

Parker, James N., 1961-
Parker, Philip M., 1960-

   The Official Patient's Sourcebook on Muscular Dystrophy: A Revised and Updated Directory for the Internet Age/James N. Parker and Philip M. Parker, editors
            p.   cm.
   Includes bibliographical references, glossary and index.
   ISBN: 0-497-01000-3
   1. Muscular Dystrophy-Popular works.   I. Title.

Disclaimer

This publication is not intended to be used for the diagnosis or treatment of a health problem or as a substitute for consultation with licensed medical professionals. It is sold with the understanding that the publisher, editors, and authors are not engaging in the rendering of medical, psychological, financial, legal, or other professional services.

References to any entity, product, service, or source of information that may be contained in this publication should not be considered an endorsement, either direct or implied, by the publisher, editors or authors. ICON Group International, Inc., the editors, or the authors are not responsible for the content of any Web pages nor publications referenced in this publication.

Copyright Notice

Dedication

To the healthcare professionals dedicating their time and efforts to the study of muscular dystrophy.

Acknowledgements

The collective knowledge generated from academic and applied research summarized in various references has been critical in the creation of this sourcebook which is best viewed as a comprehensive compilation and collection of information prepared by various official agencies which directly or indirectly are dedicated to muscular dystrophy. All of the *Official Patient's Sourcebooks* draw from various agencies and institutions associated with the United States Department of Health and Human Services, and in particular, the Office of the Secretary of Health and Human Services (OS), the Administration for Children and Families (ACF), the Administration on Aging (AOA), the Agency for Healthcare Research and Quality (AHRQ), the Agency for Toxic Substances and Disease Registry (ATSDR), the Centers for Disease Control and Prevention (CDC), the Food and Drug Administration (FDA), the Healthcare Financing Administration (HCFA), the Health Resources and Services Administration (HRSA), the Indian Health Service (IHS), the institutions of the National Institutes of Health (NIH), the Program Support Center (PSC), and the Substance Abuse and Mental Health Services Administration (SAMHSA). In addition to these sources, information gathered from the National Library of Medicine, the United States Patent Office, the European Union, and their related organizations has been invaluable in the creation of this sourcebook. Some of the work represented was financially supported by the Research and Development Committee at INSEAD. This support is gratefully acknowledged. Finally, special thanks are owed to Tiffany Freeman for her excellent editorial support.

About the Editors

James N. Parker, M.D.

Dr. James N. Parker received his Bachelor of Science degree in Psychobiology from the University of California, Riverside and his M.D. from the University of California, San Diego. In addition to authoring numerous research publications, he has lectured at various academic institutions. Dr. Parker is the medical editor for the *Official Patient's Sourcebook* series published by ICON Health Publications.

Philip M. Parker, Ph.D.

Philip M. Parker is the Eli Lilly Chair Professor of Innovation, Business and Society at INSEAD (Fontainebleau, France and Singapore). Dr. Parker has also been Professor at the University of California, San Diego and has taught courses at Harvard University, the Hong Kong University of Science and Technology, the Massachusetts Institute of Technology, Stanford University, and UCLA. Dr. Parker is the associate editor for the *Official Patient's Sourcebook* series published by ICON Health Publications.

About ICON Health Publications

In addition to muscular dystrophy, *Official Patient's Sourcebooks* are available for the following related topics:

- The Official Patient's Sourcebook on Avascular Necrosis
- The Official Patient's Sourcebook on Growth Plate Fractures
- The Official Patient's Sourcebook on Osteogenesis Imperfecta
- The Official Patient's Sourcebook on Osteoporosis
- The Official Patient's Sourcebook on Scoliosis
- The Official Patient's Sourcebook on Sjogren's Syndrome
- The Official Patient's Sourcebook on Spinal Stenosis

To discover more about ICON Health Publications, simply check with your preferred online booksellers, including Barnes&Noble.com and Amazon.com which currently carry all of our titles. Or, feel free to contact us directly for bulk purchases or institutional discounts:

ICON Group International, Inc.
4370 La Jolla Village Drive, Fourth Floor
San Diego, CA 92122 USA
Fax: 858-546-4341
Web site: **www.icongrouponline.com/health**

Table of Contents

INTRODUCTION

Overview

Dr. C. Everett Koop, former U.S. Surgeon General, once said, "The best prescription is knowledge."[1] The Agency for Healthcare Research and Quality (AHRQ) of the National Institutes of Health (NIH) echoes this view and recommends that every patient incorporate education into the treatment process. According to the AHRQ:

> Finding out more about your condition is a good place to start. By contacting groups that support your condition, visiting your local library, and searching on the Internet, you can find good information to help guide your treatment decisions. Some information may be hard to find—especially if you don't know where to look.[2]

As the AHRQ mentions, finding the right information is not an obvious task. Though many physicians and public officials had thought that the emergence of the Internet would do much to assist patients in obtaining reliable information, in March 2001 the National Institutes of Health issued the following warning:

> The number of Web sites offering health-related resources grows every day. Many sites provide valuable information, while others may have information that is unreliable or misleading.[3]

---

[1] Quotation from **http://www.drkoop.com**.
[2] The Agency for Healthcare Research and Quality (AHRQ):
http://www.ahcpr.gov/consumer/diaginfo.htm.
[3] From the NIH, National Cancer Institute (NCI):
http://cancertrials.nci.nih.gov/beyond/evaluating.html.

Since the late 1990s, physicians have seen a general increase in patient Internet usage rates. Patients frequently enter their doctor's offices with printed Web pages of home remedies in the guise of latest medical research. This scenario is so common that doctors often spend more time dispelling misleading information than guiding patients through sound therapies. *The Official Patient's Sourcebook on Muscular Dystrophy* has been created for patients who have decided to make education and research an integral part of the treatment process. The pages that follow will tell you where and how to look for information covering virtually all topics related to muscular dystrophy, from the essentials to the most advanced areas of research.

The title of this book includes the word "official." This reflects the fact that the sourcebook draws from public, academic, government, and peer-reviewed research. Selected readings from various agencies are reproduced to give you some of the latest official information available to date on muscular dystrophy.

Given patients' increasing sophistication in using the Internet, abundant references to reliable Internet-based resources are provided throughout this sourcebook. Where possible, guidance is provided on how to obtain free-of-charge, primary research results as well as more detailed information via the Internet. E-book and electronic versions of this sourcebook are fully interactive with each of the Internet sites mentioned (clicking on a hyperlink automatically opens your browser to the site indicated). Hard copy users of this sourcebook can type cited Web addresses directly into their browsers to obtain access to the corresponding sites. Since we are working with ICON Health Publications, hard copy *Sourcebooks* are frequently updated and printed on demand to ensure that the information provided is current.

In addition to extensive references accessible via the Internet, every chapter presents a "Vocabulary Builder." Many health guides offer glossaries of technical or uncommon terms in an appendix. In editing this sourcebook, we have decided to place a smaller glossary within each chapter that covers terms used in that chapter. Given the technical nature of some chapters, you may need to revisit many sections. Building one's vocabulary of medical terms in such a gradual manner has been shown to improve the learning process.

We must emphasize that no sourcebook on muscular dystrophy should affirm that a specific diagnostic procedure or treatment discussed in a research study, patent, or doctoral dissertation is "correct" or your best option. This sourcebook is no exception. Each patient is unique. Deciding on appropriate options is always up to the patient in consultation with their physician and healthcare providers.

Organization

This sourcebook is organized into three parts. Part I explores basic techniques to researching muscular dystrophy (e.g. finding guidelines on diagnosis, treatments, and prognosis), followed by a number of topics, including information on how to get in touch with organizations, associations, or other patient networks dedicated to muscular dystrophy. It also gives you sources of information that can help you find a doctor in your local area specializing in treating muscular dystrophy. Collectively, the material presented in Part I is a complete primer on basic research topics for patients with muscular dystrophy.

Part II moves on to advanced research dedicated to muscular dystrophy. Part II is intended for those willing to invest many hours of hard work and study. It is here that we direct you to the latest scientific and applied research on muscular dystrophy. When possible, contact names, links via the Internet, and summaries are provided. It is in Part II where the vocabulary process becomes important as authors publishing advanced research frequently use highly specialized language. In general, every attempt is made to recommend "free-to-use" options.

Part III provides appendices of useful background reading for all patients with muscular dystrophy or related disorders. The appendices are dedicated to more pragmatic issues faced by many patients with muscular dystrophy. Accessing materials via medical libraries may be the only option for some readers, so a guide is provided for finding local medical libraries which are open to the public. Part III, therefore, focuses on advice that goes beyond the biological and scientific issues facing patients with muscular dystrophy.

Scope

While this sourcebook covers muscular dystrophy, your doctor, research publications, and specialists may refer to your condition using a variety of terms. Therefore, you should understand that muscular dystrophy is often considered a synonym or a condition closely related to the following:

- Distal Muscular Dystrophy
- Duchenne's Muscular Dystrophy

- Erb's Muscular Dystrophy
- Facioscapulohumeral Disease
- Fukuyama Syndrome
- Gower's Syndrome
- Inherited Myopathy
- Landouzy-Dejerine Disease
- Landouzy-Dejerine Dystrophy
- Landouzy-Déjèrine Dystrophy
- Limb-Girdle Muscular Dystrophy
- Myotonic Muscular Dystrophy
- Ocular Muscular Dystrophy
- Oculopharyngeal Muscular Dystrophy
- Pseudohypertrophic Muscular Dystrophy
- Steinert's Disease

In addition to synonyms and related conditions, physicians may refer to muscular dystrophy using certain coding systems. The International Classification of Diseases, 9th Revision, Clinical Modification (ICD-9-CM) is the most commonly used system of classification for the world's illnesses. Your physician may use this coding system as an administrative or tracking tool. The following classification is commonly used for muscular dystrophy:[4]

- 359 muscular dystrophies and other myopathies
- 359.0 congenital muscular dystrophy
- 359.1 hereditary progressive muscular dystrophy
- 359.2 myotonic dystrophy

For the purposes of this sourcebook, we have attempted to be as inclusive as possible, looking for official information for all of the synonyms relevant to muscular dystrophy. You may find it useful to refer to synonyms when accessing databases or interacting with healthcare professionals and medical librarians.

---

[4] This list is based on the official version of the World Health Organization's 9th Revision, International Classification of Diseases (ICD-9). According to the National Technical Information Service, "ICD-9CM extensions, interpretations, modifications, addenda, or errata other than those approved by the U.S. Public Health Service and the Health Care Financing Administration are not to be considered official and should not be utilized. Continuous maintenance of the ICD-9-CM is the responsibility of the federal government."

Moving Forward

Since the 1980s, the world has seen a proliferation of healthcare guides covering most illnesses. Some are written by patients or their family members. These generally take a layperson's approach to understanding and coping with an illness or disorder. They can be uplifting, encouraging, and highly supportive. Other guides are authored by physicians or other healthcare providers who have a more clinical outlook. Each of these two styles of guide has its purpose and can be quite useful.

As editors, we have chosen a third route. We have chosen to expose you to as many sources of official and peer-reviewed information as practical, for the purpose of educating you about basic and advanced knowledge as recognized by medical science today. You can think of this sourcebook as your personal Internet age reference librarian.

Why "Internet age"? All too often, patients diagnosed with muscular dystrophy will log on to the Internet, type words into a search engine, and receive several Web site listings which are mostly irrelevant or redundant. These patients are left to wonder where the relevant information is, and how to obtain it. Since only the smallest fraction of information dealing with muscular dystrophy is even indexed in search engines, a non-systematic approach often leads to frustration and disappointment. With this sourcebook, we hope to direct you to the information you need that you would not likely find using popular Web directories. Beyond Web listings, in many cases we will reproduce brief summaries or abstracts of available reference materials. These abstracts often contain distilled information on topics of discussion.

While we focus on the more scientific aspects of muscular dystrophy, there is, of course, the emotional side to consider. Later in the sourcebook, we provide a chapter dedicated to helping you find peer groups and associations that can provide additional support beyond research produced by medical science. We hope that the choices we have made give you the most options available in moving forward. In this way, we wish you the best in your efforts to incorporate this educational approach into your treatment plan.

The Editors

PART I: THE ESSENTIALS

ABOUT PART I

Part I has been edited to give you access to what we feel are "the essentials" on muscular dystrophy. The essentials of a disease typically include the definition or description of the disease, a discussion of who it affects, the signs or symptoms associated with the disease, tests or diagnostic procedures that might be specific to the disease, and treatments for the disease. Your doctor or healthcare provider may have already explained the essentials of muscular dystrophy to you or even given you a pamphlet or brochure describing muscular dystrophy. Now you are searching for more in-depth information. As editors, we have decided, nevertheless, to include a discussion on where to find essential information that can complement what your doctor has already told you. In this section we recommend a process, not a particular Web site or reference book. The process ensures that, as you search the Web, you gain background information in such a way as to maximize your understanding.

Chapter 1. The Essentials on Muscular Dystrophy: Guidelines

Overview

Official agencies, as well as federally funded institutions supported by national grants, frequently publish a variety of guidelines on muscular dystrophy. These are typically called "Fact Sheets" or "Guidelines." They can take the form of a brochure, information kit, pamphlet, or flyer. Often they are only a few pages in length. The great advantage of guidelines over other sources is that they are often written with the patient in mind. Since new guidelines on muscular dystrophy can appear at any moment and be published by a number of sources, the best approach to finding guidelines is to systematically scan the Internet-based services that post them.

The National Institutes of Health (NIH)[5]

The National Institutes of Health (NIH) is the first place to search for relatively current patient guidelines and fact sheets on muscular dystrophy. Originally founded in 1887, the NIH is one of the world's foremost medical research centers and the federal focal point for medical research in the United States. At any given time, the NIH supports some 35,000 research grants at universities, medical schools, and other research and training institutions, both nationally and internationally. The rosters of those who have conducted research or who have received NIH support over the years include the world's most illustrious scientists and physicians. Among them are 97 scientists who have won the Nobel Prize for achievement in medicine.

---

[5] Adapted from the NIH: **http://www.nih.gov/about/NIHoverview.html**.

There is no guarantee that any one Institute will have a guideline on a specific disease, though the National Institutes of Health collectively publish over 600 guidelines for both common and rare diseases. The best way to access NIH guidelines is via the Internet. Although the NIH is organized into many different Institutes and Offices, the following is a list of key Web sites where you are most likely to find NIH clinical guidelines and publications dealing with muscular dystrophy and associated conditions:

- Office of the Director (OD); guidelines consolidated across agencies available at **http://www.nih.gov/health/consumer/conkey.htm**

- National Library of Medicine (NLM); extensive encyclopedia (A.D.A.M., Inc.) with guidelines available at **http://www.nlm.nih.gov/medlineplus/healthtopics.html**

- National Institute of Arthritis and Musculoskeletal and Skin Diseases (NIAMS); fact sheets and guidelines at **http://www.nih.gov/niams/healthinfo/**

Among those listed above, the National Institute of Arthritis and Musculoskeletal and Skin Diseases (NIAMS) is especially noteworthy. The mission of NIAMS, a part of the National Institutes of Health (NIH), is to support research into the causes, treatment, and prevention of arthritis and musculoskeletal and skin diseases, the training of basic and clinical scientists to carry out this research, and the dissemination of information on research progress in these diseases. The National Institute of Arthritis and Musculoskeletal and Skin Diseases Information Clearinghouse is a public service sponsored by the NIAMS that provides health information and information sources. The NIAMS provides the following guideline concerning muscular dystrophy.[6]

What Is Muscular Dystrophy (MD)?[7]

Muscular dystrophy (MD) refers to a group of genetic diseases characterized by progressive weakness and degeneration of the skeletal or voluntary muscles which control movement. The muscles of the heart and some other involuntary muscles are also affected in some forms of MD, and a few forms involve other organs as well. The major forms of MD include myotonic, Duchenne, Becker, limb-girdle, facioscapulohumeral, congenital,

---

[6] This and other passages are adapted from the NIH and NIAMS (**http://www.niams.nih.gov/hi/index.htm**). "Adapted" signifies that the text is reproduced with attribution, with some or no editorial adjustments.

[7] Adapted from the National Institute of Arthritis and Musculoskeletal and Skin Diseases (NIAMS): **http://www.ninds.nih.gov/health_and_medical/disorders/md.htm**.

oculopharyngeal, distal and Emery-Dreifuss. Duchenne is the most common form of MD affecting children, and myotonic MD is the most common form affecting adults. MD can affect people of all ages. Although some forms first become apparent in infancy or childhood, others may not appear until middle age or later.

Is There Any Treatment?

There is no specific treatment for any of the forms of MD. Physical therapy to prevent contractures (a condition in which shortened muscles around joints cause abnormal and sometimes painful positioning of the joints), orthoses (orthopedic appliances used for support) and corrective orthopedic surgery may be needed to improve the quality of life in some cases. The cardiac problems that occur with Emery-Dreifuss MD and myotonic MD may require a pacemaker. The myotonia (delayed relaxation of a muscle after a strong contraction) occurring in myotonic MD may be treated with medications such as phenytoin or quinine.

What Is the Prognosis?

The prognosis of MD varies according to the type of MD and the progression of the disorder. Some cases may be mild and very slowly progressive, with normal lifespan, while other cases may have more marked progression of muscle weakness, functional disability and loss of ambulation. Life expectancy may depend on the degree of progression and late respiratory deficit. In Duchenne MD, death usually occurs in the late teens to early 20s.

What Research Is Being Done?

The NINDS supports a broad program of research on MD. The goals of these studies are to increase understanding of MD and its cause(s), develop better therapies, and, ultimately, find ways to prevent and cure the disorder.

Selected References

Dubowitz V.
What's in a name? Muscular dystrophy revisited. European Journal of Paediatric Neurology. 1998;2(6):279-84

Laing NG, Mastaglia FL.
Inherited skeletal muscle disorders Annals of Human Biology. 1999 Nov-Dec;26(6):507-25

Moore DP, Kowalske KJ.
Neuromuscular rehabilitation and electrodiagnosis 5. Myopathy. Archives of Physical Medicine and Rehabilitation. 2000 Mar;81(3 Suppl 1):S32-5; quiz S36-44

Tsao CY, Mendell JR.
The childhood muscular dystrophies: making order out of chaos Seminars in Neurology. 1999;19(1):9-23

Urtizberea JA.
Therapies in muscular dystrophy: current concepts and future prospects European Neurology. 2000;43(3):127-32

Organizations

Facioscapulohumeral Dystrophy (FSHD) Society
3 Westwood Road
Lexington, MA 02420
info@fshsociety.org
http://www.fshsociety.org
Tel: 781-860-0501
Fax: 781-860-0599

Muscular Dystrophy Association
3300 East Sunrise Drive
Tucson, AZ 85718-3208
mda@mdausa.org
http://www.mdausa.org/
Tel: 520-529-2000 800-572-1717
Fax: 520-529-5300

Muscular Dystrophy Family Foundation
2330 North Meridien Street
Indianapolis, IN 46208
mdff@mdff.org
http://www.mdff.org
Tel: 317-923-6333 800-544-1213
Fax: 317-923-6334

Parent Project for Muscular Dystrophy Research
1012 North University Blvd.
Middletown, OH 45042
ParentProject@aol.com
http://www.parentprojectmd.org
Tel: 413-424-0696 800-714-KIDS (5437)
Fax: 513-425-9907

More Guideline Sources

The guideline above on muscular dystrophy is only one example of the kind of material that you can find online and free of charge. The remainder of this chapter will direct you to other sources which either publish or can help you find additional guidelines on topics related to muscular dystrophy. Many of the guidelines listed below address topics that may be of particular relevance to your specific situation or of special interest to only some patients with muscular dystrophy. Due to space limitations these sources are listed in a concise manner. Do not hesitate to consult the following sources by either using the Internet hyperlink provided, or, in cases where the contact information is provided, contacting the publisher or author directly.

Topic Pages: MEDLINEplus

For patients wishing to go beyond guidelines published by specific Institutes of the NIH, the National Library of Medicine has created a vast and patient-oriented healthcare information portal called MEDLINEplus. Within this Internet-based system are "health topic pages." You can think of a health topic page as a guide to patient guides. To access this system, log on to **http://www.nlm.nih.gov/medlineplus/healthtopics.html**. From there you can either search using the alphabetical index or browse by broad topic areas. Recently, MEDLINEplus listed the following as being relevant to muscular dystrophy:

Bell's Palsy
http://www.nlm.nih.gov/medlineplus/bellspalsy.html

Charcot-Marie-Tooth Disease
http://www.nlm.nih.gov/medlineplus/charcotmarietoothdisease.html

Genetic Brain Disorders
http://www.nlm.nih.gov/medlineplus/geneticbraindisorders.html

Laser Eye Surgery
http://www.nlm.nih.gov/medlineplus/lasereyesurgery.html

Movement Disorders
http://www.nlm.nih.gov/medlineplus/movementdisorders.html

Muscle Disorders
http://www.nlm.nih.gov/medlineplus/muscledisorders.html

Muscular Dystrophy
http://www.nlm.nih.gov/medlineplus/musculardystrophy.html

Myasthenia Gravis
http://www.nlm.nih.gov/medlineplus/myastheniagravis.html

Neuromuscular Disorders
http://www.nlm.nih.gov/medlineplus/neuromusculardisorders.htm
l

Spinal Muscular Atrophy
http://www.nlm.nih.gov/medlineplus/spinalmuscularatrophy.html

Tourette Syndrome
http://www.nlm.nih.gov/medlineplus/tourettesyndrome.html

Within the health topic page dedicated to muscular dystrophy, the following was recently recommended to patients:

- Diagnosis/Symptoms

   Accurate and Affordable Diagnosis of Duchenne Muscular Dystrophy
   Source: National Institute of Neurological Disorders and Stroke
   http://www.ninds.nih.gov/news_and_events/news_article_dmd_tes
   t.htm

   Creatine Kinase Test
   Source: Muscular Dystrophy Association
   http://www.mdausa.org/publications/Quest/q71ss-cktest.html

   Electromyography and Nerve Conduction Velocities
   Source: Muscular Dystrophy Association
   http://www.mdausa.org/publications/Quest/q75ss.html

   Muscle Biopsies
   Source: Muscular Dystrophy Association
   http://www.mdausa.org/publications/Quest/q74ss.html

- Treatment

  Steroids / Nutritional Supplements / Antibiotics
  Source: Parent Project for Muscular Dystrophy Research
  http://www.parentprojectmd.org/treatment/supplements.html

- Coping

  101 Hints to "Help-with-Ease" for Patients with Neuromuscular Disease
  Source: Muscular Dystrophy Association
  http://www.mdausa.org/publications/101hints/

  Learning to Live with Neuromuscular Disease: A Message for Parents
  Source: Muscular Dystrophy Association
  http://www.mdausa.org/publications/learning/index.html

- Children

  Meaning of Muscular Dystrophy
  Source: Nemours Foundation
  http://kidshealth.org/kid/health_problems/bone/muscular_dystrophy.html

- From the National Institutes of Health

  Muscular Dystrophy (MD)
  Source: National Institute of Neurological Disorders and Stroke
  http://www.ninds.nih.gov/health_and_medical/disorders/md.htm

- Organizations

  Muscular Dystrophy Association
  http://www.mdausa.org/

  National Institute of Arthritis and Musculoskeletal and Skin Diseases
  http://www.niams.nih.gov/

  National Institute of Neurological Disorders and Stroke
  http://www.ninds.nih.gov/

  Parent Project for Muscular Dystrophy Research
  http://www.parentprojectmd.org/

- Research

Faulty Muscle Repair Implicated in Muscular Dystrophies
Source: National Institute of Neurological Disorders and Stroke
http://www.ninds.nih.gov/news_and_events/news_article_md_rep air.htm

Gene Therapy Reaches All Damaged Muscles in Muscular Dystrophy Mouse
Source: National Institute of Arthritis and Musculoskeletal and Skin Diseases
http://www.niams.nih.gov/ne/highlights/spotlight/2004/gene_mu scle_mouse.htm

MDA Research Advances Rapidly
Source: Muscular Dystrophy Association
http://www.mdausa.org/publications/resdev.html

Protein May Hold Key to Repair of Damaged Muscles
Source: National Institute of Arthritis and Musculoskeletal and Skin Diseases
http://www.niams.nih.gov/ne/highlights/spotlight/2004/follistatin .htm

- Teenagers

Muscular Dystrophy
Source: Nemours Foundation
http://kidshealth.org/teen/diseases_conditions/bones/muscular_dy strophy.html

You may also choose to use the search utility provided by MEDLINEplus at the following Web address: **http://www.nlm.nih.gov/medlineplus/**. Simply type a keyword into the search box and click "Search." This utility is similar to the NIH search utility, with the exception that it only includes materials that are linked within the MEDLINEplus system (mostly patient-oriented information). It also has the disadvantage of generating unstructured results. We recommend, therefore, that you use this method only if you have a very targeted search.

The Combined Health Information Database (CHID)

CHID Online is a reference tool that maintains a database directory of thousands of journal articles and patient education guidelines on muscular dystrophy and related conditions. One of the advantages of CHID over other sources is that it offers summaries that describe the guidelines available, including contact information and pricing. CHID's general Web site is **http://chid.nih.gov/**. To search this database, go to **http://chid.nih.gov/detail/detail.html**. In particular, you can use the advanced search options to look up pamphlets, reports, brochures, and information kits. The following was recently posted in this archive:

- **Facts About Friedreich's Ataxia**

  Source: Tucson, AZ: Muscular Dystrophy Association. 1999. 16 p.

  Contact: Available from Muscular Dystrophy Association. Publications Department, 3300 East Sunrise Drive, Tucson, AZ 85718. (800) 572-1717 or (520) 529-2000. Website: www.mdausa.org. PRICE: Single copy free.

  Summary: This brochure describes Friedreich's ataxia (FRDA), an inherited progressive disorder of the nervous system that affects balance, coordination, movement, and sensation. Ataxia refers to a loss of coordination and is usually the earliest and most prominent characteristic of the disease. Increasing impairment of balance and movement eventually lead to the loss of the ability to walk; speech and swallowing difficulties may occur as well. The brochure is written in a question and answer format and covers incidence, heredity, recessive inheritance, symptoms, treatment options, disease progression, speech and swallowing problems associated with FRDA, how FRDA affects the heart, genetic testing, and the role of the **Muscular Dystrophy** Association (MDA). The brochure concludes with a brief description of the purpose and programs of the MDA. 7 figures.

- **Augmentative Communication: Consumers**

  Source: Rockville, MD: American Speech-Language-Hearing Association (ASHA). 199x. 36 p.

  Contact: Available from American Speech-Language-Hearing Association (ASHA). Product Sales, 10801 Rockville Pike, Rockville, MD 20852. (888) 498-6699. TTY (301) 897-0157. Website: www.asha.org. PRICE: $1.50 per booklet. Item Number 0210251.

  Summary: This consumer information booklet describes the use of augmentative communication for people who can hear but have little or no usable speech. Such severe communication disabilities can result from severe language delay, cerebral palsy, mental retardation, autism, traumatic brain injury (TBI), or stroke. In addition, a variety of specific neuromuscular disorders, such as amyotrophic lateral sclerosis (ALS), dystonia, Huntington's disease, multiple sclerosis, and **muscular dystrophy** can also cause severe speech problems. Augmentative communication is defined as any method other than speech, to send a message from one person to another. Techniques of augmentative communication range from specialized gestures and sign language to communication aids such as sign boards to highly specialized computer-based techniques. The booklet emphasizes the implementation of an effective augmentative communication system, regardless of level of sophistication, requires a detailed multidisciplinary assessment, training for the user(s), and regular re-evaluation. The booklet outlines the roles of members of the patient care team, including the speech language pathologist, the occupational therapist, the physical therapist, physicians, the educator, social worker, psychologist, rehabilitation engineer, computer programmer, vocational counselor, audiologist, orthotist, and manufacturers or distributors of communication devices. The author encourages readers to become active partners in their own care or the care of their children with communication disorders. The booklet includes a resource list of professional and consumer groups concerned with augmentative communication. An appendix provides a glossary of some of the terms used in augmentative communication. The booklet is illustrated with black and white photographs.

Healthfinder™

Healthfinder™ is an additional source sponsored by the U.S. Department of Health and Human Services which offers links to hundreds of other sites that contain healthcare information. This Web site is located at **http://www.healthfinder.gov**. Again, keyword searches can be used to find guidelines. The following was recently found in this database:

- **Facts About Limb-Girdle Muscular Dystrophy (LGMD)**

  Source: Muscular Dystrophy Association

  http://www.healthfinder.gov/scripts/recordpass.asp?RecordType=0&RecordID=8135

The NIH Search Utility

After browsing the references listed at the beginning of this chapter, you may want to explore the NIH search utility. This allows you to search for documents on over 100 selected Web sites that comprise the NIH-WEB-SPACE. Each of these servers is "crawled" and indexed on an ongoing basis. Your search will produce a list of various documents, all of which will relate in some way to muscular dystrophy. The drawbacks of this approach are that the information is not organized by theme and that the references are often a mix of information for professionals and patients. Nevertheless, a large number of the listed Web sites provide useful background information. We can only recommend this route, therefore, for relatively rare or specific disorders, or when using highly targeted searches. To use the NIH search utility, visit the following Web page: **http://search.nih.gov/index.html**.

Additional Web Sources

A number of Web sites that often link to government sites are available to the public. These can also point you in the direction of essential information. The following is a representative sample:

- AOL: **http://search.aol.com/cat.adp?id=168&layer=&from=subcats**

- Family Village: **http://www.familyvillage.wisc.edu/specific.htm**

- Google: **http://directory.google.com/Top/Health/Conditions_and_Diseases/**

- Med Help International: **http://www.medhelp.org/HealthTopics/A.html**

- Open Directory Project: **http://dmoz.org/Health/Conditions_and_Diseases/**

- Yahoo.com: **http://dir.yahoo.com/Health/Diseases_and_Conditions/**

- WebMD®Health: **http://my.webmd.com/health_topics**

Vocabulary Builder

The material in this chapter may have contained a number of unfamiliar words. The following Vocabulary Builder introduces you to terms used in this chapter that have not been covered in the previous chapter:

Audiologist: Study of hearing including treatment of persons with hearing defects. [NIH]

Bell's palsy: Paralysis of the upper and lower muscles of the face on one side, due to inflammation of the facial nerve within the stylomastoid foramen. [NIH]

Chaos: Complex behavior that seems random but actually has some hidden order. [NIH]

Impairment: In the context of health experience, an impairment is any loss or abnormality of psychological, physiological, or anatomical structure or function. [NIH]

Infancy: The period of complete dependency prior to the acquisition of competence in walking, talking, and self-feeding. [NIH]

Involuntary: Reaction occurring without intention or volition. [NIH]

Nerve: A cordlike structure of nervous tissue that connects parts of the nervous system with other tissues of the body and conveys nervous impulses to, or away from, these tissues. [NIH]

Refer: To send or direct for treatment, aid, information, de decision. [NIH]

CHAPTER 2. SEEKING GUIDANCE

Overview

Some patients are comforted by the knowledge that a number of organizations dedicate their resources to helping people with muscular dystrophy. These associations can become invaluable sources of information and advice. Many associations offer aftercare support, financial assistance, and other important services. Furthermore, healthcare research has shown that support groups often help people to better cope with their conditions.[8] In addition to support groups, your physician can be a valuable source of guidance and support. Therefore, finding a physician that can work with your unique situation is a very important aspect of your care.

In this chapter, we direct you to resources that can help you find patient organizations and medical specialists. We begin by describing how to find associations and peer groups that can help you better understand and cope with muscular dystrophy. The chapter ends with a discussion on how to find a doctor that is right for you.

Associations and Muscular Dystrophy

As mentioned by the Agency for Healthcare Research and Quality, sometimes the emotional side of an illness can be as taxing as the physical side.[9] You may have fears or feel overwhelmed by your situation. Everyone has different ways of dealing with disease or physical injury. Your attitude, your expectations, and how well you cope with your condition can all

---

[8] Churches, synagogues, and other houses of worship might also have groups that can offer you the social support you need.
[9] This section has been adapted from **http://www.ahcpr.gov/consumer/diaginf5.htm**.

influence your well-being. This is true for both minor conditions and serious illnesses. For example, a study on female breast cancer survivors revealed that women who participated in support groups lived longer and experienced better quality of life when compared with women who did not participate. In the support group, women learned coping skills and had the opportunity to share their feelings with other women in the same situation.

In addition to associations or groups that your doctor might recommend, we suggest that you consider the following list (if there is a fee for an association, you may want to check with your insurance provider to find out if the cost will be covered):

- **Muscular Dystrophy Association**

  Telephone: (520) 529-2000 Toll-free: (800) 572-1717

  Fax: (520) 529-5300

  Email: mda@mdausa.org

  Web Site: http://www.mdausa.org

  Background: Established in 1950, the **Muscular Dystrophy** Association (MDA) is a non-profit, voluntary health agency dedicated to providing comprehensive medical services to individuals affected by over 40 neuromuscular diseases. MDA provides these services at some 230 hospital-affiliated clinics across the United States. The Association's worldwide research program allocates more than $28 million a year, seeking cures and treatments for neuromuscular disorders. MDA funds some 400 individual scientific investigations each year at a cost of $57 a minute, around the clock. This represents the largest single initiative to advance current knowledge of neuromuscular diseases and to find cures and treatments for this group of diseases.

  Relevant area(s) of interest: Muscular Dystrophy

- **Muscular Dystrophy Association (Australia)**

  Telephone: 61 3 9320 9555 Toll-free: 1 800 656 632

  Fax: 61 3 9320 9595

  Email: info@mda.org.au

  Web Site: http://www.mda.org.au

  Background: The **Muscular Dystrophy** Association (MDA) is a not-for-profit organization in Australia that was founded in the early 1970s by a group of people affected by **muscular dystrophy** (MD). **Muscular dystrophy** refers to a group of genetic disorders characterized by progressive degeneration of muscle fibers, resulting in associated weakness, disability, and deformity. The different forms of **muscular dystrophy** may be categorized based upon age at onset, specific muscle groups affected, rate of disease progression, and mode of inheritance. The **Muscular Dystrophy** Association is committed to improving the quality of life of individuals with **muscular dystrophy** and other neuromuscular diseases. To fulfill its mission and objectives, the Association provides a variety of educational materials, conducts MDA camps for children and adults with neuromuscular disorders, and promotes and supports research. The Association's materials include information sheets on different forms of **muscular dystrophy,** parents guides, glossaries, and materials discussing the various aspects of these disorders. The Association also maintains a web site on the Internet that provides understandable information on **muscular dystrophy,** a FAQ ('frequently asked questions') area, a guestbook area for online visitors, and links to additional sources of information and support. In 1985, the Association established the **Muscular Dystrophy** Research Foundation to help ensure sufficient funding to accelerate research and to provide funds required for treatment programs. The MDA, in association with St. Vincents Hospital and the Department of Medicine, Melbourne University, is also affiliated with the Melbourne Neuromuscular Research Centre, and sponsors scientific research seminars and conferences.

Relevant area(s) of interest: Muscular Dystrophy

- **Muscular Dystrophy Association of Canada**
  Telephone: 416-488-0030 Toll-free: (800) 567-2873
  Fax: 416-488-7523
  Email: info@mdac.ca
  Web Site: http://www.mdac.ca

Background: The **Muscular Dystrophy** Association of Canada (MDAC) is not-for-profit voluntary organization dedicated to eliminating neuromuscular disorders and alleviating the associated symptoms. Neuromuscular disorders are a group of diseases affecting the body s ability to move due to an underlying neurological disease. Whether the problem originates within the motor nerve cell, the nerve, or the muscle, the most commonly experienced symptoms are varying degrees of progressive muscle weakness and wasting. There are over 40 nerve and muscle disorders covered under the umbrella of the **Muscular Dystrophy** Association of Canada. Founded in 1954, the Association s three main goals are funding research that will ultimately result in discovering the causes, treatments, and cures for **muscular dystrophy** and other neuromuscular disorders; providing support services that assist individuals and families affected by neuromuscular disorders; and providing information to affected individuals, their families, health care professionals, educators, and the general public as to the nature and management of neuromuscular disorders. Services provided by MDAC include the dissemination of information, advocacy, referrals, travel assistance, and some financial assistance with mobility equipment. MDAC also houses donated equipment for use by clients upon request. Informational brochures include 'What Is Spinal Muscular Atrophy?,' 'What Is Myotonic Dystrophy?,' and 'What Is Muscular Dystrophy?'. MDAC also publishes a news magazine entitled 'CONNECTIONS'. Additionally, the organization provides advocacy services in resolving individual or community problems.

Relevant area(s) of interest: Muscular Dystrophy

- **Parent Project Muscular Dystrophy**
  Telephone: (513) 424-0696 Toll-free: (800) 714-5437

  Fax: (513) 425-9907

  Email: Pat@parentprojectmd.org

  Web Site: http://www.parentprojectmd.org

  Background: Parent Project **Muscular Dystrophy** (formerly the Parent Project for Duchenne Muscular Dystrophy) is a not-for-profit national health organization founded in 1994 by parents of children with Duchenne and Becker **Muscular Dystrophy.** Today, its work focuses in five areas: It identifies, funds, and disseminates informaiton about promising Duchenne and Becker **Muscular Dystrophy** research and its applications. It seeks to ensure that all families, caregivers, health care professionals and others have access to current information about treatment and care options for children with Duchenne and Becker MD. It seeks to ensure that health and human services policymakers afford the same priority to Duchenne and Becker MD as to other disorders of similar incidence and prevalence. It seeks to ensure that the voices of people with and affected by these diseases are heard, and it seeks collaboration with other international organizations addressing these diseases.

  Relevant area(s) of interest: Muscular Dystrophy

- **Society for Muscular Dystrophy Information International**
  Telephone: 902-685-3961
  Fax: 902-685-3962

Email: smdi@auracom.com

Web Site: None

Background: The Society for **Muscular Dystrophy** Information International (SMDI) is a not-for-profit registered Canadian charity dedicated to assisting people in helping themselves by reducing the national and international isolation of individuals and organizations concerned with neuromuscular disorders/disabilities (e.g., **muscular dystrophy** and over 50 allied disorders). In general, 'neuromuscular disorder' is a term used to describe a group of over 50 diseases affecting the body s motor neurons (nerves and muscles). Symptoms may include varying degrees of progressive muscle weakness and loss of muscle mass (wasting). SMDI was established in 1983 to provide a non-technical information link for individuals with neuromuscular disorders and for organizations around the world; to link people with other people and organizations concerned with their disorder; to share information to assist people in helping themselves; and to create increased public awareness of this group of disorders. The Society publishes two bi-annual newsletters entitled 'SMDI International Newsletter,' a publication for those concerned with **muscular dystrophy** or the allied disorders and 'Access - Able Information,' a quarterly disability information resource publication. In addition to educational materials, brochures and referrals are available.

Relevant area(s) of interest: Muscular Dystrophy

Finding Associations

There are a several Internet directories that provide lists of medical associations with information on or resources relating to muscular dystrophy. By consulting all of associations listed in this chapter, you will have nearly exhausted all sources for patient associations concerned with muscular dystrophy.

The National Health Information Center (NHIC)

The National Health Information Center (NHIC) offers a free referral service to help people find organizations that provide information about muscular dystrophy. For more information, see the NHIC's Web site at **http://www.health.gov/NHIC/** or contact an information specialist by calling 1-800-336-4797.

DIRLINE

A comprehensive source of information on associations is the DIRLINE database maintained by the National Library of Medicine. The database comprises some 10,000 records of organizations, research centers, and government institutes and associations which primarily focus on health and biomedicine. DIRLINE is available via the Internet at the following Web site: **http://dirline.nlm.nih.gov/**. Simply type in "muscular dystrophy" (or a synonym) or the name of a topic, and the site will list information contained in the database on all relevant organizations.

The Combined Health Information Database

Another comprehensive source of information on healthcare associations is the Combined Health Information Database. Using the "Detailed Search" option, you will need to limit your search to "Organizations" and "muscular dystrophy". Type the following hyperlink into your Web browser: **http://chid.nih.gov/detail/detail.html**. To find associations, use the drop boxes at the bottom of the search page where "You may refine your search by." For publication date, select "All Years." Then, select your preferred language and the format option "Organization Resource Sheet." By making these selections and typing in "muscular dystrophy" (or synonyms) into the "For these words:" box, you will only receive results on organizations dealing with muscular dystrophy. You should check back periodically with this database since it is updated every 3 months.

The National Organization for Rare Disorders, Inc.

The National Organization for Rare Disorders, Inc. has prepared a Web site that provides, at no charge, lists of associations organized by specific diseases. You can access this database at the following Web site: **http://www.rarediseases.org/search/orgsearch.html**. Type "muscular dystrophy" (or a synonym) in the search box, and click "Submit Query."

Online Support Groups

In addition to support groups, commercial Internet service providers offer forums and chat rooms for people with different illnesses and conditions. WebMD®, for example, offers such a service at its Web site: **http://boards.webmd.com/roundtable**. These online self-help communities can help you connect with a network of people whose concerns are similar to yours. Online support groups are places where people can talk informally. If you read about a novel approach, consult with your doctor or other healthcare providers, as the treatments or discoveries you hear about may not be scientifically proven to be safe and effective.

Finding Doctors

One of the most important aspects of your treatment will be the relationship between you and your doctor or specialist. All patients with muscular dystrophy must go through the process of selecting a physician. While this process will vary from person to person, the Agency for Healthcare Research and Quality makes a number of suggestions, including the following:[10]

- If you are in a managed care plan, check the plan's list of doctors first.

- Ask doctors or other health professionals who work with doctors, such as hospital nurses, for referrals.

- Call a hospital's doctor referral service, but keep in mind that these services usually refer you to doctors on staff at that particular hospital. The services do not have information on the quality of care that these doctors provide.

- Some local medical societies offer lists of member doctors. Again, these lists do not have information on the quality of care that these doctors provide.

Additional steps you can take to locate doctors include the following:

- Check with the associations listed earlier in this chapter.

- Information on doctors in some states is available on the Internet at **http://www.docboard.org**. This Web site is run by "Administrators in Medicine," a group of state medical board directors.

- The American Board of Medical Specialties can tell you if your doctor is board certified. "Certified" means that the doctor has completed a training program in a specialty and has passed an exam, or "board," to assess his or her knowledge, skills, and experience to provide quality patient care in that specialty. Primary care doctors may also be certified as specialists. The AMBS Web site is located at

---

[10] This section has been adapted from the AHRQ: www.ahrq.gov/consumer/qntascii/qntdr.htm.

http://www.abms.org/newsearch.asp.[11] You can also contact the ABMS by phone at 1-866-ASK-ABMS.

- You can call the American Medical Association (AMA) at 800-665-2882 for information on training, specialties, and board certification for many licensed doctors in the United States. This information also can be found in "Physician Select" at the AMA's Web site: **http://www.ama-assn.org/aps/amahg.htm**.

If the previous sources did not meet your needs, you may want to log on to the Web site of the National Organization for Rare Disorders (NORD) at **http://www.rarediseases.org/**. NORD maintains a database of doctors with expertise in various rare diseases. The Metabolic Information Network (MIN), 800-945-2188, also maintains a database of physicians with expertise in various metabolic diseases.

Selecting Your Doctor[12]

When you have compiled a list of prospective doctors, call each of their offices. First, ask if the doctor accepts your health insurance plan and if he or she is taking new patients. If the doctor is not covered by your plan, ask yourself if you are prepared to pay the extra costs. The next step is to schedule a visit with your chosen physician. During the first visit you will have the opportunity to evaluate your doctor and to find out if you feel comfortable with him or her. Ask yourself, did the doctor:

- Give me a chance to ask questions about muscular dystrophy?
- Really listen to my questions?
- Answer in terms I understood?
- Show respect for me?
- Ask me questions?
- Make me feel comfortable?
- Address the health problem(s) I came with?
- Ask me my preferences about different kinds of treatments for muscular dystrophy?

---

[11] While board certification is a good measure of a doctor's knowledge, it is possible to receive quality care from doctors who are not board certified.
[12] This section has been adapted from the AHRQ: www.ahrq.gov/consumer/qntascii/qntdr.htm.

- Spend enough time with me?

Trust your instincts when deciding if the doctor is right for you. But remember, it might take time for the relationship to develop. It takes more than one visit for you and your doctor to get to know each other.

Working with Your Doctor[13]

Research has shown that patients who have good relationships with their doctors tend to be more satisfied with their care and have better results. Here are some tips to help you and your doctor become partners:

- You know important things about your symptoms and your health history. Tell your doctor what you think he or she needs to know.

- It is important to tell your doctor personal information, even if it makes you feel embarrassed or uncomfortable.

- Bring a "health history" list with you (and keep it up to date).

- Always bring any medications you are currently taking with you to the appointment, or you can bring a list of your medications including dosage and frequency information. Talk about any allergies or reactions you have had to your medications.

- Tell your doctor about any natural or alternative medicines you are taking.

- Bring other medical information, such as x-ray films, test results, and medical records.

- Ask questions. If you don't, your doctor will assume that you understood everything that was said.

- Write down your questions before your visit. List the most important ones first to make sure that they are addressed.

- Consider bringing a friend with you to the appointment to help you ask questions. This person can also help you understand and/or remember the answers.

- Ask your doctor to draw pictures if you think that this would help you understand.

- Take notes. Some doctors do not mind if you bring a tape recorder to help you remember things, but always ask first.

---

[13] This section has been adapted from the AHRQ:
www.ahrq.gov/consumer/qntascii/qntdr.htm.

- Let your doctor know if you need more time. If there is not time that day, perhaps you can speak to a nurse or physician assistant on staff or schedule a telephone appointment.

- Take information home. Ask for written instructions. Your doctor may also have brochures and audio and videotapes that can help you.

- After leaving the doctor's office, take responsibility for your care. If you have questions, call. If your symptoms get worse or if you have problems with your medication, call. If you had tests and do not hear from your doctor, call for your test results. If your doctor recommended that you have certain tests, schedule an appointment to get them done. If your doctor said you should see an additional specialist, make an appointment.

By following these steps, you will enhance the relationship you will have with your physician.

Broader Health-Related Resources

In addition to the references above, the NIH has set up guidance Web sites that can help patients find healthcare professionals. These include:[14]

- Caregivers:
  http://www.nlm.nih.gov/medlineplus/caregivers.html

- Choosing a Doctor or Healthcare Service:
  http://www.nlm.nih.gov/medlineplus/choosingadoctororhealthcareserv ice.html

- Hospitals and Health Facilities:
  http://www.nlm.nih.gov/medlineplus/healthfacilities.html

---

[14] You can access this information at
http://www.nlm.nih.gov/medlineplus/healthsystem.html.

PART II: ADDITIONAL RESOURCES AND ADVANCED MATERIAL

ABOUT PART II

In Part II, we introduce you to additional resources and advanced research on muscular dystrophy. All too often, patients who conduct their own research are overwhelmed by the difficulty in finding and organizing information. The purpose of the following chapters is to provide you an organized and structured format to help you find additional information resources on muscular dystrophy. In Part II, as in Part I, our objective is not to interpret the latest advances on muscular dystrophy or render an opinion. Rather, our goal is to give you access to original research and to increase your awareness of sources you may not have already considered. In this way, you will come across the advanced materials often referred to in pamphlets, books, or other general works. Once again, some of this material is technical in nature, so consultation with a professional familiar with muscular dystrophy is suggested.

CHAPTER 3. STUDIES ON MUSCULAR DYSTROPHY

Overview

Every year, academic studies are published on muscular dystrophy or related conditions. Broadly speaking, there are two types of studies. The first are peer reviewed. Generally, the content of these studies has been reviewed by scientists or physicians. Peer-reviewed studies are typically published in scientific journals and are usually available at medical libraries. The second type of studies is non-peer reviewed. These works include summary articles that do not use or report scientific results. These often appear in the popular press, newsletters, or similar periodicals.

In this chapter, we will show you how to locate peer-reviewed references and studies on muscular dystrophy. We will begin by discussing research that has been summarized and is free to view by the public via the Internet. We then show you how to generate a bibliography on muscular dystrophy and teach you how to keep current on new studies as they are published or undertaken by the scientific community.

The Combined Health Information Database

The Combined Health Information Database summarizes studies across numerous federal agencies. To limit your investigation to research studies and muscular dystrophy, you will need to use the advanced search options. First, go to **http://chid.nih.gov/index.html**. From there, select the "Detailed Search" option (or go directly to that page with the following hyperlink: **http://chid.nih.gov/detail/detail.html**). The trick in extracting studies is found in the drop boxes at the bottom of the search page where "You may refine your search by." Select the dates and language you prefer, and the format option "Journal Article." At the top of the search form, select the number of records you would like to see (we recommend 100) and check the box to display "whole records." We recommend that you type in "muscular dystrophy" (or synonyms) into the "For these words:" box. Consider using the option "anywhere in record" to make your search as broad as possible. If you want to limit the search to only a particular field, such as the title of the journal, then select this option in the "Search in these fields" drop box. The following is a sample of what you can expect from this type of search:

- **Effects of Myotonic Dystrophy and Duchenne Muscular Dystrophy on the Orofacial Muscles and Dentofacial Morphology**

  Source: Acta Odontologica Scandanavica. 56(6): 369-374. December 1998.

  Summary: This article reviews two of the less rare myopathies: myotonic dystrophy (MyD) and Duchenne **muscular dystrophy** (DMD), and their effect on the orofacial muscles and dentofacial morphology. A high prevalence of malocclusions was found among the patients affected by these diseases. The development of the malocclusions in MyD patients seems to be strongly related to the vertical aberration of their craniofacial growth due to the involvement of the masticatory muscles in association with the possibly less affected suprahyoid musculature. Thus, a new situation is established around the teeth transversely. The lowered tongue is not in a position to counterbalance the forces developed during the lowering of the mandible by the stretched facial musculature. This may affect the teeth transversely, decreasing the width of the palate and causing posterior crossbite. The lowered position of the mandible, in combination with the decreased biting forces, may permit an overeruption of the posterior teeth, with increased palatal vault height and development of anterior open bite. The development of the malocclusions in DMD patients also seems to be strongly related to the involvement of the orofacial muscles by the disease. However, the posterior crossbite is not developed owing to the narrow maxillary (upper jaw) arch, as is the case in MyD patients. On the contrary, the posterior crossbite in DMD is due to the transversal expansion of the mandibular arch, possibly because of the decreased tonus of the masseter muscle near the molars, in combination with the enlarged hypotonic tongue and the predominance of the less affected orbicularis oris muscle. 2 figures. 33 references.

Federally Funded Research on Muscular Dystrophy

The U.S. Government supports a variety of research studies relating to muscular dystrophy and associated conditions. These studies are tracked by the Office of Extramural Research at the National Institutes of Health.[15] CRISP (Computerized Retrieval of Information on Scientific Projects) is a searchable database of federally funded biomedical research projects conducted at universities, hospitals, and other institutions. Visit CRISP at **http://crisp.cit.nih.gov/crisp/crisp_query.generate_screen**. You can perform targeted searches by various criteria including geography, date, as well as topics related to muscular dystrophy and related conditions.

For most of the studies, the agencies reporting into CRISP provide summaries or abstracts. As opposed to clinical trial research using patients, many federally funded studies use animals or simulated models to explore muscular dystrophy and related conditions. In some cases, therefore, it may be difficult to understand how some basic or fundamental research could eventually translate into medical practice. The following sample is typical of the type of information found when searching the CRISP database for muscular dystrophy:

- **Project Title: 2002 GORDON RESEARCH CONF. ON INTERMEDIATE FILAMENTS**

   Principal Investigator & Institution: Coulombe, Pierre A.; Professor; Biological Chemistry; Johns Hopkins University 3400 N Charles St Baltimore, Md 21218

   Timing: Fiscal Year 2002; Project Start 30-JUN-2002; Project End 31-DEC-2002

   Summary: (provided by applicant): The purpose of this application is to generate funds to support travel, registration, and lodging for participants in the 7th Gordon Research Conference on Intermediate Filaments, which will be held June 30th-July 5th 2002 at Roger Williams University in Bristol, Rhode Island. Intermediate filaments (IFs) are prominent components of the cytoskeleton and nuclecoskeleton in higher eukaryotes. In the public draft of the human genome, there are greater than 67 functional genes encoding IF-forming polypeptides. These genes are typically regulated in a cell type-specific manner and highly

---

[15] Healthcare projects are funded by the National Institutes of Health (NIH), Substance Abuse and Mental Health Services (SAMHSA), Health Resources and Services Administration (HRSA), Food and Drug Administration (FDA), Centers for Disease Control and Prevention (CDCP), Agency for Healthcare Research and Quality (AHRQ), and Office of Assistant Secretary of Health (OASH).

conserved in mammalian genomes. A general function of IF polymers is to endow cells and tissues with the mechanical resilience they need to withstand various types of physical and non-physical stresses. Defects in IF proteins underlie a vast number of genetically determined fragility disorders involving epithelia (e.g., skin, oral, and eye blistering diseases; inflammatory bowel diseases; liver disorders), muscle (e.g., cardiomyopathies; muscular dystrophy), neural tissue (e.g., amyotrophic lateral sclerosis; Alexander's diseases), and even adipose tissue (e.g., lipodystrophy). IFs fulfill other functions in a differentiation and context-dependent fashion, including promoting specific cytoarchitecture, tissue response to injury and other forms of stress, response to apoptotic signals, signaling, and nuclear architecture and gene expression (lamins). This Gordon Research Conference (GRC) is said to represent the only regular meeting devoted to IF biology. It brings together participants of junior and senior rank from all over the world who are studying IFs from a wide variety of angles. This GRC has traditionally fostered a free-flowing exchange of novel ideas, tools, and reagents, and facilitated the establishment of productive collaborations. The Program for the 2002 edition of the Conference has been finalized. The following major themes will be covered: 1) Atomic structure of IFs: From models to reality; 2) Regulating IF assembly and dynamics in vivo; 3) IFs and cell and tissue mechanics; 4) IF-associated cytolinkers: Mechanical integration and other functions; 4) Function of IFs in C. elegans, in muscle and neurons; 5) Functions of keratins in epithelia: Beyond scaffolding?; and 6) Laminopathies, lamin functions, and the nuclear envelope. In addition, there will be a special "Perspectives" session and a platform session dedicated to the discussion of posters.

Website: http://crisp.cit.nih.gov/crisp/Crisp_Query.Generate_Screen

- **Project Title: A NOVEL HIGH THROUGHPUT ASSAY FOR ION CHANNEL MODULATORS**

Principal Investigator & Institution: Wible, Barbara A.; Assistant Professor; Chanxpress, Inc. 14656 Neo Pky Cleveland, Oh 44128

Timing: Fiscal Year 2004; Project Start 01-FEB-2004; Project End 31-JUL-2004

Summary: (provided by applicant): Ion channels comprise 10-20 percent of known drug targets for diseases including cardiac arrhythmias, stroke, hypertension, heart failure, asthma, cystic fibrosis, epilepsy, migraine, mental disorders, **muscular dystrophy,** and cancer. While ion channels provide important therapeutic targets, they are often the focal point of unwanted drug interactions leading to potentially serious side effects. The cardiac potassium channel hERG is an example of frequent unwanted drug interactions; block of hERG can predispose individuals to cardiac arrhythmias. Given the dual nature of ion channel targets, there is a need for high throughput assays that address the therapeutic potential as well as the drug safety issue. ChanTest, an ion channel company dedicated to providing technology services to the biopharmaceutical industry for drug safety testing and drug discovery involving ion channels, is developing novel high throughput screens that can address both needs. These proprietary assays monitor the level of expression of ion channels using an antibody-based chemiluminescent reaction. The goals of this proposal are to develop assays using the hERG potassium channel for two purposes: 1) HTXpress: high throughput screening of diverse chemical libraries for compounds which either increase or decrease hERG expression without affecting the kinetic properties of the channel, and 2) hERG-Lite: high throughput drug safety screening to identify drugs which block hERG using increased surface expression of mutant hERG channels as a biosensor for block. For HTXpress, the specific aim of this proposal is to optimize the assay by screening a structurally diverse chemical library of over 800 compounds. The identification of ion channel expression modulators, i.e. novel agonists and antagonists, is an untapped area of drug development and can be easily applied to channels other than hERG. With respect to hERG-Lite, the goal is to validate the use of this assay as a rapid safety test for hERG block. Eighty drugs (half known hERG blockers and half nonblockers) will be assayed for their behavior in the expression assay. Their potencies and rank order will be compared to hERG block assayed by standard electrophysiological measurements. The goal is to introduce hERG-Lite to the pharmaceutical industry as a rapid, inexpensive, and sensitive screen for hERG safety testing early in drug development.

Website: http://crisp.cit.nih.gov/crisp/Crisp_Query.Generate_Screen

- **Project Title: ACQUISITION OF A NANOFLOW ION TRAP MASS SPECTROMETER**

Principal Investigator & Institution: Wysocki, Vicki H.; Professor; Chemistry; University of Arizona P O Box 3308 Tucson, Az 857223308

Timing: Fiscal Year 2003; Project Start 01-APR-2003; Project End 31-MAR-2004

Summary: (provided by applicant): This proposal requests a Thermo Finnigan ProteomeX DECAP-51000 Integrated Workstation, an ion trap mass spectrometer equipped with LC pumps, a 10 port switching valve, strong cation and reversed phase columns for multidimensional chromatography, and a nanospray probe. This instrument will serve the needs of a number of University of Arizona bioscience researchers. The major users and their applications for the instrumentation are (1) Samuel Ward, Molecular and Cellular Biology, Study of signaling pathways during cell differentiation in the Nematode C.elegans, genes are homologeous to human disease genes linked to Alzheimer's and **muscular dystrophy;** (2) Brian Larkins, Plant Sciences, College of Agriculture and Life Sciences, Identificationand Analysis of Proteins Required for Improved Maize Protein Nutritional Quality; (3) M. Halonen/D. Vercelli/F. Martinez/M. Cusanovich, Center for Respiratory Sciences, Transcription Factors that Bind Regulatory Elements in the Immunoglobulin G4 Germline Promoter, the IL-13 Promoter, and the CD 14 Promoter; Cellular and Molecular Mechanisms of Asthma (4) Elizabeth Vierling, Molecular and Cellular Biology, Molecular chaperone function; expression and function of cytoplasmic organelle and heat shock proteins, the pathways studied are critical to normal cell function; (5) Carol Dieckmann, Biochemistry, Identification of Mutations in Genes Coding for Major Polypeptides in the Chlamydomonas Eyespot;, (6) Thomas Baldwin, Biochemistry, Pulsed Alkylation MS to Investigate Protein Folding in Bacterial Luciferase; (7) Vicki Wysocki, Chemistry, Mechanisms and Energetics of Peptide Dissociation, this work is directly applicable to the identification of proteins from biological organisms. Modern protein research cannot be accomplished without mass spectrometry. The access to a dedicated microflow LC-mass spectrometer with a nanospray probe to characterize samples that are not amenable to analysis with the current mass spectrometry facility instruments is critical to the maximum productivity and success of these projects. The University has made a strong commitment to the project by by renovating space for a new "branch" mass spectrometry laboratory that is located in Biosciences, by hiring a full time Ph.D. biological mass spectrometry specialist (about $60,000 per year), by providing funds for a Director of Proteomics (about $80,000/year) and a technician (about $35,000/year) to help with sample preparation, and by providing cost sharing in the amount of $75,000.

Website: http://crisp.cit.nih.gov/crisp/Crisp_Query.Generate_Screen

- **Project Title: ACTININ ASSOCIATED LIM PROTEIN & FSH MUSCULAR DYSTROPHY**

Principal Investigator & Institution: Bredt, David S.; Professor; Physiology; University of California San Francisco 3333 California Street, Suite 315 San Francisco, Ca 941430962

Timing: Fiscal Year 2002; Project Start 01-FEB-1996; Project End 31-JAN-2003

Summary: Disruptions of the myofiber cytoskeleton underlie several genetic muscular dystrophies, including Duchenne and Limb-girdle muscular dystrophies. In addition to these dystrophin-related disorders, certain inherited muscular dystrophies are due to mutations in cytoskeletal proteins that do not interact with the dystrophin complex. Identification of the responsible proteins and clarification of mechanisms that regulate the myofiber cytoskeleton are therefore critical goals. Recent molecular cloning studies have identified actinin-associated LIM protein (ALP), which is a novel component of the muscle cytoskeleton. ALP contains a PDZ protein motif that is also present in certain dystrophin-associated proteins, yet ALP does not interact with dystrophin. Instead ALP binds to actinin, a structural homologue of dystrophin, and ALP associates with actinin at the Z-lines of skeletal muscle. Chromosomal mapping studies show that ALP occurs in 4q35, within 7 Mb of the telomeric region that is deleted in facioscapulohumeral **muscular dystrophy** (FSHD), the most common autosomal **muscular dystrophy.** ALP is the only muscle-specific gene yet found to map in this region. Therefore, a possible role for ALP in the pathogenesis of FSHD must be explored. We now propose to characterize the molecular interaction of ALP with actinin and to determine the composition and function of the ALP-associated complex at the Z-lines. To help assess whether ALP participates in FSHD, we will determine whether ALP expression is altered in muscle biopsies from diseased patients. Because FSHD is a dominant disease, it is likely that only one allele of the responsible gene(s) will be abnormal. To address this, we will also evaluate allele-specific expression of ALP in FSHD muscle samples. Because complex genetics underlie FSHD, studies of human tissues alone may not decisively identify the responsible gene(s). We will therefore target disruption of ALP in stem cells and breed mice that lack ALP protein. Muscle development, histology and function will be carefully evaluated in the ALP mutants. Assembly of the ALP-associated protein complex at the Z-lines will also be evaluated in the mutants. If these mutant mice manifest signs that resemble FSHD this would implicate a role for ALP in this disease and the mice would provide a unique animal model. The proposed studies will lead to a better understanding of formation and function of the myofiber cytoskeleton and may provide insight in the pathogenesis and treatment of FSHD.

Website: http://crisp.cit.nih.gov/crisp/Crisp_Query.Generate_Screen

- **Project Title: ADENO-ASSOCIATED VIRUS (AAV) VECTORS TO IMPROVE MATURE MUSCLE FUNCTION**

Principal Investigator & Institution: Xiao, Xiao; Associate Professor; University of Pittsburgh at Pittsburgh 350 Thackeray Hall Pittsburgh, Pa 15260

Timing: Fiscal Year 2002; Project Start 01-APR-2002; Project End 31-MAR-2003

Summary: Muscular dystrophies are a relatively common group of inherited degenerative muscle disease. Most types are caused by mutations in genes coding for membrane associated proteins in muscle. Duchenne **muscular dystrophy** (DMD) and **limb-girdle muscular dystrophy** (LGMD) often manifest themselves in young ages and lead to early morbidity with no currently available effective treatment. These diseases are recessive, loss-of- function of the corresponding gene product, which makes them suitable for gene replacement therapy. Recombinant adeno-associate virus (rAAV) is one promising gene replacement vector based on defective human parvoviruses. The rAAV system has attracted attention due to its non- pathogenicity, genomic integration, transduction of quiescent cells, and apparent lack of cellular immune reactions. In contrast to other viral vectors, rAAV is capable of efficiently bypassing the myofiber basal lamina and transducing mature muscle cells. We have demonstrated that rAAV vectors harboring a foreign gene can achieve highly efficient and sustained gene expression in mature muscle of immunocompetent animals for more than 1.5 years without detectable toxicity. Recently, significant improvement in vector production methodology has made it possible to generate high titer and high quality rAAV vectors completely free of helper adenovirus contamination. However, no experiments using rAAV vectors to restore the functional deficits in muscle tissue itself have been reported to date. Here, we propose to take advantage of rAAV vector system, to test two therapeutic genes (delta-sarcoglycan and a highly truncated dystrophin), under the control of two different promoter systems (viral/CMV or muscle- specific/MCK), in two relevant animal models of muscular dystrophies (Bio14.6 hamster for LGMD and mdx mouse for DMD). Two distinct vector delivery methods, local intramuscular infection versus systemic delivery will be utilized. We have the following three hypotheses to be tested. 1): muscle deficient in delta-sarcoglycan can be functionally rescued by genetic complementation using intramuscular AAV vector injection in the LGMD hamster model. 2) systemic delivery of the delta-sarcoglycan gene can be mediated by rAAV vectors through intra-artery or intra-ventricle injection. 3) a dystrophin mini-gene lacking the central rod domain will improve the function of dystrophin-deficient muscle when delivered into dystrophic mdx mice by AAV vectors.

Website: http://crisp.cit.nih.gov/crisp/Crisp_Query.Generate_Screen

- **Project Title: ANALYSIS OF TORSIN PROTEIN FUNCTION IN C. ELEGANS**

Principal Investigator & Institution: Caldwell, Guy A.; Biological Sciences; University of Alabama in Tuscaloosa Tuscaloosa, Al 35487

Timing: Fiscal Year 2003; Project Start 01-FEB-2003; Project End 31-JAN-2006

Summary: (provided by applicant): Dystonia is estimated to be six times more prevalent than Huntington's Disease, ALS, or **Muscular Dystrophy.** However, as few as 5% of the over 350,000 persons in North America estimated to be affected have been correctly diagnosed and are under treatment (NIH Budget Office). The most severe early-onset form of this disorder has been linked to a mutation in a human gene named TOR1A that encodes torsinA, a protein that is also localized to inclusions in the brains of Parkinson's patients termed Lewy bodies. While a causative genetic mutation has been identified, the cellular mechanisms of pathogenesis underlying dystonia remain unknown. We are applying the advantages of the model organism, Caenorhabditis elegans, towards a detailed analysis of two specific torsin-related gene products in this nematode. The chromosomal positioning of these genes suggests that they may represent a functionally co-expressed unit and preliminary studies from our laboratory indicate they act neuronally. Phylogenetic analysis of the torsin family indicates these proteins share distant sequence similarity with the functionally diverse AAA+ family of proteins. We have determined that ectopic overexpression of a C. elegans torsin homolog results in a reduction of polyglutamine repeat-induced protein aggregation in a manner similar to that previously reported for molecular chaperones. The suppressive effects of torsin overexpression quantitatively persisted as animals aged. Antibody staining of transgenic animals using antisera specific to TOR-2 indicated this protein was highly localized to sites of protein aggregation. We propose to extend these preliminary studies through a combination of reverse genetic approaches designed to investigate the cellular role of torsin proteins in the nematode. The specific aims of the proposed project include: 1) to determine what phenotypes are associated with C. elegans torsin homologues; 2) to define sites of C. elegans torsin protein function; and 3) to determine potential effectors of torsin activity. These studies will further our understanding of the molecular mechanisms responsible for early-onset torsion dystonia. Moreover, the aberrant protein deposition associated with diverse neurodegenerative disorders like Parkinson's Disease and those caused by polyglutamine expansion such as Huntington's Disease warrants further investigation of any putative neuroprotective effects of torsins.

Website: http://crisp.cit.nih.gov/crisp/Crisp_Query.Generate_Screen

- **Project Title: ANTISENSE OLIGONUCLEOTIDE SUPPRESSION OF DMD**

Principal Investigator & Institution: Wilton, Stephen D.; University of Western Australia Crawley, Wa, 6009

Timing: Fiscal Year 2004; Project Start 01-JAN-2004; Project End 31-DEC-2007

Summary: (provided by applicant): The ultimate goal of this project is to develop an antisense oligonucleotide (AO) therapy for Duchenne **muscular dystrophy** (DMD). Antisense oligonucleotides (AOs) can be used to reduce the severity of DMD by removing specific exons during pre-mRNA splicing, to either by-pass nonsense mutations or restore the reading frame around dystrophin genomic deletions. As a result of the treatment, dystrophin expression would be restored in dystrophic tissue and DMD patients would theoretically manifest only the milder phenotype of Becker **Muscular Dystrophy** (BMD). This project will explore the design and delivery of AOs to minimize the consequences of disease-causing dystrophin gene mutations. (1) Animal models of **muscular dystrophy** will be used to develop treatment regimens and assess therapeutic benefits in vivo. (2) AOs will be designed to target the most amenable splicing motifs at relevant exons in the human dystrophin gene transcript and will be evaluated in cultured human muscle cells. Although this approach cannot permanently correct the primary genetic lesion, we propose that repeated administration, preferably through systemic delivery, should be feasible. AO chemistries or modifications to increase stability and/or uptake, optimized for in vivo induction of exon skipping, will be developed and evaluated. Only periodic administration of AOs should be required to maintain therapeutic levels of induced dystrophin in dystrophic muscle. DMD is a serious disorder for which there is no effective treatment. AOs will not cure this devastating condition, however, AO-based splicing intervention has the potential to reduce the severity of DMD so that treated boys should be able to produce some functional dystrophin. This would be expected to moderate the severity of DMD and improve the quality of life for patients and their families.

Website: http://crisp.cit.nih.gov/crisp/Crisp_Query.Generate_Screen

- **Project Title:** ASTROCYTE DYSTROGLYCAN COMPLEXES IN BRAIN DEVELOPMENT

Principal Investigator & Institution: Moore, Steven A.; Professor; Pathology; University of Iowa Iowa City, Ia 52242

Timing: Fiscal Year 2002; Project Start 20-APR-2001; Project End 31-MAR-2004

Summary: (Applicant's abstract): The dystrophin-glycoprotein complex (DGC) is a well characterized array of cytoplasmic, membrane spanning, and extracellular matrix proteins that form a critical linkage between the cytoskeleton and the basal lamina of striated muscle. Within the central nervous system (CNS), similar dystroglycan linkages to basal laminae are present at two interfaces formed by astrocytes: (1) foot processes abutting on cerebral blood vessels and (2) foot processes that form the glia limitans at the pial surface of the brain. The former interface is critical for formation and maintenance of the blood-brain barrier, while the latter is likely to play important roles in anchoring radial glia during neuronal migration. Basal lamina abnormalities at the glia limitans have been identified in some forms of congenital **muscular dystrophy** in humans (e.g. Fukuyama muscular dystrophy) and basal lamina disruption at the glia limitans leads to abnormal CNS development in animal models. In this proposal, we will focus attention on the central protein in the astrocyte-basal lamina linkage, dystroglycan. Our Specific Aims propose to identify protein elements of the astrocyte-dystroglycan complex, elucidate protein interactions within the complex, and demonstrate the importance of the astrocyte dystroglycan complex during CNS development. Through the use of Cre-lox methodology, we plan to create a novel murine model of CNS developmental disorders. This project is a cross-discipline collaboration among investigators with expertise in clinical neuropathology and in basic neuroscience, molecular biology, cell biology, and membrane physiology who are uniquely situated to carry out the proposed studies. Aim 1: To define the composition of the astrocyte-dystroglycan complex(es), we will test the hypothesis that one-or-more dystroglycan complexes are present in astrocytes using a combination of biochemical and immunohistochemical methods. These studies will utilize tissue sections and cultured astrocytes from wild type mice and mice with naturally occurring or genetically engineered mutations of one or more of the DGC components known to be expressed in astrocytes. Aim 2: To create a new model of CNS developmental abnormalities by selectively disrupting the astrocyte-dystroglycan complex. Dystroglycan +/-, dystroglycan lox/lox, and GFAP-Cre mice will be bred to produce GFAP-Cre/dystroglycan lox/- and GFAP-Cre/dystroglycan lox/lox mice. This strategy should disrupt the astrocyte DGC beginning in the latter half of embryonic development. We believe this strategy will produce mice with neuronal migration and cerebrovascular defects.

Website: http://crisp.cit.nih.gov/crisp/Crisp_Query.Generate_Screen

- **Project Title: BIOENGINEERING RESEARCH PARTNERSHIP-- MUSCULAR DYSTROPHY**

  Principal Investigator & Institution: Sweeney, Hugh Lee.; Professor and Chairman; Physiology; University of Pennsylvania 3451 Walnut Street Philadelphia, Pa 19104

  Timing: Fiscal Year 2002; Project Start 20-SEP-2000; Project End 31-AUG-2005

  Summary: (Applicant's abstract verbatim) The goal of this BRP is to utilize a number of aspects of bioengineering in order to develop tools and therapeutics for the treatment and monitoring of muscular dystrophies. The project is collaboration between three investigators and includes the following areas of bioengineering relevant to the PA: 1) cell and tissue engineering, 2) imaging and 3) therapeutics. Collectively we will delineate factors that when expressed in muscle may slow that rate of degeneration that is concomitant with either the complete (Duchenne muscular dystrophy) or partial (Becker muscular dystrophy) loss of dystrophin. These studies will utilize the mdx mouse as the animal model for dystrophin deficiency. The long-term goal is to gain the understanding and tools necessary to develop adeno-associated (AAV)-based gene therapy for Duchenne and Becker muscular dystrophies. Three parallel lines of investigation (each directed by one of the three investigators) are proposed: Section 1: a dissection the mechanical role of dystrophin and muscle adhesion proteins (directed by Dennis Discher); Section 2: an assessment of the functional benefits of restoring adhesion molecules to dystrophic muscle using recombinant adeno-associated virus gene delivery (directed by H. Lee Sweeney, Ph.D.); and Section 3: development of non-invasive methods for monitoring therapeutic benefits of dystrophin gene transfer (directed by Glenn Walter, Ph.D.).

  Website: http://crisp.cit.nih.gov/crisp/Crisp_Query.Generate_Screen

- **Project Title: CAVEOLIN-3 AND MUSCULAR DYSTROPHY**

  Principal Investigator & Institution: Lisanti, Michael P.; Professor; Molecular Pharmacology; Yeshiva University 500 W 185Th St New York, Ny 10033

  Timing: Fiscal Year 2002; Project Start 01-APR-2000; Project End 31-MAR-2005

Summary: The long-term objective of this proposal is to understand the role of muscle caveolae and caveolin-3 i) in normal muscle development; and ii) in the pathogenesis of muscle dystrophy. Caveolae are "little caves" at the surface of cells. It has been proposed that caveolae function as message centers" for regulating signal transduction. Caveolin-3, a muscle-specific caveolin-related protein, is the principal structural protein of caveolae membrane domains in striated muscle cell types (cardiac and skeletal). Recently, we identified a novel autosomal dominant form of limb girdle **muscular dystrophy** (LGMD-1C) in humans that is due to mutations within the coding sequence of the human caveolin-3 gene (3p25). The aim of this proposal is to test the hypothesis that caveolin-3 expression is important for normal muscle development and that changes in caveolin-3 expression (either up-regulation or down-regulation) can result in **muscular dystrophy** phenotype. In order to test this hypothesis,, we will use a variety of complementary in vivo approaches, such as the use of caveolin-3 anti-senses in cultured cells and the development of mouse animal models. The specific aims of the project are: 1) To determine the role of caveolin-3 mutations in the pathogenesis of LGMD- 1C. We will examine the phenotypic behavior of LGMD-1C mutations of caveolin-3 after heterologous expression in NIH 3T3 cells, as compared with wild-type caveolin-3; 2) To develop transgenic mouse models that over wild-type caveolin-3 and LGMD-1C mutant forms of caveolin-3. We will over-express wild type and LGMD-1C mutant forms of caveolin- 3 as transgenes in mice and assess their effects on skeletal muscle. As caveolin-3 levels are up-regulated in **Duchenne's muscular dystrophy,** these experiments will help us evaluate if caveolin-3 up-regulation contributes to the pathogenesis of this diseases; and 3) To examine if caveolin-3 expression is required for normal muscle development. Using an anti-sense approach, we will abrogate caveolin-3 expression in C2C12 cells, a skeletal myoblast cell line that differentiates in culture. We will then assess the effects of caveolin-3 down-regulation on C2C12 myoblast fusion and myotube formation. In addition, through a targeted gene disruption approach, we will create and characterize "knock-out" mice that lack caveolin-3 gene expression. It is expected that these studies will contribute fundamen6tal knowledge toward understanding the role of muscle cell caveolae in normal muscle development and **muscular dystrophy.**

Website: http://crisp.cit.nih.gov/crisp/Crisp_Query.Generate_Screen

- **Project Title: CELLULAR SIGNALING AND MUSCULAR DYSTROPHIES**

Principal Investigator & Institution: Rando, Thomas A.; Associate Professor; Neurology & Neurological Scis; Stanford University Stanford, Ca 94305

Timing: Fiscal Year 2002; Project Start 15-AUG-2001; Project End 31-JUL-2006

Summary: The muscular dystrophies are devastating diseases of progressive weakness due to apoptotic and necrotic death of muscle cells. The normal cellular mechanisms regulating cell survival that are disrupted in these diseases are not well understood. Several forms of **muscular dystrophy** are due to abnormalities of membrane proteins and protein complexes, such as integrins and caveolins, that are known to regulate cellular signaling pathways in general, and cell survival signaling in particular, in different cell types. Others, such as those due to dystrophin mutations, are due to abnormalities of protein complexes that are postulated to transduce signals from the extracellular matrix into the cell. We will focus on three proteins/protein complexes that cause muscular dystrophies when a component of the complex is deficient or defective - alpha5beta1 integrin, caveolin-3, and the dystrophin-glycoprotein complex (DGC). The experiments of this proposal are designed to explore the cellular signaling processes the promote cell survival via these membrane protein complexes, and the mechanisms of cell death when these complexes are disrupted. For studies of integrin signaling, we will use cells genetically deficient in alpha5 integrin to test which isoforms of protein kinase C are important in alpha5 integrin mediated muscle cell survival (based on our previous finding of the importance of protein kinase C in this process). We will explore how alpha5 integrin deficiency leads to muscle cell death by testing for dysregulation of cell survival/cell death pathways involving the Bcl family of proteins, cytochrome c release from mitochondria, and activation of the caspase cascade. We will also examine the role of activation of the PI3 kinase/Akt pathway in alpha5 integrin- mediated muscle cell survival. For studies of the DGC, we will investigate how disruption (genetically, by antibody inhibition, or by antisense expression) of the association of the complex with the extracellular matrix may lead to cell death. In these studies, we will also examine cells for dysregulation of cell survival mechanisms involving Bcl family proteins since apoptosis has been shown to be the earliest change in muscle associated with dystrophin deficiency. For studies of dystrophies due to caveolin-3 mutations, we will render muscle cells functionally deficient in caveolin-3 using both antisense methods and dominant negative inhibitors. We will study the mechanisms by which caveolin-3 deficiency lead to muscle cell death, and we will test whether these mechanisms involve the disruption of either normal integrin signaling or signaling through the DGC.

Website: http://crisp.cit.nih.gov/crisp/Crisp_Query.Generate_Screen

- **Project Title: CLINICAL AND MOLECULAR ANALYSIS OF OREGON EYE DISEASE**

Principal Investigator & Institution: Pillers, De-Ann M.; Associate Professor; Pediatrics; Oregon Health & Science University Portland, or 972393098

Timing: Fiscal Year 2002; Project Start 30-SEP-1994; Project End 31-MAY-2005

Summary: (Verbatim from applicant's abstract): The title of the application is "Clinical and molecular analysis of Oregon Eye Disease." A more current title would be "Dystrophin and the retina." During the initial application period, it was shown that dystrophin, the product of the Duchenne **muscular dystrophy** (DMD) gene, is involved in retinal electrophysiology. Three lines of evidence support this. The position of a mutation in the DMD gene predicts the ERG phenotype, and abnormal ERGs were correlated in large part with mutations of a specific isoform of dystrophin, Dp260, which was identified and cloned from retina. New data suggests that other muscular dystrophies are associated with defects in retinal electrophysiology. Specifically, mouse models with defects in laminin-2 have abnormal ERGs. Dystrophin is part of a cellular continuum from the actin cytoskeleton to laminin and the extracellular matrix via a transmembrane group of proteins known as dystrophin-associated glycoproteins (DGC). It is hypothesized that defects in the interaction between retina-specific isoforms of dystrophin and the DGC result in altered retinal electrophysiology and an abnormal ERG. It is proposed that the retinal isoform Dp260 plays an important role in retinal electrophysiology by interfacing with the DGC at the photoreceptor to bipolar synapse. It is further proposed that dystrophin isoforms with non-overlapping cellular distributions have distinct roles in retinal function. Three specific aims will be performed to test these hypotheses, involving: (1) defining genotype-phenotype correlations for the DGC performing ERGs on both mutant mice and patients with defects in these proteins; (2) defining the specific cell synapse responsible for the ERG abnormalities demonstrated in the mdxCV3 mouse by in vitro cell-specific electrophysiology; and (3) delineating the diversity of dystrophin isoform expression in retina and to determining unique aspects of isoform structure and expression that may contribute to retinal electrophysiology. The long-term goals are to delineate the pathway by which dystrophin contributes to the normal ERG. By so doing, proteins will be identified, which when mutated, will be candidate genes for inherited retinal disorders associated with abnormal electrophysiology. Dystrophin and other proteins including members of the DGC will be targets for future gene therapy approaches.

Website: http://crisp.cit.nih.gov/crisp/Crisp_Query.Generate_Screen

- **Project Title: CLONING/CHARACTERIZATING A MYOTONIC DYSTROPHY LOCUS**

Principal Investigator & Institution: Ranum, Laura P.; Professor; Neurology; University of Minnesota Twin Cities 200 Oak Street Se Minneapolis, Mn 554552070

Timing: Fiscal Year 2002; Project Start 01-JUN-1997; Project End 31-MAY-2005

Summary: Myotonic dystrophy (DM) is a multisystem disease and the most common form of **muscular dystrophy** in adults. In 1992, one form of DM was shown to be caused by an expanded CTG repeat in the 3' untranslated region of the myotonin protein kinase gene (DMPK) on chromosome 19. Although multiple theories attempt to explain how the CTG expansion causes the broad spectrum of clinical features in DM, there is no consensus about how this mutation, which does not alter the protein coding region of a gene, affects cellular function. We have identified a five-generation family (MN1) with a genetically distinct form of myotonic dystrophy. Affected members have the characteristic features of DM (myotonia, proximal and distal limb weakness, frontal balding, cataracts, and cardiac arrhythmias) but do not have the chromosome 19 mutation. We have mapped the disease locus (DM2) for the MN1 family to a small region of chromosome 3 (Nature Genetics 19:196- 198). This proposal outlines a strategy to identify and characterize the DM2 locus. Understanding what is common to chromosome 19 DM (now designated DM1 by the DM consortium) and DM2 at the molecular level should shed light on the mechanisms responsible for the broad constellation of clinical features present in both diseases. Our specific aims are: 1) to develop a high-resolution map of the DM2 region (0.5-1.0 cM) using haplotype and linkage disequilibrium analysis of 29 DM2/PROMM families from Minnesota and Germany; 2) to identify the expressed genes and repeat motifs in the region and prioritize candidates based on homology and expression patterns; 3) to identify the DM2 mutation; 4) to characterize the DM2 gene and investigate whether or not the pathogenic molecular changes found in DM2 are part of a common pathway also affected in DM1; 5) to determine whether molecular changes affecting RNA splicing,

CUG binding proteins, and apamin receptors are similar to those found in DM1.

Website: http://crisp.cit.nih.gov/crisp/Crisp_Query.Generate_Screen

- **Project Title: COMPUTATIONAL ANALYSIS OF HUMAN 'AT-RISK' DNA MOTIFS**

Principal Investigator & Institution: Stenger, Judith E.; Assistant Professor; Medicine; Duke University Durham, Nc 27710

Timing: Fiscal Year 2002; Project Start 01-JUN-2001; Project End 31-MAY-2004

Summary: (Taken from the Candidate's Abstract) At-Risk DNA Motifs (ARMS), which include repetitive elements such as Alu sequences, homonucleotide runs and triplet repeats, are potentially unstable segments of the human genome. ARMS are a factor in genetic susceptibility to disease, requiring particular combinations of genetic backgrounds and environmental triggers to express a disease phenotype. While some of the mechanisms are understood, it is not clear under what circumstances repetitive DNA elements mediate pathological mutagenesis. Although a high burden of these sequences is generally tolerated in humans, they can have an enormous impact on health by contributing to diseases that have devastating effects on afflicted individuals. For example, Alus have been linked to numerous diseases including Fanconi anemia, alphazerothalassemia, leukemia, hypertension, neurofibromatosis, breast, and colon cancers. Trinucleotide repeat expansions have been linked with Kennedy's Disease, Huntington's Disease, **myotonic muscular dystrophy,** and Friedreich ataxia. The long term objective of this proposal is to gain insight into the genetic factors that mitigate gene rearrangement in hopes of predicting when the presence of a repetitive element truly constitutes a threat to the health of an individual. The hypothesis is that the characterization of ARMS according to all possible attributes (i.e. size of repeats, separation distances between repeats, orientation, sequence similarity between repeats, nucleotide base constitution and proximity and/or containment of mutagenic and/or toxicological agent targets, DNA processive or other enzymatic target sites) can reveal largely excluded situations that can be viewed as unstable. It is also postulated that a multidimensional database of repetitive sequences characterized according to the aforementioned attributes can be used to predict repetitive elements that are most prone to mutation, ARMS, while increasing our understanding of the interactions between these genetic elements and their environment. The approach is to use a combination of computational biology and molecular genomic analysis to locate and analyze ARMS. The specific aims of this proposal are to: 1) characterize available data according to the conceivable relevant attributes of size, distance, orientation, degree of homology, base constitution and containment of known target sequences. 2) To test the hypothesis by computationally identifying loci that have already known to contain ARMS linked to a mutation resulting in disease, and then to identify specific genes that may be at-risk for mutation and experimentally testing them using molecular biological approaches. 3) To set up an interactive on-line database and program server so that the scientific community can use the information and apply it to drive experimental research.

Website: http://crisp.cit.nih.gov/crisp/Crisp_Query.Generate_Screen

- **Project Title: CONFERENCE: BIOLOGY OF CALPAINS IN HEALTH AND DISEASE**

Principal Investigator & Institution: Forsberg, Neil E.; Professor; Federation of Amer Soc for Exper Biology Bethesda, Md 208143998

Timing: Fiscal Year 2004; Project Start 03-MAY-2004; Project End 31-JUL-2004

Summary: (provided by applicant): A FASEB Summer Conference titled "Biology of Calpains in Health and Disease" is scheduled for June 12-17, 2004. The meeting will be held in Tuscon, Arizona. This will be the third FASEB-sponsored Calpain meeting. Funds are being requested from three NIH divisions (NIAMS, NIDDK and NEI) in partial support of this conference. The thematic sessions for the conference will be: 1) Calpain Gene Family, 2) Calpain Structure, 3) Physiological Roles, 4) Calpains and Signal Transduction, 5) Pathologic Involvement of Calpains, 6), Calpain Inhibitors in Treatment of Disease, 7) Agricultural Applications and 8) A Holistic View (two sessions). The latter session (A Holistic View) is designed to stimulate thoughts on how the calpains participate, in tandem with other proteases, in mediation of normal and pathological processes (e.g., apoptosis and myofibrillar protein degradation). This topic will be supported by a keynote speaker who is a leader in the biology of cysteine proteases (Dr. Alan Barrett, Babraham Institute) and by speakers who have expertise with other proteolytic systems (notably the ubiquitin/proteasome system). A meeting on the biology of the calpains is highly-relevant to the NIH because calpains are involved in both normal and pathologic processes. The activities of the house-keeping u- and m-calpains are important to normal turnover and processing of cytoskeletal and membrane proteins in all tissues. A defective muscle-specific calpain (p94) is responsible, in part, for **Limb-Girdle Muscular Dystrophy** Type IIA. Interestingly, the gene encoding p94 is also expressed as a lens-specific calpain isoform (Lp82) which, when activates, underlies cataractogenesis. Defects in calpain-10 have now been related to adult onset diabetes and to cystic ovary disease. Skeletal and cardiac muscle damage as well as cerebral ischemia have been related to pathologic activation of calpains. Three years will have passed since the last meeting on calpains. Substantial progress on the genomics, biology, structure, activation and roles of calpains has been made in the past few years. The proposed program will provide the forum by which the momentum in this field may be maintained.

Website: http://crisp.cit.nih.gov/crisp/Crisp_Query.Generate_Screen

- **Project Title: CORE--AAV VECTOR FACILITY**

Principal Investigator & Institution: Barranger, John A.; Professor; University of Pittsburgh at Pittsburgh 350 Thackeray Hall Pittsburgh, Pa 15260

Timing: Fiscal Year 2003; Project Start 30-SEP-2003; Project End 31-AUG-2008

Description (provided by applicant): The manufacture of clinical grade gene transfer vectors requires the development of efficient, large scale methods that are appropriate for the generation of safe materials to be used in human study subjects. This work involves both laboratory expertise and regulatory oversight of the safety of the products made in the Human Gene Therapy Applications Laboratory (HGTAL). Specific Aim 1: The HGTAL will work collaboratively with the AAV preclinical vector development core, Directed by Dr. Xiao Xiao, to translate laboratory AAV production techniques into a scalable and controlled manufacturing process that can be used to produce clinical grade AAV in years 2 and 3 to support the proposed clinical trial that is projected to start in year 3. Specific Aim 2: The HGTAL will manufacture and certify a lot of recombinant AAV for the support of a phase 1 dose determination study. This material will also be certified and characterized according to CBER guidelines and will be used supporting toxicology studies. Specific Aim 3: The HGTAL will refine and improve upon its AAV vector manufacturing capabilities and will produce at least two subsequent lots of recombinant AAV vector to support a phase II efficacy study. A determination of the size of the lots needed to be produced will be finalized based upon the highest dose which can be administered to patients, as determined in the phase 1 dose escalation study.

Website: http://crisp.cit.nih.gov/crisp/Crisp_Query.Generate_Screen

- **Project Title: CORE--BIOLOGIC IMAGING**

Principal Investigator & Institution: Watkins, Simon C.; Professor; University of Pittsburgh at Pittsburgh 350 Thackeray Hall Pittsburgh, Pa 15260

Timing: Fiscal Year 2003; Project Start 30-SEP-2003; Project End 31-AUG-2008

Description (provided by applicant): Visualization and localization of message, protein, or structural change resulting from gene expression is an essential step in evaluating the efficacy of successful gene transfer into cells and tissues. The goals of this program are to extend our understanding of the cellular pathology of Duchenne **Muscular Dystrophy** and to develop vector systems for dystrophin delivery using a variety of possible delivery systems, including AAV, Herpes, and stem cells. It is expected that these vectors will be used to use these vectors to generate clinically useful therapeutic regimens. In each case there is a fundamental need to define the level of incorporation of the delivered dystrophin into muscle, and to assess the effectiveness of the therapy. This identification varies from the low-resolution studies of whole tissues, defining correction of pathological phenotype, to high-resolution observations of successful subcellular passaging and presentation of protein. The Center for Biologic Imaging, in which this core service will be performed, is designed with this function in mind. It is equipped to perform a continuum of optical methods including all types of light and electron microscopy essential to this program project. Within the scope of this project at the light microscopic level these include: histological, immuno-histological and possibly live cell technologies. At the electron microscopic level we will provide fine structural and immuno-electron microscopic evaluation of specimens as a natural extension of the light microscopic analyses when needed. Furthermore, our considerable experience in computerized image processing and morphometry will allow quantitative analysis of observed phenomena to corroborate earlier, possibly quite subtle qualitative changes. This core will be used extensively by all projects, though the imaging tools used will vary from project to project. Preliminary data have shown the validity of these approaches, and we expect a very significant increase in the use of optical techniques within the formal setting of this program.

Website: http://crisp.cit.nih.gov/crisp/Crisp_Query.Generate_Screen

- **Project Title: CORE--RESEARCH RESOURCES**

Principal Investigator & Institution: Thornton, Charles A.; University of Rochester Orpa - Rc Box 270140 Rochester, Ny 14627

Timing: Fiscal Year 2003; Project Start 30-SEP-2003; Project End 31-MAY-2008

Summary: The last three years have brought remarkable progress in understanding the disease mechanisms in dominantly-inherited muscular dystrophies, myotonic dystrophy (DM), facioscapulohumeral dystrophy (FSHD), and **oculopharyngeal muscular dystrophy** (OPMD). A relatively complete pathophysiologic understanding of these disorders is within reach, and it seems likely that more attention will be devoted to developing new treatments. To maximally exploit these research opportunities it will be necessary to expand the base of basic and translational researchers who work on these disorders and give them access to critical biological and bioinformatic resources. To help accomplish this objective, the aim of this project is to develop a Repository Core for the University of Rochester **Muscular Dystrophy** Cooperative Research Center. The resources in the Repository have been built up over many years by investigators in this Center. These resources include DM and FSHD myoblasts, transgenic mouse models and cells derived from these models, plasmids for expressing expanded RNA repeats and for developing new models for repeat expansion disorders, antibodies, and tissue samples. In addition, a comprehensive database of expression profile data from normal individuals and patients with DM or FHSD will be provided to researchers interested in data mining or to serve as controls for studies of muscle gene expression that are performed at other institutions. Orderly procedures for requesting and delivering materials from the Repository are proposed. By helping to remove barriers to research, this Repository can improve the quality and quantity of research on dominantly-inherited muscular dystrophies, and stimulate the involvement of new investigators.

Website: http://crisp.cit.nih.gov/crisp/Crisp_Query.Generate_Screen

- **Project Title: CORE--TRAINING PROGRAM**

Principal Investigator & Institution: Clemens, Paula R.; Associate Professor; University of Pittsburgh at Pittsburgh 350 Thackeray Hall Pittsburgh, Pa 15260

Timing: Fiscal Year 2003; Project Start 30-SEP-2003; Project End 31-AUG-2008

Description (provided by applicant): The specific aim of this proposal is to provide advanced training to clinician scientists to pursue an academic career in translational research related to gene and stem cell based therapies for **muscular dystrophy.** The primary goal is to train physicians to conduct clinical gene therapy trials targeting muscular dystrophies. Most physicians at the completion of their medical or surgical training simply do not possess the knowledge or skills needed to implement a basic clinical trial, let alone one utilizing gene therapy vectors. Thus, a training program to accomplish these goals must provide exposure to the conduct of a clinical trial, data analysis, medical ethics, and regulatory affairs pertaining to human gene therapy, as well as basic molecular biology skills. We have designed a two-year stem and gene therapy training program for two Clinician Scientist trainees per year. We have assembled a diverse group of faculty members that include clinical investigators, molecular biologists, gene therapists, immunologists, pharmacologists, bioengineers, epidemiologists, statisticians, and bioethicists. During the first year of the training program, the Clinician Scientist trainees will participate in the NIH-funded Clinical Research Training Program (CRTP) established at the University of Pittsburgh. The CRTP aims to teach the skills necessary to design and conduct high quality clinical research. We will utilize the core curriculum and integrated seminar series of the CRTP as part of the training plan to avoid unnecessary duplication of resources and to allow for immediate implementation. Also during the first year, each trainee will be assigned to one of the ongoing MDCRC projects to get early exposure to a gene or stem cell approaches for treating DMD. During the second year of the program, the trainees will participate in the management of active clinical trials through the PCRN and the GCRC. The Pittsburgh Clinical Research Network (PCRN) is a clinical research organization that provides site management services for the conduct of industry-sponsored research. The General Clinical Research Center (GCRC) provides the infrastructure and support staff required for the conduct of clinical research and gene therapy trials at the University of Pittsburgh. The second year of training will also include three Gene Therapy Research Modules with basic coursework and laboratory experience focusing on gene therapy issues.

Website: http://crisp.cit.nih.gov/crisp/Crisp_Query.Generate_Screen

- **Project Title: CRYSTALLOGRAPHIC STUDIES OF EUKARYOTIC POLY(A)POLYMERASE**

Principal Investigator & Institution: Doublie, Sylvie; Microbiol & Molecular Genetics; University of Vermont & St Agric College 340 Waterman Building Burlington, Vt 05405

Timing: Fiscal Year 2002; Project Start 18-DEC-2000; Project End 31-MAY-2006

Summary: (From the applicant's abstract) The long-term goal of this project is to understand the molecular mechanisms of eukaryotic mRNA polyadenylation. mRNA polyadenylation plays an essential role in the initiation step of protein synthesis, in the export of mRNAs from the nucleus to the cytoplasm, and in the control of mRNA stability. Polyadenylation is a key regulatory step in the expression of many genes. Aberrant polyadenylation has been shown to cause diseases such as thalassemia and lysosomal storage disorder. Moreover, **oculopharyngeal muscular dystrophy** is the result of the insertion of short GCG repeats in the gene encoding one of the polyadenylation factors, poly(A) binding protein 2 (PABP 2). We are investigating the crystal structure of the enzyme at the heart of the polyadenylation machinery, poly(A) polymerase (PAP), its interaction with substrates, and its association with proteins playing a part in mRNA 3'-end processing. There are no structural data to date for any of the mammalian polyadenylation factors. The specific aims are as follows: 1. The X-ray crystal structure of bovine PAP with its substrates ATP and poly(A) RNA will be determined using a combination of multiwavelength anomalous diffraction (MAD) and multiple isomorphous replacement. The structure of PAP complexed with substrates will guide additional structural and functional studies. 2. PABP 2 is required for processive synthesis and control of the poly(A) tail length. PABP2 is known to bind both the poly(A) tail and PAP. We will work towards the structure determination of the ternary complex of PABP2, PAP, and poly(A), using either the intact proteins or the interacting domains of each protein. 3. Phosphorylation of target sites located in the C-terminal domain of PAP results in strong repression of PAP activity. The down regulation of PAP via hyperphosphorylation is reminiscent of the inhibitory effect of U1A, which has been shown to inhibit polyadenylation of its own mRNA by binding to PAP. We will work towards the crystallization of the complex between PAP and U1A, using either the intact proteins, or the C-termini of each protein. We will concurrently attempt to crystallize phosphorylated, full-length bovine PAP. A comparison of the phosphorylated PAP structure with that of the PAP-U1A complex should elucidate whether both situations use a similar mechanism of repression. It is expected that these results will not only provide a sound structural basis for understanding the mechanism of polyadenylation at the molecular level but will also shed light on the mechanisms of processivity and repression.

Website: http://crisp.cit.nih.gov/crisp/Crisp_Query.Generate_Screen

- **Project Title: CYTOSKELETAL INTERACTIONS OF DYSTROPHIN**

Principal Investigator & Institution: Ervasti, James M.; Professor; Physiology; University of Wisconsin Madison 750 University Ave Madison, Wi 53706

Timing: Fiscal Year 2002; Project Start 15-JUL-1994; Project End 31-MAR-2005

Summary: (Verbatim from the Applicant's Abstract): The objective of this project is to determine the cytoskeletal interactions of the dystrophin-glycoprotein complex in the skeletal muscle to understand how its absence or abnormality leads to Duchenne (DMD) and Becker (BMD) muscular dystrophies and some forms of cardiomyopathy. Rather than just simply serving to anchor its associated glycoprotein complex to the cortical actin, our previous studies lead us to hypothesize that dystrophin also plays an important role in stabilizing the cortical cytoskeleton through an extended lateral association with actin filaments. We further hypothesize that the dystrophin homologue utrophin is missing an actin binding suite important for F-actin stabilization. These hypotheses will be tested, both in vitro and in vivo, through the pursuit of 3 complementary specific aims. The F-actin binding properties of full-length and truncated forms of recombinant dystrophin and utrophin will be measured by established biochemical and spectroscopic procedures (Aim 1). Completion of this aim will yield the first direct structure/function comparison for dystrophin and utrophin up-regulation to effectively compensate for dystrophin deficiency. Recombinant dystrophin/utrophin will be visualized alone and in complex with actin filaments using electron microscopy combined with three-dimensional reconstruction techniques (Aim 2). These studies will yield important new information about the shape, dimensions and flexibility of dystrophin and utrophin and will independently determine how much (and which sub-domains) of dystrophin lie in close apposition with F-actin. Analysis by three-dimensional reconstruction will also identify changes in actin monomer and filament structure that may lead to more stable association of other costameric proteins with F-actin. Finally, we will relate the in vitro features of the dystrophin/F-actin interaction with its role in stabilizing costomeric actin in vivo (Aim 3). Sarcolemmal membranes will be mechanically isolated from muscles of transgenic mdx mice expressing dystrophin constructs deleted in different domains and the status of costameric actin determined by confocal microscopy. We will also determine whether the absence of dystrophin results in an unstable sarcolemmal association of other costameric actin binding proteins. Completion of these aims will result in a highly detailed and integrated understanding of dystrophin's role in stabilizing the muscle membrane cytoskeleton through its interaction with cortical actin.

Website: http://crisp.cit.nih.gov/crisp/Crisp_Query.Generate_Screen

- **Project Title: DERMOMYOTOME DIFFERENTIATION AND MYOTOME DEVELOPMENT**

Principal Investigator & Institution: Ordahl, Charles P.; Professor; Anatomy; University of California San Francisco 3333 California Street, Suite 315 San Francisco, Ca 941430962

Timing: Fiscal Year 2002; Project Start 01-APR-1997; Project End 31-JAN-2006

Summary: (appended verbatim from investigator's abstract): Although skeletal muscle accounts for a large fraction of the body mass, it is one of the least regenerative of tissues. Satellite cells, which reside within the basal lamina of mature skeletal muscle fibers, are capable of mitotic expansion thereby generating new adult myoblasts to effect local repair of injured or diseased muscle. Such adult myoblasts, however, are not capable of replacing large losses of muscle tissue that occur through injury or as a consequence of chronic muscle disease, such as **Duchenne's muscular dystrophy.** Even after in vitro enrichment and implantation into injured muscle sites, such adult myoblasts evidence little incorporation and integration into organized muscle tissue. Ideal cells that could be used in muscle replacement therapy should be capable of: (1) large mitotic expansion potential through stem cell activity; (2) morphogenetic capacity (involving complex intra-tissue and extra-tissue interactions); (3) migratory capacity (short and long distance). At present, neither a source of such cells nor an effective muscle replacement strategy is available. These qualities are possessed by the embryonic cells that build the muscle primordia of the body. During the previous 3 years of this project we have identified, Isolated and otherwise analyzed a novel class of embryonic muscle stem cells that we name mvogenic progenitor cells (MP cells). MP cells are distinct from satellite cells in their ability to undergo migration and morphogenetic movements. MP cells are distinct from their earlier embryonic counterparts, typically referred to as "embryonic stem cells," in that they are not multipotent but are developmentally restricted to the formation of skeletal muscle tissue only. Most importantly, after transplantation from one embryo to another, MP cells act in a semiautonomous fashion to generate organized muscle tissue, even under non-permissive conditons. Thus, MP cells retain intrinsic determined qualities that allow them to form muscle tissues even in localities that are inappropriate or even hostile. Thus, embryonic MP cells possess the qualities required for cells to be used for muscle replacement therapy. In the present proposal, we will isolate MP cells from avian embryos and analyze their cellular, tissue, and molecular properties. These studies will lead to a deeper understanding of the processes by which muscle tissue is formed in both normal and abnormal development. More important from a potential therapeutic point of view however, the properties discovered about MP cells from this study will provide a foundation for the engineering of their essential properties into other cells, such as satellite cells, for their potential use in myoblast transfer or other therapies.

Website: http://crisp.cit.nih.gov/crisp/Crisp_Query.Generate_Screen

- **Project Title: DETERMINANTS OF MYOGENIC AND NEURONAL MEMBRANE PHENOMENA**

Principal Investigator & Institution: Horwitz, Alan F.; Professor; Cell Biology; University of Virginia Charlottesville Box 400195 Charlottesville, Va 22904

Timing: Fiscal Year 2002; Project Start 01-JAN-1988; Project End 31-DEC-2002

Summary: Skeletal muscle is an ideal system with which to study adhesion molecules and the membrane-cytoskeletal linkages in which they participate as they play a central role in muscle development, structure and physiology, and pathology. Once muscle precursors have migrated to their targets, the program of terminal differentiation commences, which is regulated by the extracellular matrix. An elaborate contractile apparatus is synthesized and organized, which contains several cell surface associations including the myotendinous and costomeric junctions. Muscle cells are innervated at neuromuscular junctions. It is now clear that dystrophin, the **muscular dystrophy** gene product, has homologies to cytoskeletal proteins and is associated with adhesion molecules like integrin. The integrin family of receptors for extracellular matrix molecules are implicated in all of the above phenomena by virtue of their localization in junctional regions, their functions as dual receptors for extracellular matrix and cytoskeletal molecules, and as mediators of signal transductions. The hypothesis that guides our current research is that the integrins play a central role in organizing the surface, the extracellular matrix, and the contractile apparatus of skeletal muscle and in addition mediate signals from the extracellular matrix triggering its differentiation. Our general aims for the project period are to identify and characterize the amino acid sequences on integrin cytoplasmic and extracellular domains that determine the organization of junctional regions and determine their role in adhesion. This will be done using a recently constructed library of single-amino acid substitutions in the Beta1- cytoplasmic domain and synthetic peptides corresponding to active and mutant sequences. A similar library will be constructed for alpha subunits. Analogous, but different, methods are proposed to find extracellular matrix binding sequences in the extracellular domain. The second major aim is to identify and purify novel integrin associated cytoplasmic proteins. Previous specificity problems will be addressed using peptide sequences derived from mutant and wild type cytoplasmic domain sequences. Recently we have identified two novel integrin associated molecules. Both are cytoskeletal and one is a complex of 5 proteins. They will be characterized further for binding specificities and localization on muscle. The third objective is to elucidate the role of integrins in organizing and stabilizing junctional regions. This will be done using molecular genetic techniques to identify functional domains, alter regulation of expression, and reduce or eliminate the expression of specific integrins.

Website: http://crisp.cit.nih.gov/crisp/Crisp_Query.Generate_Screen

- **Project Title: DEVELOPING CLINICAL OUTCOMES FOR GENE TRANSFER**

Principal Investigator & Institution: Mendell, Jerry R.; Professor & Chair; University of Pittsburgh at Pittsburgh 350 Thackeray Hall Pittsburgh, Pa 15260

Timing: Fiscal Year 2003; Project Start 30-SEP-2003; Project End 31-AUG-2008

Summary: The proposed study represents a systematic approach to recruit subjects and develop outcome measures necessary to reach a phase I gene transfer trial in Duchenne **muscular dystrophy** (DMD) and in two forms of limb girdle **muscular dystrophy** [LGMD 2D or alpha-sarcoglycan (SG) deficiency, and LGMD 2E or beta-SG deficiency]. The prepatory stage will be carried out in years one through three of the proposal. In years four and five, Phase 1 clinical transfer trials will be done in these three forms of **muscular dystrophy.** The specific aims define the approach to reach the stated goals: Specific Aim 1: Identify a cohort of DMD subjects with small gene mutations to participate in Phase 1 gene transfer studies Specific Aim 2: Establish the most appropriate muscle(s) for gene transfer in a population of DMD subjects using magnetic resonance imaging (Aim 2A) and quantitative muscle strength testing (maximum voluntary isometric contraction testing or MVICT) (Aim 2B) Specific Aim 3: Identify a population of LGMD 2D (alpha-SG) and LGMD 2E (beta-SG) subjects for participation in Phase 1 gene transfer studies Specific Aim 4: Establish the most appropriate muscle(s) for gene transfer in a population of LGMD 2D and LGMD 2E subjects using magnetic resonance imaging (Aim 4A) and quantitative muscle strength testing (MVICT) (Aim 4B) Specific Aim 5: Establish appropriate delivery methods for gene transfer of adeno-associated virus (AAV) considering volume, rate, and spread of vector from the site of injection

Specific Aim 6: Perform Phase 1 gene transfer trials in DMD and two forms of LGMD (2D alpha-SG) and (2E beta-SG)

Website: http://crisp.cit.nih.gov/crisp/Crisp_Query.Generate_Screen

- **Project Title: DISINTEGRINS & METALLOPROTEINASES IN ORTHOPEDIC DISEASE**

Principal Investigator & Institution: Smith, Jeffrey W.; Staff Fellow; Burnham Institute 10901 N Torrey Pines Rd La Jolla, Ca 920371005

Timing: Fiscal Year 2002; Project Start 01-APR-1994; Project End 31-MAR-2004

Summary: (Adapted from the Applicant's Abstract): The events leading to cell-cell fusion are key to the development and homeostasis of bone and muscle. The broad objective of this study is to understand the mechanisms that lead to the differentiation and fusion of osteoclasts and myotubes. Results from the study could lead to new treatments for osteoporosis and **muscular dystrophy.** The hypothesis of the proposal is that a recently discovered family of transmembrane proteins, called ADAMs, are important in the differentiation of bone and muscle. The ADAMS contain A Disintegrin And Metalloproteinase domain. The study will initially focus on meltrin-alpha, an ADAM expressed by myoblasts and osteoclasts. One objective of the study is to perform the first characterization of the biosynthesis and cellular localization of meltrin-alpha. These experiments will determine if the metalloproteinase domain of meltrin is released from the cell surface, and whether meltrin-alpha co-localizes with integrin in focal adhesion sites. A second objective will be to determine how each domain of meltrin-alpha is involved in the fusion of myoblasts. In this analysis, site-directed mutagenesis and polyclonal antibodies will be applied to ablate the biochemical activity of domains of meltrin, and the effects of these manipulations on myogenesis will be assessed. A third objective is to examine the structure-function relationships of the metalloproteinase and disintegrin domains of meltrin-alpha. Phage-display will be used to build inhibitors of the metalloproteinase. Studies will be conducted to identify the cell surface receptor for the disintegrin domain of meltrin-alpha. A final objective is to identify the ADAM proteins present in osteoclasts and their precursors. Homology-based PCR will be used to clone osteoclast ADAMs. Antibodies against these ADAMs will be used in attempts to block osteoclast differentiation.

Website: http://crisp.cit.nih.gov/crisp/Crisp_Query.Generate_Screen

- **Project Title: DISULFIDE STRUCTURE OF BIOMEDICALLY IMPORTANT PROTEINS**

Principal Investigator & Institution: Watson, Jack T.; Associate Professor; Biochemistry; Michigan State University 301 Administration Bldg East Lansing, Mi 48824

Timing: Fiscal Year 2002; Project Start 01-FEB-2001; Project End 31-JAN-2005

Summary: Disulfide bonds are a critically important determinant of the shape and, thus, the activity of some biomedically important proteins. The common bleeding disorder, von Willebrand Disease, appears to be related to a defect in the disulfide bonding pattern among 18 cysteines (including two pairs of adjacent cysteines) of a particular protein (VWF) that disrupts the normal blood clotting cascade. Very little is known about the cysteine status of the von Willebrand protein (VWF), and such knowledge will help explain the cause of this disorder at the molecular level; however, VWF is resistant to the conventional proteolytic approach to disulfide mapping. Knowledge of the disulfide bonding pattern in the receptor- binding proteins for TGF-beta will help provide an important 'template' for the development of drugs (antagonists) for treatment of fibrotic disorders ,e.g., Duchennes **muscular dystrophy;** similarly, the development of other drugs (agonists) may serve as anti-cancer agents by promoting the negative proliferative response to TGF-beta. However, the highly knotted, cysteine-rich (up to 12 cysteines, 3 of which are adjacent) receptor-binding proteins for TGF-beta are resistant to conventional disulfide mapping. Developing a protocol for the disulfide mapping of VEGF homodimer will provide the basis for designing and monitoring the proper folding of related pharmaceutical proteins with angiogenic activity. Our novel approach to disulfide mapping, based on cyanylation of and cleavage at cysteine residues, offers new hope for determining the disulfide bonding pattern of the biomedically important cystinyl proteins described above that are refractory to conventional methodology. Cyanylation is selective for free sulfhydryls and can be accomplished at pH 3, a condition that suppresses problems with disulfide scrambling. We have demonstrated that the cyanylation/cleavage approach is applicable to proteins containing adjacent cysteines, an attribute that recommends it for successfully attacking the difficult analytical challenges posed by the proteins described herein. An algorithm will be developed to assign the connectivity of cysteines in disulfide bonds given an input of amino acid sequence and mass spectra of cyanylation/cleavage products.

Website: http://crisp.cit.nih.gov/crisp/Crisp_Query.Generate_Screen

- **Project Title: DMD GENE THERAPY USING HSV/AAV HYBRID VECTOR SYSTEM**

Principal Investigator & Institution: Wang, Yaming; Brigham and Women's Hospital 75 Francis Street Boston, Ma 02115

Timing: Fiscal Year 2002; Project Start 15-AUG-2000; Project End 31-JUL-2003

Summary: The principle investigator for this proposal, Dr. Yaming Wang, is an Instructor in Anesthesia at Brigham and Women's Hospital and Harvard Medical School. The work outlined in this proposal will serve to fund the mentored transition of Dr. Wang into gene therapy of muscular diseases and from a research associate to an independent academic investigator and application R01 level funding. The mentor in this proposal, Dr. Allen is an independent clinical scientist with extensive published experience in the area of muscle biology. A mentor committee consisting of Dr. Allen and three other scientists (Dr. Breakefield, Dr. Kunkle, and Dr. Leboulch) will serve as the advisory committee for Dr. Wang and will carefully oversee her progress. The environment in which the proposed work will be carried out (Harvard Medical School) is a world class scientific community where biomedical research is performed at the highest level with intimate associations between clinical and basic science disciplines. In this proposal, Dr. Wang will investigate the effectiveness of an exciting novel hybrid HSV/AAV amplicon virion expressing dystrophin as a possible solution to the problems facing the currently proposed and active gene therapy protocols for a common X-linked myopathy, **Duchenne's Muscular Dystrophy** (DMD). Current therapy has failed because it has been unsuccessful in obtaining durable expression of the transferred gene product. There were a number of reasons for this failure, such as cytotoxicity, immune reactions caused by with viral gene expression and virion proteins, and non-integration of vector DNA. She has demonstrated that the HSV-1 amplicon virions are capable of transducing skeletal muscle myofibers in vivo and myoblasts and myotubes in vitro using both GFP and dystrophin as the experimental marker gene. Both GFP and dystrophin virions were shown to permanently transduce myoblasts in culture at a low frequency (0.5-2 percent) suggesting their ability to integrate into the host genome. As a work in progress she has designed new amplicon vectors capable of carrying the 14kB dystrophin cDNA, GFP and an antibiotic selection marker, and has demonstrated that these amplicons can be packaged into HSV virion particles that can induce transcription of the appropriate protein in mdx myotubes. The overall aim of this project is to create a new nontoxic, high efficiency and long term transgene expression

AAV/HSV-1 hybrid vector system to express dystrophin in a mdx mouse animal model to attempt DMD phenotype correction.

Website: http://crisp.cit.nih.gov/crisp/Crisp_Query.Generate_Screen

- **Project Title: DYSTROPHIC CARDIOMYOPATHIES IN MDX**

Principal Investigator & Institution: Townsend, Dewayne; Molecular/Cell/Develop Biology; University of Michigan at Ann Arbor 3003 South State, Room 1040 Ann Arbor, Mi 481091274

Timing: Fiscal Year 2004; Project Start 01-AUG-2004; Project End 31-JUL-2007

Summary: (provided by applicant): Cardiomyopathies are very common in patients with **Duchenne's Muscular Dystrophy** (DMD), occurring in 90% patients. DMD results from the absence of dystrophin, a large protein found primarily in striated muscle. The effects of DMD on skeletal muscle have been well documented, but the effects on cardiac muscle are largely unexplored. The mdx mouse is a model of DMD, displaying only mild pathology, although the diaphragm is severely affected in older mice. Recent evidence suggests that the heart of the mdx mouse is particularly susceptible to damage with an increase in workload. This study examines this phenomenon through the specific aims testing the following hypotheses: 1) Stressing the heart will result in a cardiomyopathy in the mdx heart, while wild type mice remain unaffected. This decline in cardiac function will be monitored by both invasive and non-invasive techniques. 2) The dystrophic cardiomyopathy of the mdx mouse can be prevented or reversed following genetic manipulations, by either transgenic or by adenoviral vectors, that express functional dystrophin in cardiomyocytes.

Website: http://crisp.cit.nih.gov/crisp/Crisp_Query.Generate_Screen

- **Project Title: DYSTROPHIN-GLYCOPROTEIN COMPLEX IN CARDIOMYOPATHY**

Principal Investigator & Institution: Michele, Daniel E.; Physiology and Biophysics; University of Iowa Iowa City, Ia 52242

Timing: Fiscal Year 2003; Project Start 01-MAY-2003; Project End 31-MAR-2004

Summary: (provided by applicant): The long term objective of this proposal is to understand the molecular basis of inherited cardiomyopathies, particular those associated with mutations in components of the dystroglycan-glycoprotein complex. The dystroglycan-glycoprotein complex provides a link from the cytoskeleton to the extracellular matrix. Mutations in components of this complex, such as delta sarcoglycan, cause recessive forms of **muscular dystrophy.** Interestingly, heterozygous mutations in the same delta sarcoglycan can also cause dilated cardiomyopathy without **muscular dystrophy.** The basis for the tissue specificity of these mutations and the mechanism behind sarcoglycan associated dilated cardiomyopathy is unclear. Furthermore, **muscular dystrophy** patients with mutations in enzymes that glycosylate dystroglycan and whose activity is necessary for dystroglycan to bind extracellular ligands, also have a high prevalence of cardiomyopathy. This proposal tests the hypothesis that the link between the cytoskeleton and the extracellular matrix 'through dystroglycan, specifically in cardiac myocytes, is critical 'to the development of cardiomyopathy. The proposed research will test the dominant-negative and tissue specific effects of delta sarcoglycan mutations on the attachment of alpha-dystroglycan to the transmembrane complex using isolated muscle cell gene transfer. In addition, the tissue specific role of dystroglycan glycosylation in the link to the extracellular matrix and the development of cardiomyopathy will be tested in the myodystrophy mouse. Finally, tissue specific gene targeted mice will be generated to determine if the link from cytoskeleton to matrix through dystroglycan, is necessary and sufficient in a tissue specific manner, to cause and explain the development of DGC associated cardiomyopathy.

Website: http://crisp.cit.nih.gov/crisp/Crisp_Query.Generate_Screen

- **Project Title: EXCITATION-CONTRACTION COUPLING IN DYSTROPHIC MUSCLE**

Principal Investigator & Institution: Vergara, Julio L.; Professor; Physiology; University of California Los Angeles 10920 Wilshire Blvd., Suite 1200 Los Angeles, Ca 90024

Timing: Fiscal Year 2003; Project Start 01-APR-2003; Project End 31-MAR-2008

Summary: (provided by applicant): Abnormalities in the mechanisms of calcium regulation and excitation-contraction (EC) coupling that may be linked to the degeneration of skeletal muscle fibers in Becker **Muscular Dystrophy** (BMD) and in Duchenne **Muscular Dystrophy** (DMD) will be investigated using isolated muscle fibers from mdx mice. Cells from this animal model, like those of dystrophic patients, have deficiencies in the expression of the protein dystrophin. Although there is substantial biochemical evidence demonstrating the association of the dystrophin-glycoprotein complex with transmembrane- and membrane-bound muscle proteins, little is known about its specific role in the physiological aspects of a muscle fiber. The main goal of this proposal is to obtain critical experimental evidence linking the absence of dystrophin with specific alterations in the electrical propagation in the transverse tubular system and calcium signaling machinery. Several possibilities that may explain these observations will be explored experimentally. Changes in intracellular calcium concentration triggered by electrical activity of the muscle fibers will be recorded with the aid of low affinity calcium sensitive fluorescent indicators and membrane potential changes in the transverse tubules will be monitored with potentiometric indicators. The investigations will be carried out using high-resolution optical methods that permit to assess the functional state of these critical steps of the EC coupling process, not only at the cellular level, but also within sub-regions of the muscle fiber and even within a single sarcomere. We will perform these measurements across three different age groups of the mdx mouse in order to understand the progression of the disease with time. We will also test if muscle fibers from a utrophin/dystrophin-lacking double mutant mouse, which exhibits a harsher pathology (similar to DMD), show signs of more pronounced defects in EC coupling. These types of experiments are necessary to unravel the mysterious role that dystrophin may play in the normal regulation of calcium metabolism in skeletal muscle. The knowledge gained in the proposed studies will help to elucidate the functional role of dystrophin in mammalian skeletal muscle, to this date the most fundamental and elusive problem in **muscular dystrophy** research. The enhanced methods proposed to detect defective steps in the EC coupling mechanisms within localized submicroscopic regions of mammalian muscle fibers may become the optimal choice for the future evaluation of genetic therapeutic procedures in sub-regions of a single muscle cell.

Website: http://crisp.cit.nih.gov/crisp/Crisp_Query.Generate_Screen

- **Project Title: FUNCTION OF THE WW DOMAIN OF DYSTROPHIN**

Principal Investigator & Institution: Sudol, Marius; Molecular, Cellular & Dev Biol; Mount Sinai School of Medicine of Nyu of New York University New York, Ny 10029

Timing: Fiscal Year 2002; Project Start 15-AUG-2000; Project End 31-JUL-2003

Summary: (appended verbatim from investigator's abstract): Duchenne and Becker muscular dystrophies are caused by genetic lesions of the dystrophin gene. These mutations result in the production of an abnormal protein or its absence. The long term goal of our research is to fully characterize the function of dystrophin to facilitate early detection, treatment and perhaps prevention of **muscular dystrophy.** During the last three years, we have identified and characterized a protein module, the WW domain, which binds proline rich ligands. The WW domain is present within the carboxyterminal region of dystrophin. Dystrophin interacts with several proteins including B-dystroglycan, which spans the membrane and communicates with the extracellular matrix. The overall hypothesis to be evaluated is that the WW domain, EF hands and the ZZ domain of dystrophin mediate interaction with B-dystroglycan in vivo, and that without this interaction, a partial or complete dystrophic phenotype results at the level of organism. Our specific aims are: 1. To characterize the specificity of the interaction between the WW domain of dystrophin and the proline rich core of B-dystroglycan using site directed mutagenesis, phage displayed peptide repertoires, the SPOT technique of peptide synthesis, and immunoprecipitation. 2. To elucidate the role of the cysteine rich region of dystrophin in modulating the interaction between the WW domain, EF hands plus the Z domain of dystrophin and B-dystroglycan by mutational analysis and x-ray crystallography. 3. To provide evidence of the biological role of modular protein domains of dystrophin (the WW domain, EF hands, the Z domain) by showing that dystrophin transgenes in which any of the four domains alone or in combination with other modules is point mutated can only partially complement the mdx phenotype (muscular dystrophy in mice), in contrast to the control, a wild type transgene, which fully complements the mdx phenotype. These studies will provide insight into molecular function of dystrophin and could point towards potential therapies for Duchenne and Becker muscular dystrophies.

Website: http://crisp.cit.nih.gov/crisp/Crisp_Query.Generate_Screen

- **Project Title: FUNCTIONAL ANALYSIS OF CALCIUM STORES IN TETRAHYMENA**

Principal Investigator & Institution: Turkewitz, Aaron P.; Associate Professor; Molecular Genetics & Cell Biol; University of Chicago 5801 S Ellis Ave Chicago, Il 60637

Timing: Fiscal Year 2002; Project Start 01-FEB-2000; Project End 31-JAN-2004

Summary: Exocytosis of secretory dense-core vesicles in many cell types is triggered by a transient elevation of cytosolic calcium that is mobilized from intracellular reservoirs. The best characterized calcium reservoirs are the endoplasmic reticulum (ER) and specialized ER-like organelles. Both the structure of reservoirs as well as the organization of the proteins within them are likely to contribute to the efficiency and specificity of signaling. One indication of this is that calcium is not uniformly distributed throughout the ER, implying that sub-regions may differ in signaling potential. Calcium-rich domains may be generated by the non-random distribution of specific proteins with the membrane and lumen of these reservoirs. This has not been tested, nor are the bases for such sub-regions known. Our aim is to develop further a system in which individual proteins can be identified and analyzed both in vitro and in vivo, to address these issues. The ciliate Tetrahymena thermophila offers a host of experimental advantages for studying such mechanisms. In this proposal, we focus on an ER-like network in ciliated protists, called the alveoli, that has evolved to facilitate signaling at the cell surface. Alveolar calcium is released when cells undergo stimulation with secretagogues, and the increase in cytosolic calcium triggers exocytosis of regulated secretory vesicles. In Tetrahymena, all such vesicles are tethered at the plasma membrane and undergo synchronous membrane fusion. From the experimental perspective, this provides an ideal read-out of alveolar signaling activity. We propose to study the function of individual alveolar proteins in exocytic signaling in Tetrahymena, taking advantage of homologous recombination for in vivo analysis. To begin, we have developed a cell-free alveolar preparation that is active in calcium transport. Our first aim is to isolate biochemically the calcium buffer proteins (homologs of vertebrate calsequestrins) that reside in the alveolar lumen, and clone the corresponding genes. This will be a starting point for mutational analysis of in vivo function, using gene replacement. Other proteins that modulate calcium flux in alveoli will be identified based on direct or indirect genetic screens. The long-term aim of this work is to develop an understanding of how proteins in intracellular reservoirs contribute to calcium signaling and homeostasis. Such questions are medically important for at least two reasons. First, defects in calcium homeostasis may be a direct cause of muscle necrosis in **muscular dystrophy,** in which prolonged high cytosolic levels can trigger apoptosis. Secondly, a detailed understanding of alveoli in particular might be a basis for intervention against parasites belonging to the Alveolate lineage, including the organisms responsible for malaria, cryptosporodiosis, and toxoplasmosis.

Website: http://crisp.cit.nih.gov/crisp/Crisp_Query.Generate_Screen

- **Project Title: GALGT2, DYSTROGLYCAN, AND MUSCLE EXTRACELLULAR MATRIX**

Principal Investigator & Institution: Martin, Paul T.; Assistant Professor; Neurosciences; University of California San Diego La Jolla, Ca 920930934

Timing: Fiscal Year 2004; Project Start 15-MAR-2004; Project End 31-JAN-2009

Summary: The broad objective of this project is to define the functional roles for glycosylation in neuromuscular development and disease. This work will focus on the roles of a glycosyltransferase, Galgt2, which creates the cytotoxic T cell (CT) carbohydrate antigen. Both Galgt2 and the CT antigen are normally confined to the neuromuscular junction in mammalian skeletal muscle. The ectopic expression of the CT antigen in extrasynaptic regions of the myofiber membrane alters the expression of other normally synaptic proteins, including Synaptic laminins, utrophin, and neural cell adhesion molecule (NCAM), in transgenic mice. In addition, Galgt2 overexpression alters important aspects of muscle and neuromuscular development, and inhibits the formation of **muscular dystrophy** in mdx mice, a model for Duchenne **muscular dystrophy.** The principal protein that is glycosylated by Galgt2 in transgenic muscles is alpha dystroglycan, a major binding protein for the extracellular matrix (ECM). This grant will test a model wherein modification of dystroglycan by Galgt2 alters its properties and function. In addition, it will test mechanisms for altered laminin expression using muscle cells, transgenic mice, and gene knockout mice. These experiments will decipher mechanisms responsible for the functional roles of Galgt2 in muscle and neuromuscular development, as well as for its therapeutic role in **muscular dystrophy.**

Website: http://crisp.cit.nih.gov/crisp/Crisp_Query.Generate_Screen

- **Project Title: GENE AND CELL THERAPY OF DUCHENNE MUSCULAR DYSTROPHY**

Principal Investigator & Institution: Glorioso, Joseph C.; Professor and Chairman; Molecular Genetics & Biochem; University of Pittsburgh at Pittsburgh 350 Thackeray Hall Pittsburgh, Pa 15260

Timing: Fiscal Year 2003; Project Start 30-SEP-2003; Project End 31-AUG-2008

Summary: Muscular dystrophy is a common genetic disease that affects 1 in 3500 male births annually. The disease is characterized by early muscle hypertrophy followed by muscle degeneration and early death in adolescence resulting from failure of heart and diaphragm muscle. The disease results from mutations that affect expression or function of dystrophin, an important structural component of the subplasma membrane. Currently no treatment is available. The overall goal of the proposed research is to develop gene and cell therapeutic methods for treatment of **muscular dystrophy.** Clinical, pre-clinical and basic muscle cell development studies are described in which experts in gene transfer, muscle cell biology, animal models of **muscular dystrophy** and clinical applications are brought together in a manner to achieve the highest level of data sharing, synergy and creative solution finding will be possible. Project 1 (J Mendell) will define clinical end-points and identify cohorts of patient that would participate in a phase I dose escalation safety clinical trial using an AAV gene vector carrying the functional dystrophin minigene delivered to a single skeletal muscle and continue gene therapy clinical trials for limb girdle MD. In Project 2 (X Xiao and J Kornegay), will explore methods for improved AAV-dys gene delivery using the dog model. In Project 3 (J Huard), experiments using muscle stem cells will be carried out using dystrophic mouse models in attempts to achieve muscle delivery of normal muscle derived stem cells to engraft into diseased heart. In Project 4 (J Glorioso), a novel functional genomics approach to identify genes that participate in differentiation of mouse embryonic stem cells toward muscle cell lineages is proposed using HSV gene vector cDNA libraries obtained from muscle derived stem cells. The core programs are designed to directly support the projects in the form of Administration (Core A: J Glorioso and P Robbins), Clinical Vector Production (Core B: J Barranger), a **muscular dystrophy** dog colony (Core C: J Kornegey) and Imaging (Core D: S Watkins) to provide information on the results of gene transfer in animals and patients. Finally, our center includes a training program for residents interested in gene therapy for muscle disease. We believe this to be a timely and highly innovative proposal which is likely to provide new armroaches to the treatment of muscular dvstrophv.

Website: http://crisp.cit.nih.gov/crisp/Crisp_Query.Generate_Screen

- **Project Title: GENE CAUSING PAGET & LIMB-GIRDLE MUSCULAR DYSTROPHY**

Principal Investigator & Institution: Kimonis, Virginia E.; Associate Professor; Children's Hospital (Boston) Boston, Ma 021155737

Timing: Fiscal Year 2002; Project Start 15-FEB-2001; Project End 31-JAN-2004

Summary: (Taken from the application): **Limb-Girdle Muscular Dystrophy** (LGMD) encompasses a clinically diverse group of disorders characterized by proximal muscle weakness first affecting the hip and shoulder girdle elevated creatinine kinase values, and non-specific changes in the muscle biopsy. In addition to clinical heterogeneity within the LGMD category, genetic heterogeneity is indicated by the existence of dominant and recessive forms. We have identified a large family with autosomal dominant LGMD and early onset Paget disease of bone (PDB). These individuals have bone pain in the hips, shoulders and back from the Paget disease. Individuals eventually become bed bound and die prematurely from progressive muscle weakness +/-cardiomyopathy in their forties to sixties. Laboratory investigation indicates elevated alkaline phosphatase levels in affected individuals. CPK is normal to mildly elevated. Muscle biopsy of the oldest affected male revealed non-specific changes and vacuolated fibers. Preliminary molecular analysis excluded linkage to the known loci for the autosomal dominant and recessive forms as well as 2 loci for autosomal dominant PDB and 6 loci for cardiomyopathy. Exclusion of the candidate loci prompted a genome-wide scan of 39 family members (9 affected, 24 unaffected, 6 spouses} with 402 polymorphic microsatellite markers (Marshfield Genotyping Services). The disease locus was linked to chromosome 9p21-q21 with marker D9S301 (max LOD=3.64), thus supporting our hypothesis that this family displays a genetically distinct form of Limb-Girdle-Muscular-Dystrophy associated with Paget disease of bone and cardiomyopathy. Subsequent haplotype analysis with a high density of microsatellite markers flanking D9S301 refined the disease locus to a 3.76 cM region on chromosome 9p21-13.2. This region excludes the IBM2 locus for autosomal recessive vacuolar myopathy. Two candidate genes mapped to the critical region, NDUFB6 and IL-11RA, are being examined for disease-associated mutations. NDUFB6 encodes a subunit of Complex I of the mitochondrial respiratory chain and the IL11RA gene product influences proliferation and differentiation of skeletogenic progenitor cells. Identification of the genes involved in the LGMDs has led to the elucidation of an entire family of proteins that function in the dystrophin-glycoprotein complex. and a basis for understanding the pathophysiology of this complex. Delineation of the genetic component responsible for the LGMD/PDB phenotype should promise similar insight and facilitate in the design of novel treatment protocols for the two disorders.

Website: http://crisp.cit.nih.gov/crisp/Crisp_Query.Generate_Screen

- **Project Title: GENE EXPRESSION IN NORMAL & DISEASED MUSCLE DEVELOPMENT**

Principal Investigator & Institution: Kunkel, Louis M.; Professor; Children's Hospital (Boston) Boston, Ma 021155737

Timing: Fiscal Year 2002; Project Start 25-SEP-2001; Project End 31-AUG-2006

Summary: PROGRAM (provided by applicant): The last decade has witnessed remarkable progress in defining primary defects that cause inherited muscle disorders. The genetic heterogeneity of these diseases is enormous; mutations in more than 40 different genes are implicated. Many critical questions remain concerning the pathogenesis of muscle cell degeneration in these diseases and strategies for their treatment. This Program Project will use classical methods of gene and protein analysis and state-of-the-art gene expression array technology to study these questions. The investigators in this program have contributed importantly to the **muscular dystrophy** field. The proposed 4 projects have unique features but overlapping concepts and methodologies. Project 1 will study the dystrophin-associated complex of proteins, emphasizing the sarcoglycans and the newly described filamin-C. Project 2 will investigate the biology of dysferlin, its potential protein partners, and how these are altered by dysferlin gene mutations. Project 3 will examine the function of myotubularin in normal muscle development and the mechanisms by which its mutations cause developmental myopathies. Project 4 will study the biological and therapeutic properties of muscle stem cells. Three Cores will provide administrative oversight and services essential to the smooth progression of this program. Core B will coordinate sample acquisition and muscle RNA preparation for each project. Core C will perform the microarray analysis of gene expression and provide expertise in bioinformatics and data interpretation. The aim is to identify patterns of gene expression that are global in all dystrophies or distinct to specific sets of dystrophies and myopathies; this will provide insight into the molecular basis of normal muscle development and its dysfunction in these disease states. The long-term goal is to use this information in conjunction with the insights from studies of stem cell biology to devise new approaches to the treatment of the muscular dystrophies and related myopathies.

Website: http://crisp.cit.nih.gov/crisp/Crisp_Query.Generate_Screen

- **Project Title: GENE THERAPY FOR DUCHENNE MUSCULAR DYSTROPHY**

Principal Investigator & Institution: Wolff, Jon A.; Professor; Pediatrics; University of Wisconsin Madison 750 University Ave Madison, Wi 53706

Timing: Fiscal Year 2002; Project Start 30-SEP-2000; Project End 31-AUG-2005

Summary: (Copied from Applicant Abstract): Gene therapy promises to be a cure for the muscular dystrophies, such as Duchenne **muscular dystrophy.** Studies by my laboratory and others indicate that the transfer of the normal human dystrophin gene into dystrophic muscle (in the mouse model) prevents the death of the myofiber. The critical problem now is how to deliver the normal dystrophin gene to enough of the muscle cells and have it stably expressed in order to effect a cure. We have spectacular preliminary results that show that plasmid DNA can be delivered via a blood vessel into more than 10 percent of the muscle cells throughout the leg of a rat. This percentage of transfected muscle cells approaches the critical minimum percentage necessary to be curative in children with Duchenne **muscular dystrophy.** With this approach, multiple administrations should be possible, ensuring that a sufficient number of cells would be converted to dystrophin-positivity. Our studies also indicate that this approach should lead to stable expression of the gene. We have shown that the intravascular injection of naked plasmid DNA (pDNA) into the femoral artery of rats leads to very high foreign gene expression in skeletal muscle throughout the leg and without damaging the muscle. Previous experience with naked DNA and adenoviral vectors showed that the gene transfer efficiency decreased substantially when going from the young mouse, to adult mouse and then adult rat. The fact that we can achieve very efficient expression in an adult rat is quite encouraging. The objective of this proposal is to extend this approach to larger animals, non-human primates and the dog and its associated Duchenne model. If successful in primates and dogs, a human clinical trial in patients with Duchenne **muscular dystrophy** could begin in the near future.

Website: http://crisp.cit.nih.gov/crisp/Crisp_Query.Generate_Screen

- **Project Title: GENETIC MECHANISMS OF MUSCULAR DYSTROPHY IN MICE**

Principal Investigator & Institution: Cox, Gregory A.; Associate Staff Scientist; Jackson Laboratory 600 Main St Bar Harbor, Me 04609

Timing: Fiscal Year 2003; Project Start 01-JUN-2003; Project End 31-MAY-2008

Summary: (provided by applicant): The broad long term goals of this research are to better understand the molecular genetic mechanisms underlying neuromuscular disease using a novel mouse mutation as an experimental model. Muscular dystrophies include a diverse group of genetically heterogeneous disorders characterized by progressive muscle weakness and wasting that leads to severe disability and often premature death. There is a need to learn more about pathogenesis of the diseases and translate this knowledge into effective treatments. Toward this goal, we propose to study the mechanism of pathogenesis in the mdm mutant mouse, a novel model of progressive **muscular dystrophy** that functionally links the enormous Titin (Ttn) gene to the **limb-girdle muscular dystrophy** type 2A (LGMD2A) cysteine protease calpain 3 (Capn3). We have genetically mapped and identified the mdm mutation as a complex rearrangement that results in a small in-frame deletion within a putative CAPN3-interacting domain of TTN. The mdm mouse may also serve as a genetic model for human tibial **muscular dystrophy** (TMD) which maps to the TTN locus at 2q31. This is the first demonstration that mutations in Ttn are associated with **muscular dystrophy** and provides a novel animal model to test for functional interactions between these two disease genes. The steps we will take to elucidate the roles of titin and calpain 3 in muscle cell degeneration will be to 1) test the hypothesis that calpain 3 interactions with titin are disrupted by the mdm mutation, 2) test the alternate hypotheses that the progressive mdm **muscular dystrophy** is due to either reduced CAPN3 levels or aberrant activation of the CAPN3 protease, and 3) generate a Ttn-null allele by gene targeting and an allelic series of **muscular dystrophy** mutations at the Ttn locus using a sensitized ENU mutagenesis screen. Thus, the mdm mutant mouse provides a unique tool for understanding molecular pathways causing **muscular dystrophy** and may reveal entry points in which to intervene in the disease process.

Website: http://crisp.cit.nih.gov/crisp/Crisp_Query.Generate_Screen

- **Project Title: GENETIC STUDIES IN NEUROLOGICAL DISORDERS**

Principal Investigator & Institution: Pericak-Vance, Margaret A.; Professor; Medicine; Duke University Durham, Nc 27710

Timing: Fiscal Year 2002; Project Start 01-JAN-1989; Project End 31-MAR-2004

Summary: This Program Project involves clinical neurology, genetic linkage analyses, and molecular genetic techniques and strategies to study neurogenetic disease. The program involves three cores and three projects. Project I involves the molecular studies of autosomal dominant spastic paraplegia (SPG). Project II proposes to define the complex underlying genetic etiology in autistic disorder. project III proposes to study autosomal dominant limb- girdle **muscular dystrophy** (LGMD). Core A is the Administrative Core and oversees the overall direction of the Neurogenetics Center as well as the financial aspects of the Center. Core B is the Mutation and Candidate Gene Resources Core and provides the technical resources an physical support for the project studies. Core C is the Family Ascertainment, Linkage Analysis and Informatics Core and provides family ascertainment, statistical analysis and databasing support for Projects I through III.

Website: http://crisp.cit.nih.gov/crisp/Crisp_Query.Generate_Screen

- **Project Title: GORDON RESEARCH CONFERENCE ON BASEMENT MEMBRANES**

Principal Investigator & Institution: Kramer, James M.; Professor; Gordon Research Conferences Box 984, 512 Liberty Ln West Kingston, Ri 028920984

Timing: Fiscal Year 2002; Project Start 09-JUN-2002; Project End 31-DEC-2002

Summary: (provided by applicant): This application requests partial funding for the support of invited speakers for the 2002 Gordon Conference on Basement Membranes. This is the eleventh in a series of conferences, which have become an international forum for dissemination of new ideas and information about the structure and functions of basement membranes (BMs). These are complex, three dimensional, extracellular structures formed at epithelial mesenchymal interfaces and around mesenchymal cells, with important roles in the organization and function of most tissues and organs, e.g., blood vessels, lung, kidney, skin, peripheral nerves, and muscle. For example, basement membranes regulate the migration and organization of cells in the musculoskeletal system, as well as axons and synapses in the nervous system. Mutations in genes encoding basement membrane components result in severe inherited disorders in humans (e.g., epidermolysis bullosa of skin, congenital **muscular dystrophy** and associated nerve defects, Alport syndrome of kidney). Acquired defects in basement membranes also contribute to the pathogenesis of diabetic microvascular disease and serve as entry sites for infectious agents, such as leprosy, and for metastatic cancer cells. Traditionally, the conference has attracted scientists from a wide range of fields in basic research, including protein and carbohydrate structure, gene expression, cell and developmental biology, and neurobiology. In addition, it has been attended by clinicians and scientists involved in research and/or treatment of human disorders involving BM components of lung, blood vessels, skin, kidney, bone, muscle and immune systems. Basic studies of BM degradation and turnover are also of interest to scientists investigating dynamic processes such as angiogenesis, cancer metastasis, embryo implantation, and involution of the mammary gland and uterus. There has been substantial interest from clinicians and scientists in the pharmaceutical and biotechnology industries studying the roles of BMs in wound healing, angiogenesis, nerve regeneration, inflammation, and tissue repair. The Conference will present a diverse mixture of sessions on the basic science of basement membrane and extracellular matrix (ECM) structure, biosynthesis, assembly, turnover, and functions. Comparative studies of BM function in vertebrates and invertebrates and the roles of BM and ECM in embryonic development will also be incorporated into the program. In addition, emphasis will be given to studies on the genetic analyses of BM and ECM functions, and the generation of animal models of human BM disorders.

Website: http://crisp.cit.nih.gov/crisp/Crisp_Query.Generate_Screen

- **Project Title: INTERACTIONS BETWEEN INTERMEDIATE FILAMENTS AND NUCLEUS**

Principal Investigator & Institution: Goldman, Robert D.; Professor; Cell and Molecular Biology; Northwestern University Office of Sponsored Research Chicago, Il 60611

Timing: Fiscal Year 2004; Project Start 01-JUN-1981; Project End 31-JAN-2009

Summary: (provided by applicant): The goals of this project are to determine the structure and function of the nuclear lamins. The lamins are Type V intermediate filament proteins that are found in the nuclear lamina and in the nucleoplasm. Mutations in the nuclear lamins have been linked to many human diseases including different forms of **muscular dystrophy,** cardiomyopathies and premature aging. The specific aims of this grant are targeted towards a greater understanding of the function of the lamins in DNA replication, transcription, nuclear assembly and disassembly, and in the overall molecular architecture of the nucleus. Structural studies will be undertaken at both the light and electron microscope levels of resolution. Live cell imaging will also be used employing the jellyfish green fluorescent protein (GFP). Other methods will include the silencing of specific lamins using siRNA and a variety of biochemical and molecular methods aimed at determining the protein-protein interactions required for lamin assembly and structure. In addition, attempts will be made to identify the specific binding partners, which link the A and B-type lamins to the RNA polymerase II machinery and to the DNA replication elongation complex.

Website: http://crisp.cit.nih.gov/crisp/Crisp_Query.Generate_Screen

- **Project Title: ION CHANNELS AND CHEMICALS CONTROLLING SYNAPSE STABILITY**

Principal Investigator & Institution: Mcardle, Joseph J.; Professor; Pharmacology and Physiology; Univ of Med/Dent Nj Newark Newark, Nj 07107

Timing: Fiscal Year 2003; Project Start 01-FEB-2003; Project End 31-JAN-2007

Summary: (provided by applicant): Synapses are the major locus of information transfer within our brain as well as the target of numerous pathologies which can afflict humans from development in utero to death. Therefore, major research effort is given to understanding synapse formation and stabilization throughout life. The scientific literature concerning synapses is rich with discovery of fundamental principles derived from study of the neuromuscular junction (NMJ). In particular, proteins responsible for NMJ function, formation, and stability are relatively well understood. Nevertheless, fundamental questions remain concerning interactions between these proteins. An important experimental model suggests that heterogeneous activity of AChRs influences stability of the adult NMJ. This proposal modifies and extends that model to the developing NMJ where co-expression of immature gamma and mature epsilon AChRs during the critical phase of NMJ maturation produces heterogeneity of end-plate activity. Our model suggests that end-plate areas rich in epsilon AChR mediate Ca 2+ influx which activates co-localized nitric oxide synthase (nNOS). The nitric oxide (NO) produced diffuses to nerve terminals competing for the motor end-plate. New preliminary data suggest that NO enhances Ca2+ currents and transmitter release at adult motor nerve terminals. Thus, developing nerve terminals activating end-plate loci containing the epsilon AChR may be functionally enhanced and nurtured via NO activation of presynaptic guanylyl cyclase. In contrast, NO may repress function and stability of competing nerve terminals activating epsilon AChR poor end-plate foci. The mouse Triangularis sterni (TS) preparation facilitates exact testing of our model. Our preliminary data show that the TS preparation isolated from neonatal mice allows simultaneous recording of nerve terminal currents and post-synaptic events at end-plates receiving innervation from terminals originating in distinct nerve trunks. This allows unprecedented study of the function of, and NO-mediated cross talk between, mammalian nerve terminals competing for a postsynaptic target. The availability of epsilon subunit and nNOS knock out mice, as well as the epsilon AChR selective ligand Waglerin- 1 further strengthen experiments proposed to test our model. Additional novel preliminary data suggest that insulin, an activator of the neuronal K-ATP channel, suppresses quantal release of Ach at the adult NMJ. Therefore, a second goal of this proposal is to discover if insulin, as well as glucose, effects the function, and eventual stability, of nerve terminals competing at the developing NMJ. This will be explored in a non-obese mouse model of type I diabetes. Overall, this research is clinically relevant since NO signaling cascades are significantly altered in Duchenne **muscular dystrophy** as well as animal models of stroke. In addition, altered function of the epsilon AChR is responsible for NMJ pathology associated with slow channel congenital myasthenic syndrome. The proposed evaluation of insulin effects is novel and will enhance understanding of the neurologic consequence of adult and juvenile forms of diabetes. The knowledge gained from this research will enlighten future molecular approaches to treating pathologies which afflict children and adults.

Website: http://crisp.cit.nih.gov/crisp/Crisp_Query.Generate_Screen

- **Project Title: LAMININ INDUCED MEMBRANE COMPLEXES IN MUSCLE AND NERVE**

Principal Investigator & Institution: Yurchenco, Peter D.; Professor; Pathology & Laboratory Medicine; Univ of Med/Dent Nj-R W Johnson Med Sch Robert Wood Johnson Medical Sch Piscataway, Nj 088545635

Timing: Fiscal Year 2002; Project Start 01-APR-1999; Project End 31-MAR-2004

Summary: Null and domain-activating mutations of the basement membrane laminin alpha2 (merosin) subunit are reported to cause human and murine congenital muscular dystrophies and peripheral nerve defects. Our laboratory is studying the inductive role of laminins on myotubes and Schwann cells, and preliminary data reveal that alpha2-laminin and its alpha1-laminin homologue binding to myotube cell surfaces through laminin G protein-specific integrin and alpha-dystroglycan receptors. These cruciform laminins self-assemble into polymers through their short arms, cluster the two receptors into polygonal complexes through their anchored long arm, and induce the formation of a vinculin-rich cortical cytoskeletal lattice that mirrors the organization of laminin and its receptors. We also have evidence that alpha2-laminin bearing the dy/2.1 dystrophic deletion is defective in its ability to self-assemble, to aggregate its receptors, and to assemble this cortical architecture. Based on these and other data, our working hypothesis is that laminin-2 plays a major role in driving the assembly of the myotube and Schwann cell cytoskeleton, a process mediated by its ability to bind to the cell surface, to polymerize, and to activate and reorganize its cognate receptors. This receptor and cytoskeleton reorganization, resulting from a dynamic integration of laminin activities, may be important for the development, maintenance and stabilization of muscle and nerve sheaths. Furthermore, a loss of one or more of these functions may cause muscular dystrophies with neuropathies. We propose to explore this concept in the following specific aims: I. Laminin-Myotube and Laminin-Schwann Cell interactions: We will study the composition, architecture, and sequential assembly of laminin-induced receptor-cytoskeletal complexes in normal and receptor-deficient myotubes and Schwann cells. II. Structure and function of Recombinant alpha2-Laminins Bearing Dystrophic Mutations: We will prepare and evaluate the structure and function of recombinant laminins bearing dystrophic alpha2-subunit mutations with respect to their structure, domain stability, self-assembly, and receptor activities. III. Dystrophic Recombinant Laminin Induction of Receptor-Cytoskeletal Complexes: We plan to study engineered laminins with respect to their ability to induce membrane cytoskeletal networks in myotubes and Schwann cells.

Website: http://crisp.cit.nih.gov/crisp/Crisp_Query.Generate_Screen

- **Project Title: MECHANICAL TRANSDUCTION BY CARDIOCYTES**

Principal Investigator & Institution: Sachs, Frederick; Professor; Physiology and Biophysics; State University of New York at Buffalo Suite 211 Ub Commons Buffalo, Ny 14228

Timing: Fiscal Year 2004; Project Start 01-JUL-1995; Project End 31-AUG-2008

Summary: (provided by applicant): All cells have mechanosensitive ion channels MSCs). Their physiological roles in non-specialized sensory tissues, such as the heart, are unknown, but new tools have become available. A peptide isolated from tarantula venom specifically blocks a subset of mechanosensitive ion channels, including channels found in heart, kidney, glia and smooth muscle. This proposal addresses the fundamental biophysics of mechanosensitive channel gating, and the molecular properties of the channel viewed through the structure of peptide blockers. The work has direct clinical relevance to stretch induced cardiac arrhythmias, **muscular dystrophy** and glial tumors. The peptides have been shown to block atrial fibrillation, inhibit stretch induced Ca+2 uptake in dystrophic muscle and stretch-induced secretion of growth factors from glia. Most MSCs open with increases in membrane tension, but mechanisms of activation and inactivation are not clear. In eukaryotes, tension is distributed across the complex mechanical structure of the membrane cortex. This includes the heterogeneous lipid bilayer with transmembrane proteins, the cytoskeleton and the extracellular matrix. Measuring the mechanics of pure bilayers, and natural and simplified cell membranes will show the stresses are distributed. This will reveal new ways channels can be modulated. The major technique is patch clamping. Patch capacitance is a sensitive measure of membrane mechanics. The capacitance changes of defined lipid vesicles under stress will help calibrate the meaning of capacitance changes in natural membranes. Cytoskeleton depleted patches will help define how tension is shared. Current peptide blockers have relatively low affinity, and unknown sites of interaction with target channels. Using recombinant protein expression to exhaustively mutate the peptides we will attempt to find peptides with 1) significantly higher affinity, 2) different affinities for MSCs in different cell types. This knowledge will help pave the way for channel isolation by affinity chromatography and rational drug design.

Website: http://crisp.cit.nih.gov/crisp/Crisp_Query.Generate_Screen

- **Project Title: MENTORED PATIENT ORIENTED RESEARCH CAREER DEVELOPMENT**

Principal Investigator & Institution: Escolar, Diana M.; Associate Professor of Neurology & Pedia; Children's Research Institute Washington, D.C., Dc 20010

Timing: Fiscal Year 2002; Project Start 10-AUG-2001; Project End 31-JUL-2006

Summary: (provided by applicant): The applicant is a neurologist and has extensive clinical experience in pediatric and adult neuromuscular diseases. This award will allow her to obtain the training and mentoring to become an independent clinical investigator focusing on neuromuscular disorders. The educational plan includes didactic courses covering epidemiology, statistics, clinical trial design and health policies. DMD is a relatively common fatal genetic disease in children, with equal incidence throughout the world. The goal of this research is to conduct therapeutic human clinical trials with chemicals shown to improve muscle strength in the mdx. The aims of the proposed research plan are: 1) to conduct a double-blind, placebo-controlled, three-arm clinical trial of creatine and L-glutamine in patients with DMD and to assess the effect of these compounds on muscle strength as measured by manual muscle testing (MMT), quantitative muscle testing (QMT) and other functional measurements. Aim 2 is to conduct a double-blind, placebo- controlled clinical trial of coenzyme Q10 (CoQ10) in patients with DMD to assess its effects on: a) muscle strength, measured by QMT, compound Medical Research Council (MRC) score and functional measures; b) exercise capacity, to be measured by a fatigability protocol; and c) quality of life, to be measures by the Child Health Questionnaire. Aim 3 is to validate the specificity of the pediatric QMT system measuring maximal voluntary isometric contraction sequentially in children with DMD. The studies will be conducted at Pediatric Clinical Research Center (PCRC) at the Children's National Medical Center (CNMC), satellite to Georgetown General Clinical Research Center (GCRC). Three cores of the PCRC will be involved: the Biostatistics Core, the Genetics Core Laboratory and the Bioanalytical Core Laboratory. In addition, to increase the statistical power of this study, the applicant has assembled an international collaborative group that will conduct identical protocols and submit the data to the study center at CNMC. Future studies will test several other drugs with potential to improve muscle strength in DMD.

Website: http://crisp.cit.nih.gov/crisp/Crisp_Query.Generate_Screen

- **Project Title: MOLECULAR AND CELLULAR THERAPIES FOR MUSCULAR DYSTROPHY**

Principal Investigator & Institution: Froehner, Stanley C.; Professor and Chair; Physiology and Biophysics; University of Washington Grant & Contract Services Seattle, Wa 98105

Timing: Fiscal Year 2004; Project Start 15-APR-2004; Project End 31-MAR-2009

Summary: Duchenne **muscular dystrophy,** caused by mutations in the gene encoding dystrophin, is one of the most prevalent and devastating human genetic diseases. The goal of this application is to enhance and improve therapeutic strategies and to develop the basic biology for new innovative approaches. Jeff Chamberlain will build on his expertise in DMD gene therapy by developing novel vectors able to deliver mini-dystrophins and/or myogenic regulatory genes either to muscle cells or via hematopoietic and mesenchymal stem cells. A related goal will be exploring methods for the efficient conversion of somatic stem cells into skeletal muscle. Stan Froehner will study the role of alpha-dystrobrevin, a dystrophin-associated protein, in the degeneration process. Mice lacking alpha-dystrobrevin develop **muscular dystrophy** through a mechanism that involves alteration in cellular signaling. The key functional domains of alpha-dystrobrevin and proteins that interact with these domains will be identified. alpha-dystrobrevin, modified to target to the membrane, will be tested for its ability to alleviate the dystrophic pathology in mdx muscle. Finally, changes in gene expression induced in muscle cells per se by the absence of alpha-dystrobrevin will be analyzed. Steve Hausehka will test the in vivo tissue specificity and long-term expression of regulatory gene cassettes designed to be optimal for packaging different therapeutic cDNAs into AAV, Lentiviral, and Adenoviral vectors. These vectors will then be used to deliver micro-, mini-, and full-length dystrophin and a variety of compensatory proteins to the dystrophic muscles of mdx4cv mice. Steve Tapseott will investigate gene regulation in skeletal muscle by testing the hypothesis that subsets of co-expressed genes share common mechanisms of regulation that can be identified and.manipulated, leading to therapeutic approaches. He will determine if mutations that cause **muscular dystrophy** alter gene regulation at a subset of muscle-expressed promoters and identify the mechanism. Finally, he will develop a genetic screen to identify mutations that compensate for dystrophin deficiency. The Administrative Core will provide general support and organize the biannual Seattle **Muscular Dystrophy** Conference. The Mouse Biology Core will provide assistance with functional and pathological analyses of mouse models to each project. The results derived from this integrated program project will lead to new therapeutic approaches for DMD and other diseases of muscle degeneration.

Website: http://crisp.cit.nih.gov/crisp/Crisp_Query.Generate_Screen

- **Project Title: MOLECULAR DETERMINANTS OF EXERCISE-INDUCED MUSCLE DAMAGE**

Principal Investigator & Institution: Hubal, Monica J.; Exercise Science; University of Massachusetts Amherst 70 Butterfield Terrace Amherst, Ma 010039242

Timing: Fiscal Year 2004; Project Start 01-SEP-2004; Project End 31-AUG-2005

Summary: (provided by applicant): Skeletal muscle adapts to a novel bout of strenuous exercise with a period of degeneration followed by a period of regeneration. Following overexertion exercise, these processes manifest themselves as prolonged losses in muscle function, loss of sarcolemmal integrity, muscle pain and soreness and inflammation. These indices of damage are profoundly attenuated when a second bout of exercise is performed up to 6 months after the first bout. While this "repeated bout effect" is well documented, the molecular mechanisms underlying this adaptation have not been identified. The primary aim of this research proposal is to detail gene expression changes following a repeated exercise bout of exercise in the human vastus lateralis of research subjects. Microarray analyses of muscle biopsy tissue will be used to provide a pattern of global gene expression at 6 hours after a first and second bout of exercise, providing concurrent information concerning how thousands of genes respond to damaging stimuli before and after the muscle has been given a chance to adapt to the stimuli. Microarray results for a subset of differentially regulated genes will be confirmed via qRT-PCR and localized via immunocytochemistry. These data will provide information concerning which genes underlie muscle damage and adaptation. The long-term objective of this study is to create a molecular map of the genes involved in muscle damage and adaptation. One of the most germane applications of this knowledge would be to the field of **muscular dystrophy** research, as **muscular dystrophy** patients undergo periods of muscle damage followed by failed regeneration. Understanding these processes could lead to novel treatments for musculodystrophy and other myopathies that are characterized by muscle degradation.

Website: http://crisp.cit.nih.gov/crisp/Crisp_Query.Generate_Screen

- **Project Title: MOLECULAR GENETICS OF MUSCULAR/NEUROSENSORY MODELS**

Principal Investigator & Institution: Nishina, Patsy M.; Staff Scientist; Jackson Laboratory 600 Main St Bar Harbor, Me 04609

Timing: Fiscal Year 2002; Project Start 15-APR-2002; Project End 31-MAR-2006

Summary: (provided by applicant): We have recently identified a spontaneous mouse mutant, veils (vis), that has retinal vasculopathy, hearing loss and progressive muscle wasting, phenotypes reported for many human diseases, such as Coat's disease, syndromic and non-syndromic congenital hearing loss, and **muscular dystrophy,** respectively. We have mapped veils to a 0.19+/-0.13 cM interval on mouse Chr. 8 in a 1,072 meiotic recombinant cross and established the physical contig of the critical region. Portions of human Chrs. 2, 4q, 8, 13, 17, 18, 19p and 22 map to this region, the breakpoints of which have yet to be refined. Interestingly, veils has many, if not all of the phenotypes reported for the disease fascioscapulohumeral **muscular dystrophy** la (FSHD), the third most prevalent **muscular dystrophy** that affects 1/20,000 and maps to human Chr. 4q35. Also, a neuromyopathy associated with a highly variable age-of-onset maps to Chr. 19p13. Veils is a potential genetic and/or phenotypic model for these diseases. The veils mouse is also unique in that it shows retinal lamination abnormalities, a phenotype that has not previously been reported in the literature. In order to understand the biological mechanisms that underlie the disease processes and identify the biochemical pathways that are affected in different tissues, we will: (a) positionally clone the veils gene and identify the mutation in the second allele myd and test the hypothesis that the phenotypic differences between v/s and myd are explained by allelic heterogeneity; (b) begin to identify genes in the genetic background that can significantly alter the disease phenotypes of vis/vis mice; and (c) test the hypothesis that the observed phenotypes are the result of developmental defects rather than degenerative processes. Identification of disease causing genes and animal models is extremely important. Many diseases in humans, especially those involving the eye, if identified early enough, can be treated to attenuate the disease process. If no treatment is currently available, knowing the molecular basis of the disease may provide insights to new treatment regimens and the models can then be used to test those therapeutics. Finally, knowledge of the disease causing genes may lead to an understanding of pathways that are critical in maintaining normal function and physiology of the organism and perhaps, may identify therapeutic targets for prevention of muscle wasting, and vision or hearing loss.

Website: http://crisp.cit.nih.gov/crisp/Crisp_Query.Generate_Screen

- **Project Title: MOLECULAR GENETICS OF PRONUCLEAR FUNCTIONS IN DROSPHILA**

Principal Investigator & Institution: Wolfner, Mariana Federica.; Professor; Molecular Biology and Genetics; Cornell University Ithaca Office of Sponsored Programs Ithaca, Ny 14853

Timing: Fiscal Year 2002; Project Start 01-MAY-1991; Project End 31-AUG-2006

Summary: (provided by applicant): To initiate development, a newly fertilized egg must generate pronuclei that can combine to create a zygotic genome capable of initiating mitosis. The fertilized egg must also stimulate translation of previously quiescent, maternally deposited mRNAs. The goal of this proposal is to increase our understanding of this critical, but incompletely understood, developmental stage of "egg activation" in the model organism Drosophila. The first specific aim focuses on the function of an important player in the fertilized egg: the "Young Arrest" (Ya) gene. YA is a maternally encoded nuclear lamina protein that is essential for male and female pronuclei to initiate their first mitotic division. Our phenotypic analysis of Ya mutants suggests either that YA mediates changes in chromatin condensation needed for passage into S phase of the first mitosis, or alternatively that it replaces a meiotic protein that is inhibitory to subsequent mitotic cycles. The experiments described in this aim will test these hypotheses for YA function, and may further identify other molecules that interact with YA in fulfilling its roles. The results of these experiments will elucidate molecular changes necessary to transition frommeiosis to mitosis. We also expect these results to be of relevance to the mechanism of human diseases, such as Emery-Dreifuss **Muscular Dystrophy,** that are caused by mutations in nuclear lamina proteins. The second aim will investigate the implications of our finding that the subcellular location of YA changes during development. YA is excluded from nuclei during oogenesis, but is able to enter nuclei after egg activation. During the same transition, there are also changes in YA?s phosphorylation state. We will test whether the change in YA?s ability to enter nuclei is a direct consequence of changes in its phosphorylation state, and whether MAP kinase mediates these events. We will also identify additional components of a macromolecular complex we have identified that retains YA in the cytoplasm prior to egg activation. The third aim of the proposal is designed to achieve a broader view of the molecular events during egg activation. We will determine whether ovulation, which we have shown to trigger egg activation in Drosophila, causes a rise in calcium, parallel to findings in other systems.

We will also test whether modulation of phosphorylation state, such as we see with YA, happens to many proteins during egg activation. Such modulation could mediate the rapid, concerted changes in egg physiology that occur at that time.

Website: http://crisp.cit.nih.gov/crisp/Crisp_Query.Generate_Screen

- **Project Title: MOLECULAR IDENTIFICATION OF CANINE DYSTROPHINOPATHIES**

Principal Investigator & Institution: Smith, Bruce F.; Associate Professor; Scott-Ritchey Research Center; Auburn University at Auburn Auburn University, Al 36849

Timing: Fiscal Year 2002; Project Start 05-AUG-2002; Project End 31-JUL-2005

Summary: (provided by applicant): Duchenne **muscular dystrophy** is a common inherited disease, affecting approximately 1 in 3000 live male births. Currently, there is no effective therapy for this disease, however, new therapies are being proposed that offer hope to patients and their families. These therapies must be evaluated for their efficacy in the most stringent manner possible, and in the case of DMD, that requires an appropriate animal model. The long term GOAL of this project is to characterize the molecular defects present in 3 new canine models of dystrophin deficiency. It is hypothesized that these models accurately reflect the depth and breadth of mutations and their effects that is seen in the human population. Current murine models require that multiple genes be knocked out to show the same disease that the loss of dystrophin causes in boys. The canine model system is the only model which appropriately reflects the relentlessly progressive and ultimately fatal disease of boys. However, the complexity of the dystrophin gene and thus the variety of mutations possible, require the availability of multiple models in which to test therapies. The best source of these models continues to be spontaneously occurring canine disease. This severely handicaps the utility of these models in evaluating new therapies. This project will not only elucidate the mutation in these three new canine models, but it will also create a set of tools that will allow investigators worldwide to rapidly evaluate further spontaneous cases of canine **muscular dystrophy** for their usefulness, both in exploring new therapies and in gaining new insight into the mechanism behind Duchenne **muscular dystrophy**. Specifically, we propose to use panels of monoclonal antibodies with known specificity to dystrophin, simultaneously with PCR amplification of the coding sequence to rapidly scan for mutations. Suspicious areas will be sequenced to determine if the mutation is contained within. Once the mutations are identified, their effect on transcription, translation and the presence of dystrophin will be evaluated and compared to similar human mutations to determine if there is a pathophysiological correlation between species and their mutations. Successful completion of this project will result in the addition of three models of human dystrophin deficiency to the tools available to investigators seeking novel treatments. The correlation of these mutations with the clinical course of the disease will allow therapies to be evaluated under a variety of clinical circumstances. These mutations will provide new and different genetic backgrounds upon which various therapies, and in particular genetic therapies, may be examined in a large, outbred animal species.

Website: http://crisp.cit.nih.gov/crisp/Crisp_Query.Generate_Screen

- **Project Title: MOLECULAR PATHOGENESIS OF MYOTONIC DYSTROPHY**

Principal Investigator & Institution: Tapscott, Stephen J.; Professor; University of Washington Grant & Contract Services Seattle, Wa 98105

Timing: Fiscal Year 2003; Project Start 26-SEP-2003; Project End 31-JUL-2008

Summary: Many genetic mutations have been identified that cause human muscular dystrophies, but the mechanisms of cellular damage remain poorly understood for these diseases. In many cases a similar mutation in different individuals cause different degrees of disability. Understanding the molecular basis of the common pathophysiology and the factors that contribute to individual variance will be important for managing and treating muscular dystrophies. Our broad and long-term objective is to identify the molecular mechanisms that mediate the pathologic response to the causative mutation in myotonic. Our specific aims will: (Aim 1) Use a model system of skeletal muscle differentiation and tissue samples from individuals with myotonic dystrophy to identify defects in the molecular regulation of gene transcription in caused by the CUG repeat containing RNA. (Aim 2) Determine whether variable patterns of CpG methylation in the region of the DM 1 locus contribute to the highly variable penetrance of the disease. The significance of this proposal is that it will determine the molecular basis of gene expression changes associated with myotonic dystrophy and the contribution of methylation to the clinical phenotype. These studies will provide a basis for therapeutic intervention.

Website: http://crisp.cit.nih.gov/crisp/Crisp_Query.Generate_Screen

- **Project Title:** MOLECULAR PATHOPHYSIOLOGY OF FACIOSCAPULOHUMERAL MUSCUL*

Principal Investigator & Institution: Chen, Yi-Wen; Children's Research Institute Washington, D.C., Dc 20010

Timing: Fiscal Year 2002; Project Start 28-SEP-2001; Project End 31-MAY-2004

Summary: (provided by applicant): Facioscapulohumeral **muscular dystrophy** (FSHD) is one of the most common inherited muscle diseases following Duchenne **muscular dystrophy** and myotonic dystrophy. The disorder is autosomal dominant with nearly complete penetrance (95%) by age 20. Severity of muscle involvement in FSHD is extremely variable, ranging from elderly individuals with mild facial weakness to wheelchair bound children. Besides variability between individual patients, FSHD patients often show enigmatic asymmetry of muscle involvement. This disease feature permits a novel experimental design, where progression of the disease can be studied within a single patient at a single time point. Previous studies showed a statistically significant correlation between severity of clinical presentation and the deletion of D4Z4 repeats on chromosome 4q35 in patients with FSHD. Current hypotheses center on a position effect of telomeric sequences on genes in or near the deletion site, however the molecular mechanisms underlying this disease are far from clear. In our study, we hypothesize that FSHD patient muscle shows a disease-specific expression profile, relative to other muscle disease (Duchenne **muscular dystrophy,** alpha-sarcoglycan deficiency, juvenile dermatomyositis, and dysferlin deficiency). In addition, we hypothesize that one can identify a subset of the FSHD-specific genes will be shown to correlate with progression of-muscle involvement in FSHD muscle by comparing expression changes correlated with clinically-affected vs. unaffected muscles within single dystrophy patients. In our preliminary data, we have defined an FSHD-specific set of 29 genes that are candidates for primary involvement of disease pathogenesis by using the HuGeneFL array (-6,000 full length genes). In this proposal, we plan to broaden the number of genes studied, so that a genome-wide set of genes implicated in the primary etiology can be defined. Specifically, we will extend our truly promising preliminary data to over 60,000 genes and EST sequences included on the Human genome U95A, B, C, D, E stock chips, as well as the > 2,000 human muscle ESTs on our custom-produced MuscleChip. In addition, a custom glass slide array consisting of - 200 genes and ESTs from 4q35 and 1Oq26 will be used to identify FSHD region specific alterations in gene expression. All FHSD-specific ESTs identified will be characterized in detail. Further studies will likely include the delineation of a complete picture of the pathophysiology of

FSHD, as well as identification of functional SNPs in the refined gene list that correlate with disease severity.

Website: http://crisp.cit.nih.gov/crisp/Crisp_Query.Generate_Screen

- **Project Title: MTOR SIGNALING IN SKELETAL MYOGENESIS**

Principal Investigator & Institution: Chen, Jie; Assistant Professor; Cell and Structural Biology; University of Illinois Urbana-Champaign Henry Administration Bldg Champaign, Il 61820

Timing: Fiscal Year 2003; Project Start 01-JUN-2003; Project End 31-MAY-2008

Summary: (provided by applicant): Skeletal muscle differentiation is a well-orchestrated process regulated by autocrine, paracrine, and endocrine factors via multiple signal transduction pathways. The bacterial macrolide rapamycin inhibits a wide spectrum of cellular functions, from proliferation, growth, to differentiation, and it has served as a powerful tool to probe relevant signaling pathways. While the rapamycin-sensitive pathway is under intensive investigation in the context of cell growth and proliferation, its importance in skeletal muscle development is only beginning to be recognized. The mammalian target of rapamycin - mTOR- is a multi-functional protein that serves as a central component of multiple signaling pathways that are inhibited by rapamycin. Preliminary studies from this investigator's laboratory have revealed an essential function of mTOR in skeletal muscle differentiation and the existence of novel mechanisms of mTOR signaling. The proposed studies are designed to test the hypothesis that an mTOR pathway distinct from that in cell growth and proliferation regulates skeletal muscle satellite cell differentiation by controlling the autocrine production of IGF-I and IGF-II. With a combination of biochemical, molecular, cellular and genetic approaches, and in the systems of a tissue culture model (C2C12) and mouse primary satellite cells, the specific aims of this proposal are to investigate (1) regulation of IGF autocrine production by mTOR; (2) involvement of a phospholipase D-phosphatidic acid-mTOR pathway in myogenesis; and (3) mTOR's structure-function relationship and novel signaling partners in differentiation. Knowledge gained in these studies will not only provide invaluable insights into the signaling mechanisms of the pleiotropic mTOR pathway, but also make significant contributions to the molecular understanding of skeletal muscle development, which is tightly coupled to health-related issues such as **muscular dystrophy,** exercise-induced hypertrophy, and aging-related atrophy.

Website: http://crisp.cit.nih.gov/crisp/Crisp_Query.Generate_Screen

- **Project Title: MUSCLE STEM CELL-BASED THERAPIES FOR CARDIOMYOPATHY**

Principal Investigator & Institution: Huard, Johnny; Henry J. Mankin Associate Professor of o; University of Pittsburgh at Pittsburgh 350 Thackeray Hall Pittsburgh, Pa 15260

Timing: Fiscal Year 2003; Project Start 30-SEP-2003; Project End 31-AUG-2008

Summary: Cardiomyopathy is a serious heart disease that often leads to congestive heart failure, a condition in which the heart muscle can no longer effectively pump blood. Patients that suffer from various muscle diseases, including Duchenne **muscular dystrophy** (DMD), develop progressive cardiomyopathy. Cellular cardiomyoplasty (CCM), a procedure that involves the transplantation of exogenous cells into damaged myocardium, has been proposed as a possible therapy to regenerate diseased myocardium and deliver therapeutic genes. Although a wide variety of cell types has been used for CCM, various limitations (including ethical, biological, or technical challenges) have impeded their suitability for use in human patients. We recently have used the modified preplate technique to isolate a novel population of muscle-derived stem cells (MDSCs) that display improved transplantation capacity in skeletal muscle when compared to satellite cells. The MDSCs' ability to proliferate in vivo for an extended period of time-- combined with their strong capacity for serf-renewal, multipotent differentiation, and immune-privileged behavior--reveals, at least in part, a basis for the benefits associated with their use in cell transplantation in skeletal muscle. The proposed project will investigate the use of MDSCs as a novel cell source for cardiac cell transplantation in a cardiomyopathic murine model of **muscular dystrophy.** We already have observed that MDSCs delivered by intra-cardiac injection display good cell survival and can deliver dystrophin within the dystrophic myocardium. In this project we will investigate whether MDSCs implanted in the hearts of dystrophic mdx mice display an improved transplantation capacity when compared to conventional satellite cell implantation (Aim #1). We then will explore the relative contribution of the MDSCs' capacity for long-term proliferation and self-renewal (Aim #2) to the increased regenerative capacity of these cells after transplantation in heart muscle. Finally, we will determine the degree to which development of approaches to prevent fibrosis (Aim #3) and improve angiogenesis (Aim #4) would further enhance the regenerative capacity of muscle-derived cells in the heart. This project will increase our understanding of the basic biology of myogenic cell populations that display stem cell characteristics. This information may, in turn, unveil new techniques to improve heart regeneration and repair via the transplantation of muscle-derived stem cells.

Website: http://crisp.cit.nih.gov/crisp/Crisp_Query.Generate_Screen

- **Project Title: MUSCULAR DYSTROPHY COOPERATIVE RESEARCH CENTER**

Principal Investigator & Institution: Chamberlain, Jeffrey S.; Professor; Neurology; University of Washington Grant & Contract Services Seattle, Wa 98105

Timing: Fiscal Year 2003; Project Start 26-SEP-2003; Project End 31-JUL-2008

Summary: This MDCRC application is designed to advance our abilities to treat the muscular dystrophies by capitalizing on the breadth and depth of expertise at our collaborating institutions in the fields of neuromuscular disease research and patient care, molecular genetics, immunology, and gene therapy. The participating researchers include scientists and clinicians from the University of Washington Medical Center, Children's Hospital and Regional Medical Center, Fred Hutchinson Cancer Research Center, and the VA Medical Center, Seattle. Our goals are to provide an interactive environment that will advance knowledge of and treatments for the muscular dystrophies by promoting collaborations, providing shared resources, advancing basic research, stimulating translational research, fostering outreach activities, developing greater patient awareness of basic and clinical research and enabling their participation in clinical trials, and by facilitating the development gene therapy for the muscular dystrophies. Our Center is composed of four research projects and three Core laboratories, and includes a membership of more than 30 faculty members in the Seattle area with interests in neuromuscular disease research. The director and codirector are J Chamberlain and S Tapscott, researchers with a long history of genetic and clinical studies of the muscular dystrophies. Project 1 (J Chamberlain, S Tapscott and S Froehner) will conduct pre-clinical studies in dystrophic mice that lead to a phase I clinical tdal of gene therapy for Duchenne **muscular dystrophy** (DMD). Project2 (M-T Little and S Tapscott) will study the canine model for DMD to address pre-clinical issues related to DMD therapy by emphasizing immunological, safety and allometdc issues important for the evelopment of therapies for DMD. Project 3 (S Hauschka) explores issues important for regulating gene expression vectors in muscles of humans, mice and dogs, and will develop animal and cell culture models for human muscle gene transfer. Project 4 (S. Tapscott) will study abnormal gene expression in cells from individuals with myotonic dystrophy, and will explore the clinical significance of methylation at the DM1 locus in adult onset myotonic dystrophy. Core A (Chamberlain) is an administrative core to coordinate and organize collaborative and interactive activities within and outside of our center. Core B (Chamberlain, J Allen) is a viral vector core and a scientific research resource core that will facilitate the availability of research and clinical grade gene transfer vectors for basic research and the development of gene therapies for the muscular dystrophies. Finally, Core C (T Bird) is a genetic counseling core for patients and families with **muscular dystrophy** that will also allow increased participation of patients in studies of a variety of types of **muscular dystrophy.**

Website: http://crisp.cit.nih.gov/crisp/Crisp_Query.Generate_Screen

- **Project Title: MUSCULAR DYSTROPHY COOPERATIVE RESEARCH CENTER**

Principal Investigator & Institution: Moxley, Richard T.; Professor; Neurology; University of Rochester Orpa - Rc Box 270140 Rochester, Ny 14627

Timing: Fiscal Year 2003; Project Start 30-SEP-2003; Project End 31-MAY-2008

Summary: A major strength of the University of Rochester MDCRC is having a large group of highly motivated, well-characterized patients with myotonic dystrophy (DM1 & DM2) and facioscapulohumeral **muscular dystrophy** (FSHD), eager to support basic research and participate in clinical studies, and a group of enthusiastic investigators with a longstanding expertise in these diseases. These assets have led us to make "The Dominantly Inherited Muscular Dystrophies: Pathophysiology and Treatment" the major focus of our 3 scientific projects and 2 scientific cores. Our primary emphases are on DM1 and FSHD. Project 1 explores the "Role of RNA Toxicity and Muscleblind Proteins in the Pathophysiology of DM". Using muscleblind knockout mice and studies of alternative splicing of the skeletal muscle chloride channel Project 1 examines a toxic RNA model for the myotonic dystrophies. It tests the hypothesis that the abnormally expanded mRNA alleles in DM1 & DM2 sequester certain dsRNA-binding factors, the muscleblind proteins, and that this leads to myotonia and myopathy. Project 2 investigates a potential new treatment in DM1 and hopes to prove that SomatoKine (insulin-like growth factor-1 [IGF1] complexed with recombinant IGF binding protein-3) is safe, well-tolerated, and promising as a therapy. This project tests the hypothesis that deficient activation by IGF1 contributes to the atrophy in DM1, and that maintaining high blood levels of IGF1 will correct this deficiency. Project 3 strives to increase our knowledge of the molecular and cellular pathophysiology of FSHD. It uses microarray analysis of muscle biopsy specimens to test two hypotheses: in FSHD: a) deletion of D4Z4 heterochromatic repeats does not alter adjacent 4q35 genes; and, b) aberrant overexpression of smooth muscle genes is an important contributor to the pathophysiology. One Scientific Core is an Imaging Center. It provides specialized muscle histochemical and immunological techniques, fluorescent in situ hybridization, confocal microscopy, and electron microscopy. Projects 1 & 3 make extensive use of this Core. The other Scientific Core is a Repository of resources for research on **Muscular Dystrophy.** This Core maintains: a) myoblast cell lines for DM1 and FSHD; b) transgenic model cell lines; c) plasmids; d) antibodies; e) autopsy tissue DM1; and f) gene expression data on DM1 & FSHD patients. Projects 1, 2, & 3 interact with the Repository Core and this Core will interact with the other MDCRCs.

Website: http://crisp.cit.nih.gov/crisp/Crisp_Query.Generate_Screen

- **Project Title: MYELOID CELL FUNCTION IN MUSCULAR DYSTROPHY**

Principal Investigator & Institution: Tidball, James G.; Professor; Physiological Sciences; University of California Los Angeles 10920 Wilshire Blvd., Suite 1200 Los Angeles, Ca 90024

Timing: Fiscal Year 2002; Project Start 24-SEP-2001; Project End 31-AUG-2006

Summary: (provided by applicant): Duchenne **muscular dystrophy** (DMD) is the most common, inherited, lethal disease of childhood. Although mutations in the dystrophin gene are primarily responsible for DMD and animal models of DMD, many features of dystrophinopathies indicate that secondary processes can contribute substantially to pathology. Recent findings have indicated that the immune system can contribute significantly to the pathological progression of dystrophin-deficiency in the mdx mouse model of the disease. The long-term goal of our studies of the pathology of dystrophin-deficiency is to identify the specific immune cells and mechanisms that promote the pathology of dystrophin-deficiencies, after which we will use that information for the development of immune-based therapeutics. Although our preliminary data implicate both myeloid and lymphoid cells in promoting the dystrophic pathology, the studies proposed here will focus on cytotoxic mechanisms that are mediated by macrophages and eosinophils in dystrophic muscle. Our rationale for focusing on these specific myeloid cells is that our preliminary findings strongly implicate these cells in promoting the pathology of dystrophin-deficiency through both innate and acquired immune responses. Our general strategy will be to assess the effect on muscle pathology of depletion of specific myeloid cell populations from the dystrophic mdx mouse. In addition, the effect of those depletions on the lifespan of the dystrophic mdx/utrophin-deficient mice will be assessed because these mice die from **muscular dystrophy** at an early age. We will also test whether introducing null mutations of the inducible nitric oxide synthase gene or major basic protein gene into mdx mice will reduce muscle pathology, because our findings implicate cytotoxic pathways in the mdx pathology that involve the products of these genes. Results of the study proposed here will permit us to determine whether therapeutic approaches that are based on reducing myeloid cell mediated pathology can be productive approaches to the treatment of these forms of **muscular dystrophy.**

Website: http://crisp.cit.nih.gov/crisp/Crisp_Query.Generate_Screen

- **Project Title: MYOSIN GENE DIVERSITY AND FUNCTION**

Principal Investigator & Institution: Leinwand, Leslie A.; Professor and Chair; Molecular, Cellular & Dev Biol; University of Colorado at Boulder Boulder, Co 80309

Timing: Fiscal Year 2003; Project Start 01-SEP-1981; Project End 31-JAN-2007

Summary: (provided by applicant): The formation of skeletal muscle and its adaptation to the environment requires precise temporal and spatial regulation of a host of proteins, including the molecular motor protein, myosin. The precise adaptation of myosin heavy chain (MyHC) genes requires coordinate regulation, yet, little is known about its molecular biology. We propose to define the molecular aspects of fiber type specificity and the pathways that regulate these genes. In mammals, there are 6 characterized skeletal muscle MyHC genes. Although muscle fibers expressing each of them have unique contractile velocities, the enzymatic properties of the individual motors remain elusive. We will express the 6 human skeletal MyHC head domains in an inducible mammalian system and characterize their biochemical and biophysical properties. Despite the perception that the sarcomeric MyHC gene family had been defined, examination of the human genome revealed a novel striated MyHC that we propose to characterize. We have found that it is expressed in cardiac and skeletal muscle and that phylogenetically, it appears most closely related to the alpha and beta MyHC genes. We will compare the sequence features of the coding, regulatory regions and the intron/exon organization of this gene in mouse and human. We will also determine its expression in development and in the adult and test whether well-characterized muscle adaptations alter its pattern of expression. Until recently, there had been no diseases associated with mutations in skeletal

MyHC. However, a mutation in the MyHC IIa gene has been reported which we propose to model in transgenic mice. We are also characterizing the IId gene of a childhood myopathy patient who appears to be null for its expression. An interesting feature of the MyHC gene family that may have relevance to Duchenne **muscular dystrophy** (DMD) is that the most abundant MyHC protein in rodents, IIb, is barely detectable in normal adults. However, we find its expression is induced in DMD. Because of the potential functional consequences of expression of this fast myosin motor, we will define the molecular basis for this species difference and its induction. Finally, we will extend our studies of an unusual cell type, the myofibroblast, which has properties of both muscle and nonmuscle cells, including expression of adult fast skeletal MyHCs, to understand the pathways that define these cells and distinguish them from skeletal muscle.

Website: http://crisp.cit.nih.gov/crisp/Crisp_Query.Generate_Screen

- **Project Title: MYOSTATIN IN MUSCLE GROWTH AND REGENERATION**

Principal Investigator & Institution: Wagner, Kathryn R.; Assistant Professor; Neurology and Neurosurgery; Johns Hopkins University 3400 N Charles St Baltimore, Md 21218

Timing: Fiscal Year 2002; Project Start 15-MAY-2001; Project End 31-MAR-2006

Summary: (provided by applicant): Skeletal muscle grows and atrophies in response to environmental stimuli and has an impressive ability to regenerate following a variety of insults. The processes underlying muscle growth and regeneration are incompletely understood but are apparently governed by a number of growth and differentiation factors. Myostatin, a recently described member of the TGFbeta superfamily, appears to be a negative regulator of muscle growth. Targeted deletion of the myostatin gene in nice causes widespread and massive skeletal muscle hypertrophy and hyperplasia. This study will examine the mechanism of action of myostatin and its potential role in regeneration with three specific aims. First, the precise biological function of myostatin will be defined in vivo and in vitro. Myostatin null mice will be further characterized, particularly with respect to muscle progenitor cells. The normal, cellular pattern of myostatin expression will be determined by RNA analysis of myocytes in vitro and in situ. The biological effects of purified recombinant myostatin on myocytes will be examined in primary and established cell cultures. Second, 1he main focus of the project will be to identify the receptor to myostatin. The binding affinity and distribution of receptors will be determined by binding of radioiodinated myostatin to cultured cells, tissue membranes and embryo whole mounts. The receptor will then be cloned through an approach including expression cloning. Third, the potential role of myostatin in disease and regeneration will be explored in the null mutant mouse through models of myopathy including dystrophinopathy, crush injury and toxic insult. Understanding, and potentially modulating, the factors that influence muscle growth and regeneration. have important applications to myopathies, muscular dystrophies and muscle aging (sarcopenia). The proposed research will employ a variety of molecular biology, protein biochemistry, cell culture and histopathology techniques m order to study an apparently powerful negative regulator of muscle growth. In addition to the ultimate goal of providing clinical applications for muscle disease, this multidisciplinary approach should provide excellent training for a career integrating clinical myology and molecular neuroscience.

Website: http://crisp.cit.nih.gov/crisp/Crisp_Query.Generate_Screen

- **Project Title: MYOTENDINOUS JUNCTION FORMATION IN SKELETAL MUSCLE**

Principal Investigator & Institution: Kramer, Randall H.; Professor; Stomatology; University of California San Francisco 3333 California Street, Suite 315 San Francisco, Ca 941430962

Timing: Fiscal Year 2002; Project Start 01-FEB-1999; Project End 31-JAN-2004

Summary: (Adapted from investigator's Abstract): Craniofacial skeletal muscle defects occur in certain myopathies, such as **muscular dystrophy;** in congenital deformities, such as hemifacial microsomia and facial/palatal clefts; and as a result of surgical procedures for oral cancer or trauma. Success in the repair or replacement of muscle defects is limited by difficulty in transplantation and survival of muscle tissue. An important structure of muscle is the myotendinous junction (MTJ), which transduces force generated by muscle to its connective tissue attachment site. How this complex structure is formed in developing muscle or repaired after injury or disease is poorly understood. Attachment of the muscle fiber to the connective tissue appears to involve adhesion receptors, including the alpha7-beta1 integrin. In addition, during muscle development and repair, alpha7 integrin seems important for myoblast adhesion and motility. The long- term objective of the proposed studies is to further define the molecular mechanisms by which the laminin-binding alpha7 integrin organizes the MTJ in developing and regenerating skeletal muscle. The hypothesis is that the alternatively spliced isoforms of alpha7 not only regulate transient adhesion during myoblast motility but also form the long-lived MTJ. The specific aims are 1) to determine the expression levels and distribution of laminin-binding integrins during skeletal muscle development, 2) to analyze the functionality of alpha7,beta1 alternatively spliced isoforms, and 3) to determine the role of the alternatively spliced extracellular domain in regulating alpha7 activation. The experimental approach is first to define the developmentally complex expression patterns of the alpha7 splice variants and their ligands. Next, alpha7 isoforms will be analyzed for their role in cell motility and assembly of MTJ-like structures. Finally, the role of the extracellular domain splice variants in regulating alpha7 activity will be addressed using molecular approaches. These studies will enhance understanding of the structure and assembly of the MTJ and suggest new approaches in tissue engineering to promote reconstruction of craniofacial skeletal muscle defects caused by disease, trauma, or surgical procedures.

Website: http://crisp.cit.nih.gov/crisp/Crisp_Query.Generate_Screen

- **Project Title: NEUROBIOLOGY OF DISEASE -- TEACHING WORKSHOP**

Principal Investigator & Institution: Kriegstein, Arnold R.; Professor; Society for Neuroscience 11 Dupont Cir Nw, Ste 500 Washington, Dc 20036

Timing: Fiscal Year 2004; Project Start 01-AUG-1983; Project End 31-MAY-2006

Summary: The Society for Neuroscience (SFN) is the major professional organization for scientists who study the nervous system. An important goal of this organization is to encourage scientists in training to undertake research related to diseases of the nervous system. The objective of this grant application is to support teaching workshops that introduce young neuroscientists to current concepts about the etiology and pathogenesis of disorders of the nervous system. For each workshop, about 12 faculty are chosen by the Organizing Committee after eliciting proposals from the Society at large. Clinical presentations provide enrollees with an experience of the human dimension of particular diseases. Lectures cover both clinical research and relevant laboratory work. In addition to lectures, enrollees are given a choice of attending two of four small group workshops that emphasize either specific or methodological issues and encourage lively discussion. Since its inception, 20 workshops have been held, usually on the day prior to the start of the Society for Neuroscience meeting. Topics have included: Infections in the nervous system, epilepsy, Huntington's and Alzheimer's diseases, **muscular dystrophy,** multiple sclerosis, prion diseases, drug addiction, pain and affective disorders, stroke and excitotoxicity, neuromuscular diseases, amyotrophic lateral sclerosis, schizophrenia, migraine, mental retardation and developmental disorders, Tourette's syndrome and obsessive-compulsive disorder, and the neurobiology of brain tumors. Enrollment generally runs between 100 and 200 attendees. Most enrollees are graduate students or postdoctoral fellows. Current plans are to cover the following topics in the near future: Genes, free radicals, mitochondria and apoptosis in Parkinson's disease, AIDS dementia, peripheral neuropathy, pain, language disorders, and affective disorders. Other topics will be chosen depending on their potential interest to young neuroscientists, their impact on society and the quality of recent research related to that disease area. We are especially interested in covering diseases of the nervous system which are important clinically but which are in need of enhanced basic cellular and molecular understanding. Society members are encouraged to suggest topics in the SFN Newsletter.

Website: http://crisp.cit.nih.gov/crisp/Crisp_Query.Generate_Screen

- **Project Title: NGF AND MUSCLE DEVELOPMENT**

Principal Investigator & Institution: Wheeler, Esther F.; University of Texas San Antonio San Antonio, Tx 782490600

Timing: Fiscal Year 2003; Project Start 01-AUG-2003; Project End 31-JUL-2006

Summary: The purpose of the study proposed herein is to determine the biological function of NGF and the NGF Receptors in muscle development. The preliminary data indicate a novel role for NGF and its two receptors (p75NTR and trk A) during myoblast proliferation and differentiation. The p75NTR, a non-catalytic receptor, is expressed by proliferating myoblasts but ceases to be expressed when myoblasts fuse to form myotubes. At some point during fusion, the other NGF receptor, trk A (a tyrosine-specific kinase receptor), begins to be expressed by the fused myotubes. The expression patterns of the NGF receptors raise the possibility that NGF plays a role in myogenesis. The working hypothesis is that NGF mediates processes that mediate the viability and organization of differentiating myoblasts and the normal homeostasis of differentiated myofibers. The results of the study will hopefully reveal effects of NGF on muscle that can be exploited for therapies for preventing or treating the muscular degeneration that accompanies neurodegenerative diseases as well as Duchene's **muscular dystrophy.** To determine the biological function of NGF and its receptors during myogenesis, the change of expression of the receptors will be determined at different stages of myoblast differentiation in vitro. Once cell cultures have been established that mimic receptor expression in vivo, the signaling pathways the pathways activated by the p75NTR in myoblasts will be studied. Dominant negative mutations in two of the signal transduction molecules will be used to determine pathway interactions. The spatial/temporal expression of the the trk A receptor protein will be studied in vivo in order to determine the development time the receptor becomes active. To better characterize the NGF response in myocytes, C2C12 cells will be transfected with constructs that will make it possible to induce express the receptors at inappropriate times and the resulting cell lines will be tested for defects in development and differentiation. Finally, the muscle of null mutant mice for the two receptors will be examined in vivo and in vitro for changes in myoblast differentiation and muscle function. Taken together, the aims of the proposal will reveal new information about the role of NGF in the normal development and function of muscle.

Website: http://crisp.cit.nih.gov/crisp/Crisp_Query.Generate_Screen

- **Project Title: NON-RADIAL CELL MIGRATION IN CNS DEVELOPMENT**

Principal Investigator & Institution: Golden, Jeffrey A.; Associate Professor of Pathology; Children's Hospital of Philadelphia 34Th St and Civic Ctr Blvd Philadelphia, Pa 191044399

Timing: Fiscal Year 2003; Project Start 15-FEB-2003; Project End 31-DEC-2007

Summary: (provided by applicant): Epilepsy, mental retardation and structural anomalies of the brain often have a genetic etiology. Although they affect 3-5% of all children, the underlying pathogeneses for these disorders is poorly understood in most cases. Cell migration is a central component of normal central nervous system (CNS) development and disruptions in this process have been implicated in the development of multiple disorders such as Fukuyama **Muscular dystrophy,** Miller-Dieker Syndrome, Walker-Warburg Syndrome, and the Muscle-Eye-Brain syndrome to name just a few. Two primary patterns of cell migration are recognized during CNS development, radial and non-radial. While the cellular and molecular bases of radial cell migration, long considered the predominant mode of cell migration, have begun to be defined, the mechanisms of guidance for non-radial cell migration remain largely unexplored. Using lineage analysis, we have defined the developmental time and location where non-radial cell migration begins in the chick forebrain. Based on these data we have developed a model to explain the cellular and molecular mechanisms of non-radial cell migration. Our model is based on the hypotheses that cell surface molecules, secreted molecules, and extracellular matrix molecules guide non-radially migrating cells. This proposal will begin to address our hypothesis by 1) directly testing several components of our model, and 2) generate a mammalian model to further study one of the molecules we have identified as a component of non-radial cell migration in the chick. These data will certainly enhance our understanding of normal CNS development. Furthermore, we anticipate the data from these studies will provide insight into the pathogenesis of a variety of inherited and non-inherited conditions that afflict children such as epilepsy, mental retardation and structural malformations of the brain. This may ultimately lead to improvements in the diagnosis, management, and prevention of neurological diseases where abnormal cell migration has a pathogenetic role.

Website: http://crisp.cit.nih.gov/crisp/Crisp_Query.Generate_Screen

- **Project Title: PATHOGENESIS OF A NOVEL LIMB-GIRDLE MUSCULAR DYSTROPHY**

Principal Investigator & Institution: Hirano, Michio; Assistant Professor; Neurology; Columbia University Health Sciences Po Box 49 New York, Ny 10032

Timing: Fiscal Year 2002; Project Start 01-SEP-2001; Project End 31-JUL-2004

Summary: Since the initial identification of mutations in the dystrophin gene as the cause of Duchenne and Becker muscular dystrophies, molecular genetics has provided a plethora of new information and insights into the pathogeneses of muscle diseases. In particular, our understanding of the limb-girdle muscular dystrophies (LMGD) have been greatly enhanced. Fourteen forms of LGMD have been identified; of these, specific gene have been characterized in ten. This goal of this proposal is to identify the molecular genetic basis of a fifteenth form of LGMD which has been transmitted in an autosomal dominant fashion in a large Spanish pedigree (Spanish autosomal dominant LGMD [SAD-LGMD]). The disease locus has been mapped to a seven centimorgan region of chromosome 7q31.3-32 with a maximum two-point LOD score of 7.59 with marker D7S2519. We will attempt to reduce the size of the disease locus by fine mapping studies. Candidate genes will be screened until the disease mutation is identified. The pathogenesis of the disease will be studied by studying the expression of the gene messenger RNA and the gene product in the patients' skeletal muscle and in tissue culture using cells from patients. A mouse model of the disease will be produced to further investigate the pathogenesis. Muscle biopsies from more than 50 patients with LGMD of unknown etiology will be screened for defects of the SAD-LGMD gene product. The identification of the cause of SAD-LGMD will expand our understanding of the disease and will likely enhance our general understanding of skeletal muscle functions and structure. For the patients, achieving the proposed goals will allow more accurate prenatal diagnosis, genetic counseling, and perhaps contribute to more rational therapies in the future.

Website: http://crisp.cit.nih.gov/crisp/Crisp_Query.Generate_Screen

- **Project Title: PATHOGENESIS OF LAMININ-ALPHA2 DEFICIENCY**

Principal Investigator & Institution: Miller, Jeffrey B.; Boston Biomedical Research Institute 64 Grove St Watertown, Ma 02472

Timing: Fiscal Year 2002; Project Start 19-SEP-2002; Project End 31-AUG-2006

Summary: (provided by applicant): Pathogenesis of laminin-ot2-deficiency. Mutations in the human LAMA2 gene cause congenital **muscular dystrophy,** group 1 (CMD 1), a devastating, recessive disease of childhood. LAMA2 encodes laminin-c Beta 2, an extracellular protein that is abundant in skeletal muscle. The proposed experiments will test hypotheses about how loss of laminin-c_2 leads to the severe neuromuscular dysfunction in CMD1. For Aims 1 & 2, we will examine the role of apoptosis in CMD1 pathogenesis. In culture, laminin-cz2-deficient myotubes are unstable and die by a process that is inhibited by the antiapoptosis protein Bcl-2. It is not known, however, whether apoptosis is important in the loss of CMD1 neuromuscular function in vivo. The proposed experiments willdetermine how disease in laminin-c_2-deficient mice is affected by targeted alterations of Bcl-2 family members. For Aim 3, we will determine if muscle stem cell function is altered in CMD 1. Postnatal muscle contains multipotent stem cells, but no studies have examined these recently identified stem cells in diseased muscle. We will test the possibility that laminin- Beta 2-deficiency activates proliferation and alters the differentiation capability of these rare cells. For Aim 4, we will determine if inappropriate re-entry into the cell cycle occurs in affected tissue. Inappropriate cell cycling can lead to death of normally post-mitotic cells including neurons and myofibers. We hypothesize that laminin-cz2-deficiency alters signal transmission resulting in dysregulation of the cell cycle. To test this hypothesis, we will determine if cell cycle regulators are inappropriately induced in laminin-c beta 2-deficient cells. The results will increase our understanding of CMD 1 pathogenesis and could suggest new routes to therapy, perhaps based on apoptosis inhibition, stem cell repair, or cell cycle inhibition.

Website: http://crisp.cit.nih.gov/crisp/Crisp_Query.Generate_Screen

- **Project Title: POLYCYSTIN-1 INTERACTION WITH TSC-2 IN POLYCYSTIC KIDNEY DISEASE**

Principal Investigator & Institution: Guan, Kun-Liang; Associate Professor; University of Michigan at Ann Arbor 3003 South State, Room 1040 Ann Arbor, Mi 481091274

Timing: Fiscal Year 2003; Project Start 01-SEP-2003; Project End 31-AUG-2008

Summary: Autosomal dominant polycystic kidney disease (ADPKD) is one of the most common genetic disorders in humans. In the United States, ADPKD is more common than cystic fibrosis, Huntington's disease, and **muscular dystrophy.** ADPKD is characterized by the formation of cysts in kidney and caused by mutation in either PKD1 (85%) or PKD2 (15%) gene. Tuberous sclerosis (TSC) is an autosomal dominant inheritable genetic disorder due to mutation in either TSC1 or TSC2 gene. TSC is characterized by formation of hamartomas in various tissues. Cyst formation in kidney is also observed in TSC. The PKD1 and TSC2 genes are located adjacent to each other on human chromosome 16p and deletion of both genes results in a contiguous gene syndrome responsible for the severe infantile polycystic kidney disease. TSC2 has been implicated to play a role in the proper functions of polycystin-1, the product of PKD1 gene. The long-term goals of this project are to understand the functional relationship between TSC2 and PKD1 and to elucidate the molecular mechanism of TSC2 in regulation of PKD1 function and ADPKD. The specific aims of this proposal are to elucidate the mechanism of TSC2 regulation by osmotic stress and to investigate the function of TSC2 in regulation of the plasma membrane localization of polycystin-1.

Website: http://crisp.cit.nih.gov/crisp/Crisp_Query.Generate_Screen

- **Project Title: POSITION EFFECT AND VASCULAR ADAPTATION IN FSHD**

Principal Investigator & Institution: Twil, Rabi; University of Rochester Orpa - Rc Box 270140 Rochester, Ny 14627

Timing: Fiscal Year 2003; Project Start 30-SEP-2003; Project End 31-MAY-2008

Summary: Facioscapulohumeral **muscular dystrophy** (FSHD) is the third most common form of **muscular dystrophy.** Although the genetic lesion is well described, neither the specific gene(s) nor the cellular mechanism involved in its pathophysiology are known. We propose to investigate the molecular and cellular pathophysiology of facioscapulohumeral **muscular dystrophy** (FSHD) utilizing the techniques of microarray analysis of skeletal muscle samples with followup biological confirmation of relevant dysregulated genes using real time RT-PCR and immunohistochemical techniques. The research proposal will test the hypotheses that in FSHD (1) critical deletion in D4Z4 heterochromatic repeats results in altered expression of adjacent 4q35 genes, and that (2) aberrant overexpression of vascular genes, either as a primary or downstream effect, is involved in the pathogenesis of this disease. The ultimate goal is to identify critical, causal disruptions in cellular function that are amenable to therapeutic intervention.

Website: http://crisp.cit.nih.gov/crisp/Crisp_Query.Generate_Screen

- **Project Title: PROGRAM PROJECT GRANT**

Principal Investigator & Institution: Uitto, Jouni J.; Professor and Chair; Dermatology/Cutaneous Biology; Thomas Jefferson University Office of Research Administration Philadelphia, Pa 191075587

Timing: Fiscal Year 2002; Project Start 15-AUG-1987; Project End 31-MAR-2007

Summary: This renewal application proposes extensive and innovative studies focusing on the molecular genetics of the cutaneous basement membrane zone (BMZ) towards delineating the molecular basis of various forms of epidermolysis bullosa (EB) and other selected genodermatoses affecting the epidermis. The proposed studies are designed to test the hypothesis that genetic lesions in structural genes expressed in the epidermis underlie variants of these diseases, and that the precise phenotype and mode of inheritance depend on the types and combinations of specific mutations in distinct genes. This application is based on solid progress in this project, including (a) expansion of the molecular basis of the recessive dystrophic forms of EB allowing refinement of genotype/phenotype correlations; (b) identification of novel and de novo COL7A1 mutations in dominant DEB, with an impact on genetic counseling of the families at risk of recurrence; (c) identification of a large number of novel and recurrent mutations both Herlitz and non-Herlitz junctional EB; (d) identification of uniparental disomy of chromosome 1 as a novel mechanism for H-JEB; (e) demonstration in mutations in the genes ITGA6 and ITGB4 encoding alpha-6-beta-4 integrins subunit polypeptides in EB with pyloric atresia,; (f) cloning of the human plectin gene and demonstration of mutations in EB with late-onset **muscular dystrophy;** (g) cloning of mouse type VII collagen and desmoglein 3 genes with development of "knock-out" mice with blistering phenotype; (h) identification and characterization of several novel genes expressed into the epidermis, including periplakin, ladinin, and desmo-15; (i) refinement of RNA- DNA chimeric oligonucleotide technology for repair of the mutated genes in heritable skin diseases. This proposal details continuation of concentrated, multi-disciplinary studies in five highly interdependent projects: Project 1, "Molecular Genetics of EB and Other Heritable Disorders of the Cutaneous BMZ and Epidermis," will provide precise information on the specific mutations in the gene/protein system that are at fault in various forms of EB and other epidermal heritable disorders. Project 2, "Identification and Characterization of Candidate Genes/Protein Systems Expressed in the Skin," will provide new gene probes and information about novel genes as potential candidate genes for epidermal genodermatoses. Project 3, "Consequences of the Mutations at the Protein Structure/Function Level" will examine the structural and functional alterations that result from distinct mutations in the candidate genes, utilizing computer modeling and monitoring functional interactions in biosensor analysis system. Project 4, "Development and Testing of Animal Models for EB," will generate novel animal models for EB. Project 5, "Development of Non-Viral Gene Therapy for Cutaneous Diseases," will concentrate on testing gene therapy approaches utilizing RNA/DNA chimeric oligonucleotide strategies. These multidisciplinary studies are expected to provide precise information of critical importance for translational applications towards development of refined classification, genotype/phenotype correlations, basis for genetic counseling, and prenatal testing, as well as providing the basis for novel gene therapy approaches for this devastating group of skin diseases.

Website: http://crisp.cit.nih.gov/crisp/Crisp_Query.Generate_Screen

- **Project Title: RNA DOMINANCE IN HUMAN DISEASE**

Principal Investigator & Institution: Swanson, Maurice S.; Professor; Molecular Genetics & Microbiol; University of Florida Gainesville, Fl 32611

Timing: Fiscal Year 2002; Project Start 01-APR-2000; Project End 31-MAR-2005

Summary: (appended verbatim from investigator's abstract): Myotonic dystrophy (DM) is the most common form of adult onset **muscular dystrophy.** DM is an autosomal dominant neuromuscular disorder that is caused by a (CTG)n repeat expansion in the 3' UTR of the DM protein kinase (DMPK) gene. The long term objective of the proposed research is to elucidate how a triplet repeat expansion in the 3' UTR of a gene leads to a dominantly inherited disease. Current evidence suggests that DM pathogenesis is associated with the accumulation of DMPK mutant allele transcripts within the nucleus. Our working 'sequestration' hypothesis is that DM is an RNA dominant disease in which the (CUG)n expansion forms an exceptionally stable double stranded RNA (dsRNA) hairpin structure. This unusual RNA hairpin acts as a high affinity binding site for triplet repeat expansion dsRNA binding proteins that possibly play important roles in nucleocytoplasmic RNA export. Large repeat expansions associated with severe disease lead to sequestration of these proteins on DMPK mutant allele transcripts and a dominant negative effect on the export of other RNAs. This proposal is focused on testing this RNA dominance model using several different experimental approaches. First, the hypothesis that (CUG)n expansion RNAs have a dominant negative effect on mRNA export will be directly examined using RNA microinjection into frog oocyte and mammalian fibroblast nuclei. Second, the sequestration hypothesis predicts that expansion binding proteins should accumulate in nuclear foci together with DMPK mutant transcripts. Therefore, we will complete the characterization of several proteins that preferentially recognize large (CUG)n expansions, and determine the subcellular distribution of these proteins in normal and DM patient cells. Third, preferred RNA binding sites for these expansion binding proteins will be characterized by in vitro and in vivo analyses with particular emphasis on identifying RNAs that normally associate with these proteins. Fourth, we will determine if expansion binding proteins are involved in mRNA export by combining the use of monoclonal antibodies and recombinant proteins with the microinjection system developed in the first aim. Fifth, the relevance of RNA dominance to other neuromuscular and neurological diseases will be investigated. These studies have important implications for elucidating molecular mechanisms involved in DM pathogenesis and cellular strategies which facilitate the exchange of genetic information between the nucleus and cytoplasm.

Website: http://crisp.cit.nih.gov/crisp/Crisp_Query.Generate_Screen

- **Project Title: RNA/PROTEIN INTERACTIONS IN PREMRNA SPLICING REGULATION**

Principal Investigator & Institution: Singh, Ravinder; Molecular, Cellular & Dev Biol; University of Colorado at Boulder Boulder, Co 80309

Timing: Fiscal Year 2002; Project Start 01-AUG-1999; Project End 31-JUL-2004

Summary: Sex determination is a fundamental decision that essentially all metazoans encounter during their development. Sex determination in Drosophila melanogaster involves a hierarchy of alternative splicing decisions, and is also the best understood example of splicing regulation. Splicing is a process by which non-coding sequences (introns) are removed from the precursor messenger RNA. In higher eukaryotes, constitutive and alternative splicing are important aspects of gene regulation in many important cellular processes. Approximately 15 percent of the mutations that have been linked to human diseases affect RNA splicing signals, including cellular transformation, Duchenne **muscular dystrophy,** and tumor metastasis. Our goal is to understand how RNA-binding proteins recognize target RNAs and regulate constitutive and alternative pre-mRNA splicing. The Drosophila protein Sex-lethal (SXL) acts as a key binary switch between the male and female cell fates. In the past, we defined the mechanism by which SXL regulates alternative splicing by antagonizing the known splicing factor U2AF65. Specificity is an underlying theme in biological regulation. U2AF65 and SXL offer excellent models for specific RNA-protein interactions in the context of splicing regulation. For example, while the general splicing factor U2AF65 recognizes a wide variety of polypyrimidine-tract/3' splice sites, the highly specific splicing repressor SXL recognizes a specific sequence. Although both proteins contain a ribonucleoprotein-consensus motif, they have distinct RNA-binding specificity. However, it is not understood how these seemingly similar proteins achieve unique RNA-binding specificities. To define the structural basis for the RNA-binding specificities of U2AF65 and SXL, we will extend our analysis of the RNA and the proteins by using a combination of biochemical, molecular, and genetic approaches. Our findings will also be directly applicable to other members of this largest family that likely regulate different aspects of RNA biogenesis. In addition, SXL controls many female-specific functions. However, some of the relevant genes that are regulated by SXL remain to be identified. To identify these targets, we will use a combination of recently developed molecular approaches - genomic SELEX and subtractive hybridization/differential display. These approaches should complement genetic analysis.

Website: http://crisp.cit.nih.gov/crisp/Crisp_Query.Generate_Screen

- **Project Title: ROLE OF ELAV IN NEURONAL RNA PROCESSING**

Principal Investigator & Institution: White, Kalpana P.; Professor; Brandeis University 415 South Street Waltham, Ma 024549110

Timing: Fiscal Year 2002; Project Start 10-SEP-2002; Project End 31-JUL-2007

Summary: (provided by applicant): The long-term goal of this research project is to understand how differentially-expressed trans-acting factors in neurons can control pre-mRNA processing to precisely regulate neuronal gene expression. The powerful genetics, molecular biology and transgenic techniques of Drosophila, along with the emergent DNA microarray technology, will be utilized to study the role of ELAV in mRNA processing and its overall impact on gene expression in neurons. ELAV is the founding member of the ELAV/Hu family of RNA-binding proteins, which is conserved in both vertebrates and invertebrates. Members of the ELAV/Hu family serve diverse roles in mRNA processing, including splicing, stability and translatability. The aims of the project are: (1) elucidation of mechanisms of ELAV's interactions with RNA transcripts, (2) identification of direct targets of ELAV using immunoprecipitated ELAV-ribnucleoprotein complexes and DNA microarrays, (3) assessment of the overall impact of ELAV on gene expression using microarray technology. Together, these approaches will begin to identify networks of genes that are regulated collectively and provide a comprehensive view of how post-transcriptional regulation is utilized in neuronal gene expression. Given the evolutionary conservation between Drosophila and human genomes, insights in regulatory strategies will be directly transferable to human studies. Human members of the ELAV/Hu family have been implicated in pathogenesis of paraneoplastic cerebellar dysfunction. RNA processing defects have been documented in a large number of human diseases and inherited disorders including cancer, **muscular dystrophy** and fragile X syndrome.

Website: http://crisp.cit.nih.gov/crisp/Crisp_Query.Generate_Screen

- **Project Title: ROLE OF THE ALPHA 7 BETA 1 INTEGRIN IN MUSCLE INTEGRITY**

Principal Investigator & Institution: Kaufman, Stephen J.; Professor; Cell and Structural Biology; University of Illinois Urbana-Champaign Henry Administration Bldg Champaign, Il 61820

Timing: Fiscal Year 2002; Project Start 24-JAN-1997; Project End 31-AUG-2006

Summary: (provided by applicant): The proper association of muscle fibers with laminin in the extracellular matrix is essential for normal muscle function. The alpha7Beta1 integrin and the dystrophin-glycoprotein complex both bind laminin and appear to be complementary linkage systems between fibers and the extracellular matrix. Congenital and acquired defects in the dystrophin-glycoprotein complex underlie the pathology associated with Duchenne and other muscular dystrophies, as well as cardiomyopathies. Mutations in the human alpha7 gene cause an additional myopathy. We recently discovered that enhanced expression of the alpha7 integrin mediated linkage system can compensate for the absence of the dystrophin-glycoprotein complex. Dystrophin/utrophin null mice develop an acute **muscular dystrophy** and die prematurely. Enhanced expression of the alpha7 integrin inhibits the development of **muscular dystrophy** and restores longevity to these animals. We propose to expand on this result and determine the level of alpha7Beta1 integrin that best prevents development of skeletal muscle pathology in these animals and whether transgene expression in the heart and smooth muscle can prevent cardiovascular disease. We will also analyze whether enhanced expression of the alpha7 integrin in the heart reduces development of cardiomyopathy associated with enterovirus-induced cleavage of dystrophin. Additional skeletal muscle and cardiomyopathies result from other defects in the dystrophin-glycoprotein linkage system. We will use transgenic animals that over-express the alpha7Beta1 integrin in different genetic backgrounds to determine whether the integrin can prevent these myopathies. Whereas mutations in the sarcoglycan genes perturb the dystrophin-glycoprotein transmembrane linkage system and cause cardiomyopathy and **muscular dystrophy,** we will determine whether over-expression of the alpha7 integrin can inhibit the development of muscle disease in sarcoglycan deficient mice. Likewise, we will assess whether enhanced integrin expression will ameliorate alpha2-laminin congenital **muscular dystrophy.** Lastly, experiments are proposed that aim at understanding the mechanism by which enhanced integrin expression inhibits development of muscle pathology. This research will reveal whether increasing alpha7 integrin levels in humans may be worth pursuing in the future as treatments for Duchenne and other muscular dystrophies and cardiomyopathies.

Website: http://crisp.cit.nih.gov/crisp/Crisp_Query.Generate_Screen

- **Project Title: SATELLITE STEM CELL BIOLOGY**

Principal Investigator & Institution: Booth, Frank W.; Professor; Veterinary Biomedical Sciences; University of Missouri Columbia 310 Jesse Hall Columbia, Mo 65211

Timing: Fiscal Year 2002; Project Start 15-APR-2000; Project End 31-MAR-2004

Summary: (Adapted from the applicant's abstract): Satellite cells are muscle-specific stem cells that function to repair damaged myofibers and provide new myonuclei for muscle enlargement. Rosenblatt has shown that knocking out the proliferative capacity of satellite cells prevents hypertrophy of skeletal muscle. Blau and Wright have found that satellite cells prematurely senesce in young patients with **Duchenne's muscular dystrophy** who have many cycles of regeneration. Schultz has observed a progressive loss of the proliferative capacity of satellite cells as rats age, and similar data has just been reported in humans. Hayflick showed that normal, diploid cells have a finite proliferative lifespan and reach cellular senescence. However, Bischoff indicated that a critical evaluation of the self-maintenance criteria required to categorize the satellite cell as stem cell is yet to be undertaken. These provocative reports highlight some of the conceptual framework to pose the following specific aims. Using the well-established and validated approach of clonogenecity assays to determine a cell's proliferation potential, this proposal examines 1.) whether a physiological model of repeated cycles of atrophy-regrowth in old skeletal muscle speeds satellite cells to senescence so that their proliferative capacity is depleted prior to the lifespan of rats; 2.) determine whether the application of IGF-1 to skeletal muscle or 3.) increased contractile activity, or both aims 1 and 2 results in either a.) using up or b.) replenishing the finite population doublings in old satellite cells. These results would shed much needed insight into whether replicative senescence can be modulated by environmental factors. The information thus gleaned from these studies will provide the basis for follow-up experiments that will measure cell cycle markers to begin to explain the observations in molecular detail. As the number of individuals with frailty is rapidly increasing, it becomes a more urgent clinical, social, and economic issue to find out if and how satellite cell lifespan can be maintained/enhanced. This proposal will therefore provide novel insights into how the self-maintenance properties of satellite cells is modulated by compensatory factors (IGF-1 and exercise), thereby forming the basis for more effective interventions against senile-atrophy and frailty.

Website: http://crisp.cit.nih.gov/crisp/Crisp_Query.Generate_Screen

- **Project Title: SPIRITUALITY OF CHILDREN WITH DMD**

Principal Investigator & Institution: Pehler, Shelley-Rae; None; University of Iowa Iowa City, Ia 52242

Timing: Fiscal Year 2003; Project Start 01-JAN-2004; Project End 31-DEC-2006

Summary: (provided by applicant): This application proposes research to explore the spirituality of an 8 -12 year old child with Duchenne **Muscular Dystrophy.** Duchenne **Muscular Dystrophy** (DMD) is a progressive, genetically inherited, chronic disease with a life-threatening prognosis. Early confirmation of the type of genetic disease a child has allows interventions to be initiated that may affect the quality and longevity of life. What is not known is the spirituality of children with a genetically inherited, life threatening disease, even though the literature is clear that there is a heightened spirituality in the adult and adolescent populations with similar diseases. This heightened spirituality has provided meaning to the adult and adolescents' life to promote healing.

Healing does not mean cure in the usual use of the word, but instead a sense of health and well-being as experienced by hope, love, sense of control, relatedness with others, finding meaning and purpose in life and disease, and a sense that there is something greater than the self (Fryback, 1993; Mytko & Knight, 1999). The purpose of this study is to explore spirituality in children who are 8 -12 years of age and who have been diagnosed with the genetic, life-threatening disease of Duchenne **Muscular Dystrophy.** Giorgi's (1985) qualitative design will be used for this phenomenological study. Children 8 -12 years old with DMD will be recruited from a large, mid-western genetics clinic. Children will be invited to participate in the research until no new themes or meaning units are identified during the interviews. Interviews using open-ended questions and descriptions by the children of drawings they have made will elicit the data. Interview data will be transcribed to sheets of paper verbatim. Demographic information will be used to generate descriptive statistics for the sample population and to determine any religious belief systems that would help in the understanding of the child's responses to the questions. Analysis of the data will follow Giorgi's (1985) method of analysis. Rigor will be addressed through bracketing prior to interviewing and data analysis, using two different data collection strategies, development of a detailed Interview Schedule, using a peer debriefed, and developing an audit process for field notes and data analysis.

Website: http://crisp.cit.nih.gov/crisp/Crisp_Query.Generate_Screen

- **Project Title: STRUCTURE-FUNCTION ANALYSIS OF SARCOSPAN**

Principal Investigator & Institution: Crosbie, Rachelle H.; Duchenne Musc Dyst Res Ctr; University of California Los Angeles 10920 Wilshire Blvd., Suite 1200 Los Angeles, Ca 90024

Timing: Fiscal Year 2002; Project Start 24-SEP-2001; Project End 31-AUG-2006

Summary: (provided by applicant): The broad, long-term objectives of this proposal are to understand the structure and function of a novel tetraspanin called SARCOSPAN. Sarcospan is an integral component of the dystrophin-glycoprotein complex and is highly expressed in skeletal and cardiac muscles, as well as many non-muscle tissues (Crosbie et al., 1997; Crosbie et al., 1998; Crosbie et al., 1999). The dystrophin-glycoprotein complex (DGC) is a structural complex that spans the muscle plasma membrane and links the extracellular matrix with the intracellular cytoskeleton. This structural linkage is critical for normal muscle function as clearly demonstrated by the many forms of **muscular dystrophy** that result from mutations in the dystrophin-glycoprotein complex. Association of several signaling molecules with the DGC also suggests that this complex may play a role in mediating extracellular-intracellular communications. Furthermore, lateral associations amongst membrane components of the DGC are critical for function of this complex. It is hypothesized that sarcospan facilitates protein-protein interactions within the dystrophin-glycoprotein complex. These protein interactions are clearly important for the physical linkage between the extracellular matrix and the intracellular actin network and for the prevention of **muscular dystrophy.** Human mutations within the sarcospan gene have not been identified in known cases of autosomal recessive **muscular dystrophy** (Crosbie et al., 2000). However, these mutation searches have only examined the ubiquitous form of SSPN, which has a broad expression pattern. Preliminary data demonstrates that a novel, muscle-specific form of SSPN is expressed in skeletal and cardiac muscles. We hypothesize that mutations within muscle-SSPN may cause novel forms of **muscular dystrophy.** Identification and characterization of this muscle-sarcospan will advance our understanding of the role of the dystrophin-glycoprotein complex in normal muscle and in the pathogenesis of **muscular dystrophy.**

Website: http://crisp.cit.nih.gov/crisp/Crisp_Query.Generate_Screen

- **Project Title: SURGICAL APPROACHES TO SYSTEMIC GENE TRANSFER**

Principal Investigator & Institution: Stedman, Hansell H.; Assistant Professor; Surgery; University of Pennsylvania 3451 Walnut Street Philadelphia, Pa 19104

Timing: Fiscal Year 2002; Project Start 30-SEP-2002; Project End 31-AUG-2007

Summary: (provided by applicant): The overall aim of the proposed research is to improve the prospects for therapeutic gene transfer in Duchenne **muscular dystrophy** by addressing two essential rate-limiting issues: immunity to the transgene product and vector delivery. Using a newly described canine animal model for Duchenne **muscular dystrophy,** the German Short Haired Pointer, the experimental design takes advantage of a deletion of the dystrophin gene to evaluate the comparative immunogenicity of dystrophin and utrophin. We make exclusive use of rAAV vectors. The experimental design tests the hypothesis that in the context of the deletion, recombinant (canine) mini-dystrophin will elicit a deleterious cellular immune response. It further tests the hypothesis that substitution of a similarly designed canine mini-utrophin transgene will circumvent this immune response. Based on extensive preliminary data, the proposal also addresses the hypothesis that the endothelial barrier to systemic gene delivery can be bypassed by temporarily infusing histamine during a period of mechanical circulatory support. We propose a graded series of experiments to address the latter hypothesis, starting with isolated limb perfusion and culminating in systemic gene delivery. These studies will also make extensive use of another naturally occurring animal model, the hamster model for **limb-girdle muscular dystrophy.** Successful completion of the experimental plan will provide general information relevant to the immunological response to somatic gene delivery and the preservation of organ function during profound but rapidly reversible alterations in endothelial integrity. It will also provide specific information about the rational design of strategies for systemic gene therapy in one of the most common single-gene lethal diseases in man, Duchenne **Muscular Dystrophy.**

Website: http://crisp.cit.nih.gov/crisp/Crisp_Query.Generate_Screen

- **Project Title: TEST OF AAV VECTORS IN K9 DMD MODEL**

Principal Investigator & Institution: Little, Marie-Terese E.; University of Washington Grant & Contract Services Seattle, Wa 98105

Timing: Fiscal Year 2003; Project Start 26-SEP-2003; Project End 31-JUL-2008

Summary: Duchenne **Muscular Dystrophy** (DMD) in both humans and dogs is a fatal, X-linked, recessive muscle disease caused by a lack of dystrophin due to deletions or mutations in the dystrophin gene. The disease is inherited in a recessive pattern suggesting that gene therapy could offer an effective treatment if methods can be found to replace the defective gene in muscle. Studies in the mouse model ofDMD (mdx) have shown that delivery of mini-dystrophin adeno-associated viral (AAV) vectors, which display a remarkable ability to transduce skeletal muscle vectors to adult mdx muscle results in correction of most, but not all, features of dystrophy. Prior to launching into clinical trials with this vector system, data in a large animal model, which more closely reflects the disease phenotype in humans, are needed to assess the safety and effectiveness of this approach. Three specific hypotheses will be tested: 1) that an increase in muscle fiber integrity and function can be achieved by targeted direct injection of AAV vectors containing truncated canine dystrophin genes; 2) that wild type satellite cell transfer and vascularized muscle transplants will result in successful transfer and persistence of wild type satellite cells for the correction of the DMD phenotype; and 3) that seeding of wild type satellite cells will occur from normal to diseased muscle. Aims 1 and 2 will be conducted in recipients of marrow grafts to avoid potential rejection of wild type cells by the immune system. The canine model of DMD that is clinically and pathologically similar to human DMD will be used. These studies will provide baseline data for the development of a phase I clinical AAV gene therapy trial for DMD (Project 1). The long-term obiectives of the proposed research are to determine if direct AAV-dystrophin gene and cellular itransplant delivery ameliorates and reverses dystrophic pathology in xmd muscle and if this leads to normal myofiber morphology, histology, cell membrane integrity and function. The development of new therapies in the canine model could have immediate impact on the treatment of DMD patients.

Website: http://crisp.cit.nih.gov/crisp/Crisp_Query.Generate_Screen

- **Project Title: THE ROLE OF NUCLEAR LAMINS IN MUSCLE DISEASE**

  Principal Investigator & Institution: Burke, Brian; Professor; Anatomy and Cell Biology; University of Florida Gainesville, Fl 32611

  Timing: Fiscal Year 2002; Project Start 01-JUL-2002; Project End 31-MAR-2007

  Summary: (provided by applicant): A-type and B-type nuclear lamins form a family of nuclear envelope proteins that have an essential function in the maintenance of nuclear structure. Mutations in the human lamin A gene have been linked to several diseases which include Emery-Dreifuss **muscular dystrophy** (EDMD) and cardiomyopathy. Since the A-type lamins are found in majority of adult cell types it is extremely puzzling that defects in these proteins should be associated primarily with muscle specific disorders. The goal of this proposal is to elucidate the roles that individual lam in family members play in the organization of the cell nucleus and how in particular this relates to the maintenance of muscle integrity. The proposal will take advantage of mouse strains harboring targeted mutations in lamin genes, including a strain in which the lamin A gene has been deleted and which develops a disorder that closely resembles human EDMD. Inactivation of B-type lamin genes as well as the introduction of specific human disease-linked point mutations into the mouse lamin A gene will provide novel insight into the role of individual lamin proteins in nuclear organization and how this relates to disease processes in humans.

  Website: http://crisp.cit.nih.gov/crisp/Crisp_Query.Generate_Screen

- **Project Title: TRANSLATIONAL RESEARCH IN THE DYSTROPHINOPATHIES**

  Principal Investigator & Institution: Flanigan, Kevin M.; Associate Professor; Neurology; University of Utah Salt Lake City, Ut 84102

Timing: Fiscal Year 2002; Project Start 20-SEP-2002; Project End 31-JUL-2005

Summary: (provided by applicant): Duchenne **Muscular Dystrophy** (DMD) and Becker **Muscular Dystrophy** (BMD) are devastating disorders. Both are associated with mutations in the dystrophin gene, a huge gene with 79 exons spread over 2.4 million bases of genomic sequence. Deletions of large portions of the gene account for around 60% of all dystrophin mutations. The remainder consist of point mutations (primarily premature stop codon mutations), small deletions resulting in shift of the reading frame, and (in less than 5%) duplications. Dystrophin gene deletion testing is commercially and readily available, but point mutation testing is not. Recent studies in the mdx mouse, a model for DMD due to a premature stop codon mutation, have demonstrated the ability of aminoglycosides to increase the expression of dystrophin protein via induction of increased read-through. Recently, we and others have demonstrated some rules for the specificity of this effect, and a growing body of data suggests that aminoglycoside therapy may prove beneficial in some patients. We have developed the methodology to rapidly, robustly, and economically perform direct sequence analysis of the entire coding and regulatory regions of the dystrophin gene, greatly expediting the characterization of mutations in non-deleted dystrophinopathy patients. Using this methodology, we propose to characterize the mutations responsible for DMD and BMD in a large cohort of patients, from whom a standardized and thorough phenotypic characterization, will be obtained. Phenotype/genotype information will be compiled in a pilot dystrophinopathy registry database. Correlation of the phenotype to the sequence context of specific individual mutations will generate hypotheses of aminoglycoside-induced read-through efficiency in specific sequence contexts, which will be tested in an in vitro dual-luciferase transfection assay. This same assay will be used to systematically study other pharmaceutical compounds, which may cause read-through of premature stop codon or frameshift mutations, and to study other potential mechanisms for modifying intrinsic frame shifting and read-through. Finally, we propose to develop a dual-GFP transgenic mouse, which will allow in vivo characterization of tissue-specific variation in aminoglycoside-induced read-through. Although we do not propose to perform an aminoglycoside treatment trial at present, this proposed study will identify a cohort of patients who may be candidates for any future trials here or at other institutions, and may provide a rationale to suggest that individual compounds or dosages may need to be tailored to specific sequence variations in all future trials.

Website: http://crisp.cit.nih.gov/crisp/Crisp_Query.Generate_Screen

- **Project Title: WASHINGTON D.C. COLLABORATIVE PPRU**

Principal Investigator & Institution: Van Den Anker, John N.; Children's National Medical Center Washington, D.C., Dc 20010

Timing: Fiscal Year 2004; Project Start 25-APR-2004; Project End 31-DEC-2008

Summary: (provided by applicant): The Children's National Medical Center (CNMC) proposes to develop a Washington D.C. Pediatric Pharmacology Research Unit (W-PPRU) in collaboration with the Departments of Pediatrics of Georgetown University Medical Center and Howard University Hospital. The District of Columbia is a multiethnic, multiracial, and multicultural community with a broad socioeconomic base, ideally suited to perform clinical and translational pediatric research. This W-PPRU collaboration will bring complementary strengths and interests from the 3 institutions (i.e., broad patient base, minority recruitment of both subjects and trainees, translational and basic science programs). The PPRU will be housed within the NCRR funded Pediatric Clinical Research Center at CNMC in 3,000 sq. ft. of clinical space; it will have facilities for inpatient and outpatient studies. Although not currently a PPRU, CNMC has participated in 124 clinical trials that have enrolled 1494 children over the past 4 years. This has involved over 50 pediatric faculty in 12 subspecialties. The Principal Investigator, John van den Anker, M.D., Ph.D. is a neonatologistlclinical pharmacologist with prior experience as PI of a PPRU. The Unit will include a core laboratory that provides both mass spectrometry and molecular genetics resources and strong research pharmacy support. Additionally, there is a strong Data Management unit. The training mission will involve didactic courses, practicum experiences, and career development opportunities for a broad range of health care professionals. Proposed drug evaluation studies include pharmacokinetic/pharmacodynamic models for optimizing the treatment of neonatal pain (morphine), and the use of off-patent drugs (dopamine and dobutamine). Additional pharmacological studies will bring to the PPRLI Network new drugs used in Orphan Diseases (Duchenne **Muscular Dystrophy** and Urea Cycle Disorders) for which CNMC is an international Center.

Website: http://crisp.cit.nih.gov/crisp/Crisp_Query.Generate_Screen

E-Journals: PubMed Central[16]

PubMed Central (PMC) is a digital archive of life sciences journal literature developed and managed by the National Center for Biotechnology Information (NCBI) at the U.S. National Library of Medicine (NLM).[17] Access to this growing archive of e-journals is free and unrestricted.[18] To search, go to **http://www.ncbi.nlm.nih.gov/entrez/query.fcgi?db=Pmc**, and type "muscular dystrophy" (or synonyms) into the search box. This search gives you access to full-text articles. The following is a sample of items found for muscular dystrophy in the PubMed Central database:

- **A 230kb cosmid walk in the Duchenne muscular dystrophy gene: detection of a conserved sequence and of a possible deletion prone region..** by Heilig R, Lemaire C, Mandel JL.; 1987 Nov 25;

  http://www.pubmedcentral.gov/picrender.fcgi?tool=pmcentrez&action =stream&blobtype=pdf&artid=306457

- **A 71-kilodalton protein is a major product of the Duchenne muscular dystrophy gene in brain and other nonmuscle tissues..** by Lederfein D, Levy Z, Augier N, Mornet D, Morris G, Fuchs O, Yaffe D, Nudel U.; 1992 Jun 15;

  http://www.pubmedcentral.gov/picrender.fcgi?tool=pmcentrez&action =stream&blobtype=pdf&artid=49288

- **Abnormal expression of laminin suggests disturbance of sarcolemma-extracellular matrix interaction in Japanese patients with autosomal recessive muscular dystrophy deficient in adhalin..** by Higuchi I, Yamada H, Fukunaga H, Iwaki H, Okubo R, Nakagawa M, Osame M, Roberds SL, Shimizu T, Campbell KP, et al.; 1994 Aug;

  http://www.pubmedcentral.gov/picrender.fcgi?tool=pmcentrez&action =stream&blobtype=pdf&artid=296136

- **Adeno-associated virus vector carrying human minidystrophin genes effectively ameliorates muscular dystrophy in mdx mouse model.** by Wang B, Li J, Xiao X.; 2000 Dec 5;

  http://www.pubmedcentral.gov/articlerender.fcgi?tool=pmcentrez&arti d=17641

---

[16] Adapted from the National Library of Medicine:
http://www.pubmedcentral.nih.gov/about/intro.html.

[17] With PubMed Central, NCBI is taking the lead in preservation and maintenance of open access to electronic literature, just as NLM has done for decades with printed biomedical literature. PubMed Central aims to become a world-class library of the digital age.

[18] The value of PubMed Central, in addition to its role as an archive, lies the availability of data from diverse sources stored in a common format in a single repository. Many journals already have online publishing operations, and there is a growing tendency to publish material online only, to the exclusion of print.

- **Adhalin gene mutations in patients with autosomal recessive childhood onset muscular dystrophy with adhalin deficiency..** by Kawai H, Akaike M, Endo T, Adachi K, Inui T, Mitsui T, Kashiwagi S, Fujiwara T, Okuno S, Shin S, et al.; 1995 Sep; http://www.pubmedcentral.gov/picrender.fcgi?tool=pmcentrez&action=stream&blobtype=pdf&artid=185739

- **Complementary DNA probes for the Duchenne muscular dystrophy locus demonstrate a previously undetectable deletion in a patient with dystrophic myopathy, glycerol kinase deficiency, and congenital adrenal hypoplasia..** by McCabe ER, Towbin J, Chamberlain J, Baumbach L, Witkowski J, van Ommen GJ, Koenig M, Kunkel LM, Seltzer WK.; 1989 Jan; http://www.pubmedcentral.gov/picrender.fcgi?tool=pmcentrez&action=stream&blobtype=pdf&artid=303648

- **Congenital nutritional muscular dystrophy in a beef calf.** by Abutarbush SM, Radostits OM.; 2003 Sep; http://www.pubmedcentral.gov/articlerender.fcgi?tool=pmcentrez&artid=340271

- **Cultured muscle from myotonic muscular dystrophy patients: altered membrane electrical properties..** by Merickel M, Gray R, Chauvin P, Appel S.; 1981 Jan; http://www.pubmedcentral.gov/picrender.fcgi?tool=pmcentrez&action=stream&blobtype=pdf&artid=319112

- **Deficiency of dystrophin-associated proteins in Duchenne muscular dystrophy patients lacking COOH-terminal domains of dystrophin..** by Matsumura K, Tome FM, Ionasescu V, Ervasti JM, Anderson RD, Romero NB, Simon D, Recan D, Kaplan JC, Fardeau M, et al.; 1993 Aug; http://www.pubmedcentral.gov/picrender.fcgi?tool=pmcentrez&action=stream&blobtype=pdf&artid=294925

- **Deletion screening of the Duchenne muscular dystrophy locus via multiplex DNA amplification..** by Chamberlain JS, Gibbs RA, Ranier JE, Nguyen PN, Caskey CT.; 1988 Dec 9; http://www.pubmedcentral.gov/picrender.fcgi?tool=pmcentrez&action=stream&blobtype=pdf&artid=339001

- **Differential degradation of [35S]methionine polypeptides in Duchenne muscular dystrophy skin fibroblasts in vitro..** by Rodemann HP, Bayreuther K.; 1986 Apr; http://www.pubmedcentral.gov/picrender.fcgi?tool=pmcentrez&action=stream&blobtype=pdf&artid=323235

- **Direct PCR from CVS and blood lysates for detection of cystic fibrosis and Duchenne muscular dystrophy deletions..** by Balnaves ME, Nasioulas S, Dahl HH, Forrest S.; 1991 Mar 11;
  http://www.pubmedcentral.gov/picrender.fcgi?tool=pmcentrez&action=stream&blobtype=pdf&artid=333801

- **DNA amplification of a further exon of Duchenne muscular dystrophy locus increase possibilities for deletion screening.** by Speer A, Rosenthal A, Billwitz H, Hanke R, Forrest SM, Love D, Davies KE, Coutelle C.; 1989 Jun 26;
  http://www.pubmedcentral.gov/picrender.fcgi?tool=pmcentrez&action=stream&blobtype=pdf&artid=318056

- **Duchenne and Becker muscular dystrophy mutations: analysis using 2.6 kb of muscle cDNA from the 5' end of the gene..** by Smith TJ, Forrest SM, Cross GS, Davies KE.; 1987 Dec 10;
  http://www.pubmedcentral.gov/picrender.fcgi?tool=pmcentrez&action=stream&blobtype=pdf&artid=306529

- **Duchenne muscular dystrophy (DMD) gene cDNA 8 PstI and TaqI polymorphisms involve exon 51 of the HindIII map..** by Laing NG, Akkari PA, Chandler DC, Thomas HE, Layton MG, Mears ME, Kakulas BA.; 1990 Jul 25;
  http://www.pubmedcentral.gov/picrender.fcgi?tool=pmcentrez&action=stream&blobtype=pdf&artid=331223

- **Erythrocyte membrane abnormalities in Duchenne muscular dystrophy monitored by saturation transfer electron paramagnetic resonance spectroscopy..** by Wilkerson LS, Perkins RC Jr, Roelofs R, Swift L, Dalton LR, Park JH.; 1978 Feb;
  http://www.pubmedcentral.gov/picrender.fcgi?tool=pmcentrez&action=stream&blobtype=pdf&artid=411352

- **Exon skipping during splicing of dystrophin mRNA precursor due to an intraexon deletion in the dystrophin gene of Duchenne muscular dystrophy kobe..** by Matsuo M, Masumura T, Nishio H, Nakajima T, Kitoh Y, Takumi T, Koga J, Nakamura H.; 1991 Jun;
  http://www.pubmedcentral.gov/picrender.fcgi?tool=pmcentrez&action=stream&blobtype=pdf&artid=296970

- **Expression and localization of nuclear proteins in autosomal-dominant Emery-Dreifuss muscular dystrophy with LMNA R377H mutation.** by Reichart B, Klafke R, Dreger C, Kruger E, Motsch I, Ewald A, Schafer J, Reichmann H, Muller CR, Dabauvalle MC.; 2004;
  http://www.pubmedcentral.gov/articlerender.fcgi?tool=pmcentrez&artid=407848

- **Expression of a Mutant Lamin A That Causes Emery-Dreifuss Muscular Dystrophy Inhibits In Vitro Differentiation of C2C12 Myoblasts.** by Favreau C, Higuet D, Courvalin JC, Buendia B.; 2004 Feb 15; http://www.pubmedcentral.gov/articlerender.fcgi?tool=pmcentrez&arti d=344177

- **Gene expression comparison of biopsies from Duchenne muscular dystrophy (DMD) and normal skeletal muscle.** by Haslett JN, Sanoudou D, Kho AT, Bennett RR, Greenberg SA, Kohane IS, Beggs AH, Kunkel LM.; 2002 Nov 12; http://www.pubmedcentral.gov/articlerender.fcgi?tool=pmcentrez&arti d=137534

- **Immunohistochemical analysis of dystrophin-associated proteins in Becker/Duchenne muscular dystrophy with huge in-frame deletions in the NH2-terminal and rod domains of dystrophin..** by Matsumura K, Burghes AH, Mora M, Tome FM, Morandi L, Cornello F, Leturcq F, Jeanpierre M, Kaplan JC, Reinert P, et al.; 1994 Jan; http://www.pubmedcentral.gov/picrender.fcgi?tool=pmcentrez&action =stream&blobtype=pdf&artid=293741

- **Immunological identification of a high molecular weight protein as a candidate for the product of the Duchenne muscular dystrophy gene..** by Kao L, Krstenansky J, Mendell J, Rammohan KW, Gruenstein E.; 1988 Jun; http://www.pubmedcentral.gov/picrender.fcgi?tool=pmcentrez&action =stream&blobtype=pdf&artid=280456

- **Increased membrane permeability to chloride in Duchenne muscular dystrophy fibroblasts and its relationship to muscle function..** by Pato CN, Davis MH, Doughty MJ, Bryant SH, Gruenstein E.; 1983 Aug; http://www.pubmedcentral.gov/picrender.fcgi?tool=pmcentrez&action =stream&blobtype=pdf&artid=384118

- **Isolation of a conserved sequence deleted in Duchenne muscular dystrophy patients..** by Smith TJ, Wilson L, Kenwrick SJ, Forrest SM, Speer A, Coutelle C, Davies KE.; 1987 Mar 11; http://www.pubmedcentral.gov/picrender.fcgi?tool=pmcentrez&action =stream&blobtype=pdf&artid=340624

- **Linkage analysis of two cloned DNA sequences flanking the Duchenne muscular dystrophy locus on the short arm of the human X chromosome..** by Davies KE, Pearson PL, Harper PS, Murray JM, O'Brien T, Sarfarazi M, Williamson R.; 1983 Apr 25; http://www.pubmedcentral.gov/picrender.fcgi?tool=pmcentrez&action =stream&blobtype=pdf&artid=325885

- **Long-term persistence of donor nuclei in a Duchenne muscular dystrophy patient receiving bone marrow transplantation.** by Gussoni E, Bennett RR, Muskiewicz KR, Meyerrose T, Nolta JA, Gilgoff I, Stein J, Chan YM, Lidov HG, Bonnemann CG, von Moers A, Morris GE, den Dunnen JT, Chamberlain JS, Kunkel LM, Weinberg K.; 2002 Sep 15; http://www.pubmedcentral.gov/articlerender.fcgi?tool=pmcentrez&arti d=151133

- **Modulation of Myoblast Fusion by Caveolin-3 in Dystrophic Skeletal Muscle Cells: Implications for Duchenne Muscular Dystrophy and Limb-Girdle Muscular Dystrophy-1C.** by Volonte D, Peoples AJ, Galbiati F.; 2003 Oct; http://www.pubmedcentral.gov/articlerender.fcgi?tool=pmcentrez&arti d=207001

- **Molecular and functional analysis of the muscle-specific promoter region of the Duchenne muscular dystrophy gene..** by Klamut HJ, Gangopadhyay SB, Worton RG, Ray PN.; 1990 Jan; http://www.pubmedcentral.gov/picrender.fcgi?tool=pmcentrez&action =stream&blobtype=pdf&artid=360727

- **MspI RFLP for Duchenne muscular dystrophy cDNA subclone 9..** by Wagner M, Reiss J, Hentemann M, Thies U.; 1989 Apr 25; http://www.pubmedcentral.gov/picrender.fcgi?tool=pmcentrez&action =stream&blobtype=pdf&artid=317767

- **Overexpression of the cytotoxic T cell GalNAc transferase in skeletal muscle inhibits muscular dystrophy in mdx mice.** by Nguyen HH, Jayasinha V, Xia B, Hoyte K, Martin PT.; 2002 Apr 16; http://www.pubmedcentral.gov/articlerender.fcgi?tool=pmcentrez&arti d=122819

- **Rapid mapping by transposon mutagenesis of epitopes on the muscular dystrophy protein, dystrophin.** by Sedgwick SG, Nguyen TM, Ellis JM, Crowne H, Morris GE.; 1991 Nov 11; http://www.pubmedcentral.gov/picrender.fcgi?tool=pmcentrez&action =stream&blobtype=pdf&artid=329043

- **Recovery of induced mutations for X chromosome-linked muscular dystrophy in mice.** by Chapman VM, Miller DR, Armstrong D, Caskey CT.; 1989 Feb; http://www.pubmedcentral.gov/picrender.fcgi?tool=pmcentrez&action =stream&blobtype=pdf&artid=286674

- **RFLP for Duchenne muscular dystrophy cDNA clone 30-2.** by Walker AP, Bartlett RJ, Laing NG, Siddique T, Yamaoka LH, Chen JC, Hung WY, Roses AD.; 1988 Sep 26;
  http://www.pubmedcentral.gov/picrender.fcgi?tool=pmcentrez&action=stream&blobtype=pdf&artid=338682

- **RFLP for Duchenne muscular dystrophy cDNA clone 44-1.** by Laing NG, Siddique T, Bartlett RJ, Yamaoka LH, Chen JC, Walker AP, Hung WY, Roses AD.; 1988 Jul 25;
  http://www.pubmedcentral.gov/picrender.fcgi?tool=pmcentrez&action=stream&blobtype=pdf&artid=338389

- **RFLP for HindIII at the Duchenne muscular dystrophy gene.** by Prior TW, Friedman KJ, Silverman LM.; 1989 Mar 25;
  http://www.pubmedcentral.gov/picrender.fcgi?tool=pmcentrez&action=stream&blobtype=pdf&artid=317618

- **Sodium Channel and Sodium Pump in Normal and Pathological Muscles from Patients with Myotonic Muscular Dystrophy and Lower Motor Neuron Impairment.** by Desnuelle C, Lombet A, Serratrice G, Lazdunski M.; 1982 Feb;
  http://www.pubmedcentral.gov/picrender.fcgi?tool=pmcentrez&action=stream&blobtype=pdf&artid=370985

- **Successful treatment of murine muscular dystrophy with the proteinase inhibitor leupeptin..** by Sher JH, Stracher A, Shafiq SA, Hardy-Stashin J.; 1981 Dec;
  http://www.pubmedcentral.gov/picrender.fcgi?tool=pmcentrez&action=stream&blobtype=pdf&artid=349346

- **Transgenic overexpression of caveolin-3 in skeletal muscle fibers induces a Duchenne-like muscular dystrophy phenotype.** by Galbiati F, Volonte D, Chu JB, Li M, Fine SW, Fu M, Bermudez J, Pedemonte M, Weidenheim KM, Pestell RG, Minetti C, Lisanti MP.; 2000 Aug 15;
  http://www.pubmedcentral.gov/articlerender.fcgi?tool=pmcentrez&artid=16926

- **Two human cDNA molecules coding for the Duchenne muscular dystrophy (DMD) locus are highly homologous.** by Rosenthal A, Speer A, Billwitz H, Cross GS, Forrest SM, Davies KE.; 1989 Jul 11;
  http://www.pubmedcentral.gov/picrender.fcgi?tool=pmcentrez&action=stream&blobtype=pdf&artid=318130

- **Ullrich scleroatonic muscular dystrophy is caused by recessive mutations in collagen type VI.** by Camacho Vanegas O, Bertini E, Zhang RZ, Petrini S, Minosse C, Sabatelli P, Giusti B, Chu ML, Pepe G.; 2001 Jun 19;
  http://www.pubmedcentral.gov/articlerender.fcgi?tool=pmcentrez&artid=34700

- **X chromosome-linked muscular dystrophy (mdx) in the mouse..** by Bulfield G, Siller WG, Wight PA, Moore KJ.; 1984 Feb;
  http://www.pubmedcentral.gov/picrender.fcgi?tool=pmcentrez&action=stream&blobtype=pdf&artid=344791

The National Library of Medicine: PubMed

One of the quickest and most comprehensive ways to find academic studies in both English and other languages is to use PubMed, maintained by the National Library of Medicine. The advantage of PubMed over previously mentioned sources is that it covers a greater number of domestic and foreign references. It is also free to the public.[19] If the publisher has a Web site that offers full text of its journals, PubMed will provide links to that site, as well as to sites offering other related data. User registration, a subscription fee, or some other type of fee may be required to access the full text of articles in some journals.

To generate your own bibliography of studies dealing with muscular dystrophy, simply go to the PubMed Web site at **www.ncbi.nlm.nih.gov/pubmed**. Type "muscular dystrophy" (or synonyms) into the search box, and click "Go." The following is the type of output you can expect from PubMed for "muscular dystrophy" (hyperlinks lead to article summaries):

---

[19] PubMed was developed by the National Center for Biotechnology Information (NCBI) at the National Library of Medicine (NLM) at the National Institutes of Health (NIH). The PubMed database was developed in conjunction with publishers of biomedical literature as a search tool for accessing literature citations and linking to full-text journal articles at Web sites of participating publishers. Publishers that participate in PubMed supply NLM with their citations electronically prior to or at the time of publication.

- **A case of Bartter's syndrome, gout and Becker's muscular dystrophy.**
  Author(s): Fishel B, Zhukovsky G, Legum C, Jossiphov J, Alon M, Peer G, Iaina A, Nevo Y.
  Source: Clin Exp Rheumatol. 2000 May-June; 18(3): 426-7. No Abstract Available.
  http://www.ncbi.nlm.nih.gov/entrez/query.fcgi?cmd=Retrieve&db=pubmed&dopt=Abstract&list_uids=10895394

- **A first missense mutation in the delta sarcoglycan gene associated with a severe phenotype and frequency of limb-girdle muscular dystrophy type 2F (LGMD2F) in Brazilian sarcoglycanopathies.**
  Author(s): Moreira ES, Vainzof M, Marie SK, Nigro V, Zatz M, Passos-Bueno MR.
  Source: Journal of Medical Genetics. 1998 November; 35(11): 951-3.
  http://www.ncbi.nlm.nih.gov/entrez/query.fcgi?cmd=Retrieve&db=pubmed&dopt=Abstract&list_uids=9832045

- **A gene related to Caenorhabditis elegans spermatogenesis factor fer-1 is mutated in limb-girdle muscular dystrophy type 2B.**
  Author(s): Bashir R, Britton S, Strachan T, Keers S, Vafiadaki E, Lako M, Richard I, Marchand S, Bourg N, Argov Z, Sadeh M, Mahjneh I, Marconi G, Passos-Bueno MR, Moreira Ede S, Zatz M, Beckmann JS, Bushby K.
  Source: Nature Genetics. 1998 September; 20(1): 37-42.
  http://www.ncbi.nlm.nih.gov/entrez/query.fcgi?cmd=Retrieve&db=pubmed&dopt=Abstract&list_uids=9731527

- **A mitochondrial DNA mutation in a patient with an extensive family history of Duchenne muscular dystrophy.**
  Author(s): Wong LJ, Wladyka C, Mardach-Verdon R.
  Source: Muscle & Nerve. 2004 July; 30(1): 118-22.
  http://www.ncbi.nlm.nih.gov/entrez/query.fcgi?cmd=Retrieve&db=pubmed&dopt=Abstract&list_uids=15221888

- **A multicenter, double-blind, randomized trial of deflazacort versus prednisone in Duchenne muscular dystrophy.**
  Author(s): Bonifati MD, Ruzza G, Bonometto P, Berardinelli A, Gorni K, Orcesi S, Lanzi G, Angelini C.
  Source: Muscle & Nerve. 2000 September; 23(9): 1344-7.
  http://www.ncbi.nlm.nih.gov/entrez/query.fcgi?cmd=Retrieve&db=pubmed&dopt=Abstract&list_uids=10951436

- **A new mutation of the lamin A/C gene leading to autosomal dominant axonal neuropathy, muscular dystrophy, cardiac disease, and leuconychia.**
  Author(s): Goizet C, Yaou RB, Demay L, Richard P, Bouillot S, Rouanet M, Hermosilla E, Le Masson G, Lagueny A, Bonne G, Ferrer X.
  Source: Journal of Medical Genetics. 2004 March; 41(3): E29.
  http://www.ncbi.nlm.nih.gov/entrez/query.fcgi?cmd=Retrieve&db=pubmed&dopt=Abstract&list_uids=14985400

- **A novel form of recessive limb girdle muscular dystrophy with mental retardation and abnormal expression of alpha-dystroglycan.**
  Author(s): Dincer P, Balci B, Yuva Y, Talim B, Brockington M, Dincel D, Torelli S, Brown S, Kale G, Haliloglu G, Gerceker FO, Atalay RC, Yakicier C, Longman C, Muntoni F, Topaloglu H.
  Source: Neuromuscular Disorders: Nmd. 2003 December; 13(10): 771-8.
  http://www.ncbi.nlm.nih.gov/entrez/query.fcgi?cmd=Retrieve&db=pubmed&dopt=Abstract&list_uids=14678799

- **A synonymous codon change in the LMNA gene alters mRNA splicing and causes limb girdle muscular dystrophy type 1B.**
  Author(s): Todorova A, Halliger-Keller B, Walter MC, Dabauvalle MC, Lochmuller H, Muller CR.
  Source: Journal of Medical Genetics. 2003 October; 40(10): E115.
  http://www.ncbi.nlm.nih.gov/entrez/query.fcgi?cmd=Retrieve&db=pubmed&dopt=Abstract&list_uids=14569138

- **Acute heart failure during spinal surgery in a boy with Duchenne muscular dystrophy.**
  Author(s): Hayes JA, Ames WA.
  Source: British Journal of Anaesthesia. 2004 January; 92(1): 149; Author Reply 149-50.
  http://www.ncbi.nlm.nih.gov/entrez/query.fcgi?cmd=Retrieve&db=pubmed&dopt=Abstract&list_uids=14714277

- **Acute heart failure during spinal surgery in a boy with Duchenne muscular dystrophy.**
  Author(s): Schummer W, Schummer C.
  Source: British Journal of Anaesthesia. 2004 January; 92(1): 149; Author Reply 149-50.
  http://www.ncbi.nlm.nih.gov/entrez/query.fcgi?cmd=Retrieve&db=pubmed&dopt=Abstract&list_uids=14665570

- **Alterations of the retino-cortical conduction in patients affected by classical congenital muscular dystrophy (CI-CMD) with merosin deficiency.**
  Author(s): Tormene AP, Trevisan C, Martinello F, Riva C, Pastorello E.
  Source: Documenta Ophthalmologica. Advances in Ophthalmology. 1999; 98(2): 127-38.
  http://www.ncbi.nlm.nih.gov/entrez/query.fcgi?cmd=Retrieve&db=pubmed&dopt=Abstract&list_uids=10946999

- **An attempt of gene therapy in Duchenne muscular dystrophy: overexpression of utrophin in transgenic mdx mice.**
  Author(s): Gillis JM.
  Source: Acta Neurol Belg. 2000 September; 100(3): 146-50. Review.
  http://www.ncbi.nlm.nih.gov/entrez/query.fcgi?cmd=Retrieve&db=pubmed&dopt=Abstract&list_uids=11098286

- **An autosomal dominant early adult-onset distal muscular dystrophy.**
  Author(s): Zimprich F, Djamshidian A, Hainfellner JA, Budka H, Zeitlhofer J.
  Source: Muscle & Nerve. 2000 December; 23(12): 1876-9.
  http://www.ncbi.nlm.nih.gov/entrez/query.fcgi?cmd=Retrieve&db=pubmed&dopt=Abstract&list_uids=11102913

- **Analyses of beta-1 syntrophin, syndecan 2 and gem GTPase as candidates for chicken muscular dystrophy.**
  Author(s): Yoshizawa K, Inaba K, Mannen H, Kikuchi T, Mizutani M, Tsuji S.
  Source: Experimental Animals / Japanese Association for Laboratory Animal Science. 2003 October; 52(5): 391-6.
  http://www.ncbi.nlm.nih.gov/entrez/query.fcgi?cmd=Retrieve&db=pubmed&dopt=Abstract&list_uids=14625404

- **Androgen response to hypothalamic-pituitary-adrenal stimulation with naloxone in women with myotonic muscular dystrophy.**
  Author(s): Buyalos RP, Jackson RV, Grice GI, Hockings GI, Torpy DJ, Fox LM, Boots LR, Azziz R.
  Source: The Journal of Clinical Endocrinology and Metabolism. 1998 September; 83(9): 3219-24.
  http://www.ncbi.nlm.nih.gov/entrez/query.fcgi?cmd=Retrieve&db=pubmed&dopt=Abstract&list_uids=9745431

- **Antisense-induced multiexon skipping for Duchenne muscular dystrophy makes more sense.**
  Author(s): Aartsma-Rus A, Janson AA, Kaman WE, Bremmer-Bout M, van Ommen GJ, den Dunnen JT, van Deutekom JC.
  Source: American Journal of Human Genetics. 2004 January; 74(1): 83-92. Epub 2003 December 16.
  http://www.ncbi.nlm.nih.gov/entrez/query.fcgi?cmd=Retrieve&db=pubmed&dopt=Abstract&list_uids=14681829

- **Are Dp71 and Dp140 brain dystrophin isoforms related to cognitive impairment in Duchenne muscular dystrophy?**
  Author(s): Moizard MP, Billard C, Toutain A, Berret F, Marmin N, Moraine C.
  Source: American Journal of Medical Genetics. 1998 October 30; 80(1): 32-41.
  http://www.ncbi.nlm.nih.gov/entrez/query.fcgi?cmd=Retrieve&db=pubmed&dopt=Abstract&list_uids=9800909

- **Assembly of the sarcoglycan complex. Insights for muscular dystrophy.**
  Author(s): Holt KH, Campbell KP.
  Source: The Journal of Biological Chemistry. 1998 December 25; 273(52): 34667-70.
  http://www.ncbi.nlm.nih.gov/entrez/query.fcgi?cmd=Retrieve&db=pubmed&dopt=Abstract&list_uids=9856984

- **Asymptomatic carriers and gender differences in facioscapulohumeral muscular dystrophy (FSHD).**
  Author(s): Tonini MM, Passos-Bueno MR, Cerqueira A, Matioli SR, Pavanello R, Zatz M.
  Source: Neuromuscular Disorders: Nmd. 2004 January; 14(1): 33-8.
  http://www.ncbi.nlm.nih.gov/entrez/query.fcgi?cmd=Retrieve&db=pubmed&dopt=Abstract&list_uids=14659410

- **Atypical phenotypes in patients with facioscapulohumeral muscular dystrophy 4q35 deletion.**
  Author(s): Krasnianski M, Eger K, Neudecker S, Jakubiczka S, Zierz S.
  Source: Archives of Neurology. 2003 October; 60(10): 1421-5.
  http://www.ncbi.nlm.nih.gov/entrez/query.fcgi?cmd=Retrieve&db=pubmed&dopt=Abstract&list_uids=14568813

- **Becker muscular dystrophy associated with focal myositis on bone scintigraphy.**
  Author(s): Minshew PT, Silverman ED, Samuels-Botts C.
  Source: Clinical Nuclear Medicine. 2000 December; 25(12): 1010-2.
  http://www.ncbi.nlm.nih.gov/entrez/query.fcgi?cmd=Retrieve&db=pubmed&dopt=Abstract&list_uids=11129135

- **Becker muscular dystrophy combined with X-linked Charcot-Marie-Tooth neuropathy.**
  Author(s): Bergmann C, Senderek J, Hermanns B, Jauch A, Janssen B, Schroder JM, Karch D.
  Source: Muscle & Nerve. 2000 May; 23(5): 818-23.
  http://www.ncbi.nlm.nih.gov/entrez/query.fcgi?cmd=Retrieve&db=pubmed&dopt=Abstract&list_uids=10797409

- **Becker muscular dystrophy in a patient with Hodgkin's disease.**
  Author(s): Cereda S, Cefalo G, Terenziani M, Catania S, Fossati-Bellani F.
  Source: Journal of Pediatric Hematology/Oncology: Official Journal of the American Society of Pediatric Hematology/Oncology. 2004 January; 26(1): 72-3.
  http://www.ncbi.nlm.nih.gov/entrez/query.fcgi?cmd=Retrieve&db=pubmed&dopt=Abstract&list_uids=14707720

- **Becker muscular dystrophy-related cardiomyopathy: a favorable response to medical therapy.**
  Author(s): Doing AH, Renlund DG, Smith RA.
  Source: The Journal of Heart and Lung Transplantation: the Official Publication of the International Society for Heart Transplantation. 2002 April; 21(4): 496-8.
  http://www.ncbi.nlm.nih.gov/entrez/query.fcgi?cmd=Retrieve&db=pubmed&dopt=Abstract&list_uids=11927228

- **Bethlem myopathy (BETHLEM) and Ullrich scleroatonic muscular dystrophy: 100th ENMC international workshop, 23-24 November 2001, Naarden, The Netherlands.**
  Author(s): Pepe G, Bertini E, Bonaldo P, Bushby K, Giusti B, de Visser M, Guicheney P, Lattanzi G, Merlini L, Muntoni F, Nishino I, Nonaka I, Yaou RB, Sabatelli P, Sewry C, Topaloglu H, van der Kooi A.
  Source: Neuromuscular Disorders: Nmd. 2002 December; 12(10): 984-93.
  http://www.ncbi.nlm.nih.gov/entrez/query.fcgi?cmd=Retrieve&db=pubmed&dopt=Abstract&list_uids=12467756

- **Bethlem myopathy: a slowly progressive congenital muscular dystrophy with contractures.**
  Author(s): Jobsis GJ, Boers JM, Barth PG, de Visser M.
  Source: Brain; a Journal of Neurology. 1999 April; 122 (Pt 4): 649-55.
  http://www.ncbi.nlm.nih.gov/entrez/query.fcgi?cmd=Retrieve&db=pubmed&dopt=Abstract&list_uids=10219778

- **Biochemical characterization of muscle tissue of limb girdle muscular dystrophy: an 1H and 13C NMR study.**
  Author(s): Sharma U, Atri S, Sharma MC, Sarkar C, Jagannathan NR.
  Source: Nmr in Biomedicine. 2003 June; 16(4): 213-23.
  http://www.ncbi.nlm.nih.gov/entrez/query.fcgi?cmd=Retrieve&db=pubmed&dopt=Abstract&list_uids=14558119

- **Bladder dysfunction in Duchenne muscular dystrophy.**
  Author(s): MacLeod M, Kelly R, Robb SA, Borzyskowski M.
  Source: Archives of Disease in Childhood. 2003 April; 88(4): 347-9.
  http://www.ncbi.nlm.nih.gov/entrez/query.fcgi?cmd=Retrieve&db=pubmed&dopt=Abstract&list_uids=12651768

- **Blood loss in Duchenne muscular dystrophy: vascular smooth muscle dysfunction?**
  Author(s): Noordeen MH, Haddad FS, Muntoni F, Gobbi P, Hollyer JS, Bentley G.
  Source: Journal of Pediatric Orthopaedics. Part B / European Paediatric Orthopaedic Society, Pediatric Orthopaedic Society of North America. 1999 July; 8(3): 212-5.
  http://www.ncbi.nlm.nih.gov/entrez/query.fcgi?cmd=Retrieve&db=pubmed&dopt=Abstract&list_uids=10399127

- **Body composition and energy expenditure in Duchenne muscular dystrophy.**
  Author(s): Zanardi MC, Tagliabue A, Orcesi S, Berardinelli A, Uggetti C, Pichiecchio A.
  Source: European Journal of Clinical Nutrition. 2003 February; 57(2): 273-8.
  http://www.ncbi.nlm.nih.gov/entrez/query.fcgi?cmd=Retrieve&db=pubmed&dopt=Abstract&list_uids=12571659

- **Bone mineral density and bone metabolism in Duchenne muscular dystrophy.**
  Author(s): Bianchi ML, Mazzanti A, Galbiati E, Saraifoger S, Dubini A, Cornelio F, Morandi L.
  Source: Osteoporosis International: a Journal Established As Result of Cooperation between the European Foundation for Osteoporosis and the National Osteoporosis Foundation of the Usa. 2003 September; 14(9): 761-7. Epub 2003 July 29.
  http://www.ncbi.nlm.nih.gov/entrez/query.fcgi?cmd=Retrieve&db=pubmed&dopt=Abstract&list_uids=12897980

- **Bone mineral density and fractures in boys with Duchenne muscular dystrophy.**
  Author(s): Larson CM, Henderson RC.
  Source: Journal of Pediatric Orthopedics. 2000 January-February; 20(1): 71-4.
  http://www.ncbi.nlm.nih.gov/entrez/query.fcgi?cmd=Retrieve&db=pubmed&dopt=Abstract&list_uids=10641693

- **Botulinum toxin for amelioration of knee contracture in Duchenne muscular dystrophy.**
  Author(s): von Wendt LO, Autti-Ramo IS.
  Source: European Journal of Paediatric Neurology: Ejpn: Official Journal of the European Paediatric Neurology Society. 1999; 3(4): 175-6.
  http://www.ncbi.nlm.nih.gov/entrez/query.fcgi?cmd=Retrieve&db=pubmed&dopt=Abstract&list_uids=10476367

- **Brain biochemistry in Duchenne muscular dystrophy: a 1H magnetic resonance and neuropsychological study.**
  Author(s): Rae C, Scott RB, Thompson CH, Dixon RM, Dumughn I, Kemp GJ, Male A, Pike M, Styles P, Radda GK.
  Source: Journal of the Neurological Sciences. 1998 October 8; 160(2): 148-57.
  http://www.ncbi.nlm.nih.gov/entrez/query.fcgi?cmd=Retrieve&db=pubmed&dopt=Abstract&list_uids=9849797

- **Brain function in Duchenne muscular dystrophy.**
  Author(s): Anderson JL, Head SI, Rae C, Morley JW.
  Source: Brain; a Journal of Neurology. 2002 January; 125(Pt 1): 4-13. Review.
  http://www.ncbi.nlm.nih.gov/entrez/query.fcgi?cmd=Retrieve&db=pubmed&dopt=Abstract&list_uids=11834588

- **Brain magnetic resonance imaging abnormalities in merosin-positive congenital muscular dystrophy.**
  Author(s): Philpot J, Pennock J, Cowan F, Sewry CA, Dubowitz V, Bydder G, Muntoni F.
  Source: European Journal of Paediatric Neurology: Ejpn: Official Journal of the European Paediatric Neurology Society. 2000; 4(3): 109-14.
  http://www.ncbi.nlm.nih.gov/entrez/query.fcgi?cmd=Retrieve&db=pubmed&dopt=Abstract&list_uids=10872105

- **Brain MR in Fukuyama congenital muscular dystrophy.**
  Author(s): Aida N, Tamagawa K, Takada K, Yagishita A, Kobayashi N, Chikumaru K, Iwamoto H.
  Source: Ajnr. American Journal of Neuroradiology. 1996 April; 17(4): 605-13.
  http://www.ncbi.nlm.nih.gov/entrez/query.fcgi?cmd=Retrieve&db=pubmed&dopt=Abstract&list_uids=8730178

- **Breached cerebral glia limitans-basal lamina complex in Fukuyama-type congenital muscular dystrophy.**
  Author(s): Saito Y, Murayama S, Kawai M, Nakano I.
  Source: Acta Neuropathologica. 1999 October; 98(4): 330-6.
  http://www.ncbi.nlm.nih.gov/entrez/query.fcgi?cmd=Retrieve&db=pubmed&dopt=Abstract&list_uids=10502035

- **Broader clinical spectrum of Fukuyama-type congenital muscular dystrophy manifested by haplotype analysis.**
  Author(s): Yoshioka M, Toda T, Kuroki S, Hamano K.
  Source: Journal of Child Neurology. 1999 November; 14(11): 711-5. Review.
  http://www.ncbi.nlm.nih.gov/entrez/query.fcgi?cmd=Retrieve&db=pubmed&dopt=Abstract&list_uids=10593547

- **Building the French Muscular Dystrophy Association: the role of doctor/patient interactions.**
  Author(s): Bach MA.
  Source: Social History of Medicine: the Journal of the Society for the Social History of Medicine / Sshm. 1998 August; 11(2): 233-53.
  http://www.ncbi.nlm.nih.gov/entrez/query.fcgi?cmd=Retrieve&db=pubmed&dopt=Abstract&list_uids=11620429

- **Cardiac features of Emery-Dreifuss muscular dystrophy caused by lamin A/C gene mutations.**
  Author(s): Sanna T, Dello Russo A, Toniolo D, Vytopil M, Pelargonio G, De Martino G, Ricci E, Silvestri G, Giglio V, Messano L, Zachara E, Bellocci F.
  Source: European Heart Journal. 2003 December; 24(24): 2227-36.
  http://www.ncbi.nlm.nih.gov/entrez/query.fcgi?cmd=Retrieve&db=pubmed&dopt=Abstract&list_uids=14659775

- **Cardiac involvement in genetically confirmed facioscapulohumeral muscular dystrophy.**
  Author(s): Laforet P, de Toma C, Eymard B, Becane HM, Jeanpierre M, Fardeau M, Duboc D.
  Source: Neurology. 1998 November; 51(5): 1454-6.
  http://www.ncbi.nlm.nih.gov/entrez/query.fcgi?cmd=Retrieve&db=pubmed&dopt=Abstract&list_uids=9818880

- **Carrier detection in Duchenne and Becker muscular dystrophy Argentine families.**
  Author(s): Baranzini SE, Giliberto F, Dalamon V, Barreiro C, Garcia-Erro M, Grippo J, Szijan I.
  Source: Clinical Genetics. 1998 December; 54(6): 503-11.
  http://www.ncbi.nlm.nih.gov/entrez/query.fcgi?cmd=Retrieve&db=pubmed&dopt=Abstract&list_uids=9894797

- **Carrier detection of Duchenne/Becker muscular dystrophy by using fluorescent linkage analysis in Taiwan.**
  Author(s): Lee CC, Wu MC, Wu JY, Li TC, Tsai FJ, Tsai CH.
  Source: Acta Paediatr Taiwan. 2000 March-April; 41(2): 69-74.
  http://www.ncbi.nlm.nih.gov/entrez/query.fcgi?cmd=Retrieve&db=pubmed&dopt=Abstract&list_uids=10927942

- **Changes in motor cortex excitability in facioscapulohumeral muscular dystrophy.**
  Author(s): Di Lazzaro V, Oliviero A, Tonali PA, Felicetti L, De Marco MB, Saturno E, Pilato F, Pescatori M, Dileone M, Pasqualetti P, Ricci E.
  Source: Neuromuscular Disorders: Nmd. 2004 January; 14(1): 39-45.
  http://www.ncbi.nlm.nih.gov/entrez/query.fcgi?cmd=Retrieve&db=pubmed&dopt=Abstract&list_uids=14659411

- **Characterization of monoclonal antibodies to calpain 3 and protein expression in muscle from patients with limb-girdle muscular dystrophy type 2A.**
  Author(s): Anderson LV, Davison K, Moss JA, Richard I, Fardeau M, Tome FM, Hubner C, Lasa A, Colomer J, Beckmann JS.
  Source: American Journal of Pathology. 1998 October; 153(4): 1169-79.
  http://www.ncbi.nlm.nih.gov/entrez/query.fcgi?cmd=Retrieve&db=pubmed&dopt=Abstract&list_uids=9777948

- **Clinical and histopathological heterogeneity in patients with 4q35 facioscapulohumeral muscular dystrophy (FSHD).**
  Author(s): Wood-Allum C, Brennan P, Hewitt M, Lowe J, Tyfield L, Wills A.
  Source: Neuropathology and Applied Neurobiology. 2004 April; 30(2): 188-91.
  http://www.ncbi.nlm.nih.gov/entrez/query.fcgi?cmd=Retrieve&db=pubmed&dopt=Abstract&list_uids=15043716

- **Clinical and molecular genetic spectrum of autosomal dominant Emery-Dreifuss muscular dystrophy due to mutations of the lamin A/C gene.**
  Author(s): Bonne G, Mercuri E, Muchir A, Urtizberea A, Becane HM, Recan D, Merlini L, Wehnert M, Boor R, Reuner U, Vorgerd M, Wicklein EM, Eymard B, Duboc D, Penisson-Besnier I, Cuisset JM, Ferrer X, Desguerre I, Lacombe D, Bushby K, Pollitt C, Toniolo D, Fardeau M, Schwartz K, Muntoni F.
  Source: Annals of Neurology. 2000 August; 48(2): 170-80.
  http://www.ncbi.nlm.nih.gov/entrez/query.fcgi?cmd=Retrieve&db=pubmed&dopt=Abstract&list_uids=10939567

- **Clinical, pathological, and genetic features of limb-girdle muscular dystrophy type 2A with new calpain 3 gene mutations in seven patients from three Japanese families.**
  Author(s): Kawai H, Akaike M, Kunishige M, Inui T, Adachi K, Kimura C, Kawajiri M, Nishida Y, Endo I, Kashiwagi S, Nishino H, Fujiwara T, Okuno S, Roudaut C, Richard I, Beckmann JS, Miyoshi K, Matsumoto T.
  Source: Muscle & Nerve. 1998 November; 21(11): 1493-501.
  http://www.ncbi.nlm.nih.gov/entrez/query.fcgi?cmd=Retrieve&db=pubmed&dopt=Abstract&list_uids=9771675

- **Cloning of cDNA encoding a regeneration-associated muscle protease whose expression is attenuated in cell lines derived from Duchenne muscular dystrophy patients.**
  Author(s): Nakayama Y, Nara N, Kawakita Y, Takeshima Y, Arakawa M, Katoh M, Morita S, Iwatsuki K, Tanaka K, Okamoto S, Kitamura T, Seki N, Matsuda R, Matsuo M, Saito K, Hara T.
  Source: American Journal of Pathology. 2004 May; 164(5): 1773-82.
  http://www.ncbi.nlm.nih.gov/entrez/query.fcgi?cmd=Retrieve&db=pubmed&dopt=Abstract&list_uids=15111323

- **Coexistence of X-linked recessive Emery-Dreifuss muscular dystrophy with inclusion body myositis-like morphology.**
  Author(s): Fidzianska A, Rowinska-Marcinska K, Hausmanowa-Petrusewicz I.
  Source: Acta Neuropathologica. 2004 March; 107(3): 197-203. Epub 2004 January 08.
  http://www.ncbi.nlm.nih.gov/entrez/query.fcgi?cmd=Retrieve&db=pubmed&dopt=Abstract&list_uids=14712398

- **Collagen VI status and clinical severity in Ullrich congenital muscular dystrophy: phenotype analysis of 11 families linked to the COL6 loci.**
  Author(s): Demir E, Ferreiro A, Sabatelli P, Allamand V, Makri S, Echenne B, Maraldi M, Merlini L, Topaloglu H, Guicheney P.
  Source: Neuropediatrics. 2004 April; 35(2): 103-12.
  http://www.ncbi.nlm.nih.gov/entrez/query.fcgi?cmd=Retrieve&db=pubmed&dopt=Abstract&list_uids=15127309

- **Comparison of oxygen consumption measurements in children with cerebral palsy to children with muscular dystrophy.**
  Author(s): Bowen TR, Miller F, Mackenzie W.
  Source: Journal of Pediatric Orthopedics. 1999 January-February; 19(1): 133-6.
  http://www.ncbi.nlm.nih.gov/entrez/query.fcgi?cmd=Retrieve&db=pubmed&dopt=Abstract&list_uids=9890302

- **Complete atrioventricular block in Becker muscular dystrophy.**
  Author(s): Akdemir R, Ozhan H, Gunduz H, Yazici M, Erbilen E, Uyan C, Imirzalioglu N.
  Source: N Z Med J. 2004 May 21; 117(1194): U895. No Abstract Available.
  http://www.ncbi.nlm.nih.gov/entrez/query.fcgi?cmd=Retrieve&db=pubmed&dopt=Abstract&list_uids=15156213

- **Congenital muscular dystrophy with merosin deficiency: MRI findings in five patients.**
  Author(s): Farina L, Morandi L, Milanesi I, Ciceri E, Mora M, Moroni I, Pantaleoni C, Savoiardo M.
  Source: Neuroradiology. 1998 December; 40(12): 807-11.
  http://www.ncbi.nlm.nih.gov/entrez/query.fcgi?cmd=Retrieve&db=pubmed&dopt=Abstract&list_uids=9877136

- **Congenital muscular dystrophy, white-matter abnormalities, and neuronal migration disorders: the expanding concept.**
  Author(s): Mackay MT, Kornberg AJ, Shield L, Phelan E, Kean MJ, Coleman LT, Dennett X.
  Source: Journal of Child Neurology. 1998 October; 13(10): 481-7.
  http://www.ncbi.nlm.nih.gov/entrez/query.fcgi?cmd=Retrieve&db=pubmed&dopt=Abstract&list_uids=9796753

- **Congenital muscular dystrophy--a case report.**
  Author(s): Shashikiran ND, Subba Reddy VV, Patil R.
  Source: J Indian Soc Pedod Prev Dent. 2003 June; 21(2): 49-54.
  http://www.ncbi.nlm.nih.gov/entrez/query.fcgi?cmd=Retrieve&db=pubmed&dopt=Abstract&list_uids=14700336

- **Congo red, doxycycline, and HSP70 overexpression reduce aggregate formation and cell death in cell models of oculopharyngeal muscular dystrophy.**
  Author(s): Bao YP, Sarkar S, Uyama E, Rubinsztein DC.
  Source: Journal of Medical Genetics. 2004 January; 41(1): 47-51.
  http://www.ncbi.nlm.nih.gov/entrez/query.fcgi?cmd=Retrieve&db=pubmed&dopt=Abstract&list_uids=14729833

- **Continuous remodeling of adult extraocular muscles as an explanation for selective craniofacial vulnerability in oculopharyngeal muscular dystrophy.**
  Author(s): Wirtschafter JD, Ferrington DA, McLoon LK.
  Source: Journal of Neuro-Ophthalmology: the Official Journal of the North American Neuro-Ophthalmology Society. 2004 March; 24(1): 62-7. Review.
  http://www.ncbi.nlm.nih.gov/entrez/query.fcgi?cmd=Retrieve&db=pubmed&dopt=Abstract&list_uids=15206442

- **Contrasting evolutionary histories of two introns of the duchenne muscular dystrophy gene, Dmd, in humans.**
  Author(s): Nachman MW, Crowell SL.
  Source: Genetics. 2000 August; 155(4): 1855-64.
  http://www.ncbi.nlm.nih.gov/entrez/query.fcgi?cmd=Retrieve&db=pubmed&dopt=Abstract&list_uids=10924480

- **D4F104S1 deletion in facioscapulohumeral muscular dystrophy: phenotype, size, and detection.**
  Author(s): Lemmers RJ, Osborn M, Haaf T, Rogers M, Frants RR, Padberg GW, Cooper DN, van der Maarel SM, Upadhyaya M.
  Source: Neurology. 2003 July 22; 61(2): 178-83.
  http://www.ncbi.nlm.nih.gov/entrez/query.fcgi?cmd=Retrieve&db=pubmed&dopt=Abstract&list_uids=12874395

- **De novo mutations in sporadic deletional Duchenne muscular dystrophy (DMD) cases.**
  Author(s): Mukherjee M, Chaturvedi LS, Srivastava S, Mittal RD, Mittal B.
  Source: Experimental & Molecular Medicine. 2003 April 30; 35(2): 113-7.
  http://www.ncbi.nlm.nih.gov/entrez/query.fcgi?cmd=Retrieve&db=pubmed&dopt=Abstract&list_uids=12754415

- **Deflazacort treatment of Duchenne muscular dystrophy.**
  Author(s): Biggar WD, Gingras M, Fehlings DL, Harris VA, Steele CA.
  Source: The Journal of Pediatrics. 2001 January; 138(1): 45-50.
  http://www.ncbi.nlm.nih.gov/entrez/query.fcgi?cmd=Retrieve&db=pubmed&dopt=Abstract&list_uids=11148511

- **Deletion analysis & calpain status for carrier detection in a family with Duchenne muscular dystrophy.**
  Author(s): Hussain T, Devi NG, Kumari CK, Anandaraj MP.
  Source: The Indian Journal of Medical Research. 1998 September; 108: 93-7.
  http://www.ncbi.nlm.nih.gov/entrez/query.fcgi?cmd=Retrieve&db=pubmed&dopt=Abstract&list_uids=9798335

- **Deletion analysis of the dystrophin gene in Duchenne and Becker muscular dystrophy patients: use in carrier diagnosis.**
  Author(s): Kumari D, Mital A, Gupta M, Goyle S.
  Source: Neurology India. 2003 June; 51(2): 223-6.
  http://www.ncbi.nlm.nih.gov/entrez/query.fcgi?cmd=Retrieve&db=pubmed&dopt=Abstract&list_uids=14571009

- **Dermatomyositis developing in a Duchenne muscular dystrophy carrier.**
  Author(s): Bennett AN, Sangle SR, Hughes GR, D'Cruz DP.
  Source: Rheumatology (Oxford, England). 2004 May; 43(5): 668-9.
  http://www.ncbi.nlm.nih.gov/entrez/query.fcgi?cmd=Retrieve&db=pubmed&dopt=Abstract&list_uids=15103031

- **DGGE-based whole-gene mutation scanning of the dystrophin gene in Duchenne and Becker muscular dystrophy patients.**
  Author(s): Hofstra RM, Mulder IM, Vossen R, de Koning-Gans PA, Kraak M, Ginjaar IB, van der Hout AH, Bakker E, Buys CH, van Ommen GJ, van Essen AJ, den Dunnen JT.
  Source: Human Mutation. 2004 January; 23(1): 57-66.
  http://www.ncbi.nlm.nih.gov/entrez/query.fcgi?cmd=Retrieve&db=pubmed&dopt=Abstract&list_uids=14695533

- **Direct detection of exon deletions/duplications in female carriers of and male patients with Duchenne/Becker muscular dystrophy.**
  Author(s): Frisso G, Carsana A, Tinto N, Calcagno G, Salvatore F, Sacchetti L.
  Source: Clinical Chemistry. 2004 August; 50(8): 1435-8.
  http://www.ncbi.nlm.nih.gov/entrez/query.fcgi?cmd=Retrieve&db=pubmed&dopt=Abstract&list_uids=15277355

- **Distal muscular dystrophy of the Miyoshi type.**
  Author(s): Yildiz H, Emre U, Coskun O, Ergun U, Atasoy HT, Inan LE.
  Source: Clin Neuropathol. 2003 July-August; 22(4): 204-8.
  http://www.ncbi.nlm.nih.gov/entrez/query.fcgi?cmd=Retrieve&db=pubmed&dopt=Abstract&list_uids=12908758

- **Do some genetic mutations predict the development of dilated cardiomyopathy in patients with Becker's muscular dystrophy?**
  Author(s): Ozdemir O, Arda K, Soylu M, Kutuk E.
  Source: Angiology. 2003 May-June; 54(3): 383-4.
  http://www.ncbi.nlm.nih.gov/entrez/query.fcgi?cmd=Retrieve&db=pubmed&dopt=Abstract&list_uids=12785035

- **Drug treatment for facioscapulohumeral muscular dystrophy.**
  Author(s): Rose MR, Tawil R.
  Source: Cochrane Database Syst Rev. 2004; (2): Cd002276. Review.
  http://www.ncbi.nlm.nih.gov/entrez/query.fcgi?cmd=Retrieve&db=pubmed&dopt=Abstract&list_uids=15106171

- **Duchenne and Becker muscular dystrophy.**
  Author(s): Kneppers AL, Ginjaar IB, Bakker E.
  Source: Methods in Molecular Medicine. 2004; 92: 311-41.
  http://www.ncbi.nlm.nih.gov/entrez/query.fcgi?cmd=Retrieve&db=pubmed&dopt=Abstract&list_uids=14733319

- **Duchenne muscular dystrophy in monozygotic twins.**
  Author(s): Kulkarni ML, Keshavamurthy KS.
  Source: Indian Pediatrics. 2004 March; 41(3): 290-1.
  http://www.ncbi.nlm.nih.gov/entrez/query.fcgi?cmd=Retrieve&db=pubmed&dopt=Abstract&list_uids=15064524

- **Duchenne muscular dystrophy: hopes for the sesquicentenary.**
  Author(s): Byrne E, Kornberg AJ, Kapsa R.
  Source: The Medical Journal of Australia. 2003 November 3; 179(9): 463-4.
  http://www.ncbi.nlm.nih.gov/entrez/query.fcgi?cmd=Retrieve&db=pubmed&dopt=Abstract&list_uids=14583075

- **Duchenne's muscular dystrophy: animal models used to investigate pathogenesis and develop therapeutic strategies.**
  Author(s): Collins CA, Morgan JE.
  Source: International Journal of Experimental Pathology. 2003 August; 84(4): 165-72. Review.
  http://www.ncbi.nlm.nih.gov/entrez/query.fcgi?cmd=Retrieve&db=pubmed&dopt=Abstract&list_uids=14632630

- **Dysferlin and muscular dystrophy.**
  Author(s): Bushby KM.
  Source: Acta Neurol Belg. 2000 September; 100(3): 142-5. Review.
  http://www.ncbi.nlm.nih.gov/entrez/query.fcgi?cmd=Retrieve&db=pubmed&dopt=Abstract&list_uids=11098285

- **Dysferlin, a novel skeletal muscle gene, is mutated in Miyoshi myopathy and limb girdle muscular dystrophy.**
  Author(s): Liu J, Aoki M, Illa I, Wu C, Fardeau M, Angelini C, Serrano C, Urtizberea JA, Hentati F, Hamida MB, Bohlega S, Culper EJ, Amato AA, Bossie K, Oeltjen J, Bejaoui K, McKenna-Yasek D, Hosler BA, Schurr E, Arahata K, de Jong PJ, Brown RH Jr.
  Source: Nature Genetics. 1998 September; 20(1): 31-6.
  http://www.ncbi.nlm.nih.gov/entrez/query.fcgi?cmd=Retrieve&db=pubmed&dopt=Abstract&list_uids=9731526

- **Dystrophin deletions and cognitive impairment in Duchenne/Becker muscular dystrophy.**
  Author(s): Giliberto F, Ferreiro V, Dalamon V, Szijan I.
  Source: Neurological Research. 2004 January; 26(1): 83-7.
  http://www.ncbi.nlm.nih.gov/entrez/query.fcgi?cmd=Retrieve&db=pubmed&dopt=Abstract&list_uids=14977063

- **Dystrophin gene deletions in South Indian Duchenne muscular dystrophy patients.**
  Author(s): Mallikarjuna Rao GN, Hussain T, Geetha Devi N, Jain S, Chandak GR, Ananda Raj MP.
  Source: Indian Journal of Medical Sciences. 2003 January; 57(1): 1-6.
  http://www.ncbi.nlm.nih.gov/entrez/query.fcgi?cmd=Retrieve&db=pubmed&dopt=Abstract&list_uids=14514278

- **Early onset, autosomal recessive muscular dystrophy with Emery-Dreifuss phenotype and normal emerin expression.**
  Author(s): Taylor J, Sewry CA, Dubowitz V, Muntoni F.
  Source: Neurology. 1998 October; 51(4): 1116-20.
  http://www.ncbi.nlm.nih.gov/entrez/query.fcgi?cmd=Retrieve&db=pubmed&dopt=Abstract&list_uids=9781539

- **Early prednisone treatment in Duchenne muscular dystrophy.**
  Author(s): Merlini L, Cicognani A, Malaspina E, Gennari M, Gnudi S, Talim B, Franzoni E.
  Source: Muscle & Nerve. 2003 February; 27(2): 222-7.
  http://www.ncbi.nlm.nih.gov/entrez/query.fcgi?cmd=Retrieve&db=pubmed&dopt=Abstract&list_uids=12548530

- **Effect of intrapulmonary percussive ventilation on mucus clearance in duchenne muscular dystrophy patients: a preliminary report.**
  Author(s): Toussaint M, De Win H, Steens M, Soudon P.
  Source: Respiratory Care. 2003 October; 48(10): 940-7.
  http://www.ncbi.nlm.nih.gov/entrez/query.fcgi?cmd=Retrieve&db=pubmed&dopt=Abstract&list_uids=14525630

- **Effects of deflazacort on left ventricular function in patients with Duchenne muscular dystrophy.**
  Author(s): Silversides CK, Webb GD, Harris VA, Biggar DW.
  Source: The American Journal of Cardiology. 2003 March 15; 91(6): 769-72.
  http://www.ncbi.nlm.nih.gov/entrez/query.fcgi?cmd=Retrieve&db=pubmed&dopt=Abstract&list_uids=12633823

- **Effects of expressing lamin A mutant protein causing Emery-Dreifuss muscular dystrophy and familial partial lipodystrophy in HeLa cells.**
  Author(s): Bechert K, Lagos-Quintana M, Harborth J, Weber K, Osborn M.
  Source: Experimental Cell Research. 2003 May 15; 286(1): 75-86.
  http://www.ncbi.nlm.nih.gov/entrez/query.fcgi?cmd=Retrieve&db=pubmed&dopt=Abstract&list_uids=12729796

- **Emerin binding to Btf, a death-promoting transcriptional repressor, is disrupted by a missense mutation that causes Emery-Dreifuss muscular dystrophy.**
  Author(s): Haraguchi T, Holaska JM, Yamane M, Koujin T, Hashiguchi N, Mori C, Wilson KL, Hiraoka Y.
  Source: European Journal of Biochemistry / Febs. 2004 March; 271(5): 1035-45.
  http://www.ncbi.nlm.nih.gov/entrez/query.fcgi?cmd=Retrieve&db=pubmed&dopt=Abstract&list_uids=15009215

- **Emery-Dreifuss muscular dystrophy in the evaluation of decreased spinal mobility and joint contractures.**
  Author(s): Goncu K, Guzel R, Guler-Uysal F.
  Source: Clinical Rheumatology. 2003 December; 22(6): 456-60. Epub 2003 October 21.
  http://www.ncbi.nlm.nih.gov/entrez/query.fcgi?cmd=Retrieve&db=pubmed&dopt=Abstract&list_uids=14677028

- **Emery-Dreifuss muscular dystrophy.**
  Author(s): De Smet L.
  Source: Genet Couns. 2004; 15(1): 91-4.
  http://www.ncbi.nlm.nih.gov/entrez/query.fcgi?cmd=Retrieve&db=pubmed&dopt=Abstract&list_uids=15083706

- **Emery-Dreifuss muscular dystrophy: anatomical-clinical correlation (case report).**
  Author(s): Carvalho AA, Levy JA, Gutierrez PS, Marie SK, Sosa EA, Scanavaca M.
  Source: Arquivos De Neuro-Psiquiatria. 2000 December; 58(4): 1123-7.
  http://www.ncbi.nlm.nih.gov/entrez/query.fcgi?cmd=Retrieve&db=pubmed&dopt=Abstract&list_uids=11105084

- **EMG and nerve conduction studies in children with congenital muscular dystrophy.**
  Author(s): Quijano-Roy S, Renault F, Romero N, Guicheney P, Fardeau M, Estournet B.
  Source: Muscle & Nerve. 2004 February; 29(2): 292-9.
  http://www.ncbi.nlm.nih.gov/entrez/query.fcgi?cmd=Retrieve&db=pubmed&dopt=Abstract&list_uids=14755496

- **Enhanced expression of the P2X4 receptor in Duchenne muscular dystrophy correlates with macrophage invasion.**
  Author(s): Yeung D, Kharidia R, Brown SC, Gorecki DC.
  Source: Neurobiology of Disease. 2004 March; 15(2): 212-20.
  http://www.ncbi.nlm.nih.gov/entrez/query.fcgi?cmd=Retrieve&db=pubmed&dopt=Abstract&list_uids=15006691

- **Enzymatic diagnostic test for Muscle-Eye-Brain type congenital muscular dystrophy using commercially available reagents.**
Author(s): Zhang W, Vajsar J, Cao P, Breningstall G, Diesen C, Dobyns W, Herrmann R, Lehesjoki AE, Steinbrecher A, Talim B, Toda T, Topaloglu H, Voit T, Schachter H.
Source: Clinical Biochemistry. 2003 July; 36(5): 339-44.
http://www.ncbi.nlm.nih.gov/entrez/query.fcgi?cmd=Retrieve&db=pubmed&dopt=Abstract&list_uids=12849864

- **Epiphora as a presenting sign of facioscapulohumeral muscular dystrophy.**
Author(s): Funnell CL, George ND.
Source: Journal of Pediatric Ophthalmology and Strabismus. 2003 March-April; 40(2): 113-4.
http://www.ncbi.nlm.nih.gov/entrez/query.fcgi?cmd=Retrieve&db=pubmed&dopt=Abstract&list_uids=12691238

- **ERG in Duchenne/Becker muscular dystrophy.**
Author(s): Fitzgerald KM, Cibis GW, White RA.
Source: Pediatric Neurology. 1998 November; 19(5): 400-1.
http://www.ncbi.nlm.nih.gov/entrez/query.fcgi?cmd=Retrieve&db=pubmed&dopt=Abstract&list_uids=9880152

- **Evaluation of dysrhythmia in children with muscular dystrophy.**
Author(s): Oguz D, Olgunturk R, Tunaoglu FS, Gucuyener K, Kose G, Unlu M.
Source: Angiology. 2000 November; 51(11): 925-31.
http://www.ncbi.nlm.nih.gov/entrez/query.fcgi?cmd=Retrieve&db=pubmed&dopt=Abstract&list_uids=11103861

- **Evidence of early impairments in both right and left ventricular inotropic reserves in children with Duchenne's muscular dystrophy.**
Author(s): Bosser G, Lucron H, Lethor JP, Burger G, Beltramo F, Marie PY, Marcon F.
Source: The American Journal of Cardiology. 2004 March 15; 93(6): 724-7.
http://www.ncbi.nlm.nih.gov/entrez/query.fcgi?cmd=Retrieve&db=pubmed&dopt=Abstract&list_uids=15019877

- **Evidence of left ventricular dysfunction in children with merosin-deficient congenital muscular dystrophy.**
  Author(s): Spyrou N, Philpot J, Foale R, Camici PG, Muntoni F.
  Source: American Heart Journal. 1998 September; 136(3): 474-6.
  http://www.ncbi.nlm.nih.gov/entrez/query.fcgi?cmd=Retrieve&db=pubmed&dopt=Abstract&list_uids=9736139

- **Expression and distribution of a small-conductance calcium-activated potassium channel (SK3) protein in skeletal muscles from myotonic muscular dystrophy patients and congenital myotonic mice.**
  Author(s): Kimura T, Takahashi MP, Fujimura H, Sakoda S.
  Source: Neuroscience Letters. 2003 August 28; 347(3): 191-5.
  http://www.ncbi.nlm.nih.gov/entrez/query.fcgi?cmd=Retrieve&db=pubmed&dopt=Abstract&list_uids=12875918

- **Expression and localization of nuclear proteins in autosomal-dominant Emery-Dreifuss muscular dystrophy with LMNA R377H mutation.**
  Author(s): Reichart B, Klafke R, Dreger C, Kruger E, Motsch I, Ewald A, Schafer J, Reichmann H, Muller CR, Dabauvalle MC.
  Source: Bmc Cell Biology [electronic Resource]. 2004 March 30; 5(1): 12.
  http://www.ncbi.nlm.nih.gov/entrez/query.fcgi?cmd=Retrieve&db=pubmed&dopt=Abstract&list_uids=15053843

- **Expression of emerin and lamins in muscle of patients with different forms of Emery-Dreifuss muscular dystrophy.**
  Author(s): Niebroj-Dobosz I, Fidzianska A, Hausmanowa-Petrusewicz I.
  Source: Acta Myol. 2003 September; 22(2): 52-7.
  http://www.ncbi.nlm.nih.gov/entrez/query.fcgi?cmd=Retrieve&db=pubmed&dopt=Abstract&list_uids=14959564

- **Facioscapulohumeral (FSHD1) and other forms of muscular dystrophy in the same family: is there more in muscular dystrophy than meets the eye?**
  Author(s): Tonini MM, Passos-Bueno MR, Cerqueira A, Pavanello R, Vainzof M, Dubowitz V, Zatz M.
  Source: Neuromuscular Disorders: Nmd. 2002 August; 12(6): 554-7.
  http://www.ncbi.nlm.nih.gov/entrez/query.fcgi?cmd=Retrieve&db=pubmed&dopt=Abstract&list_uids=12117479

- **Facioscapulohumeral muscular dystrophy (FSHD) myoblasts demonstrate increased susceptibility to oxidative stress.**
  Author(s): Winokur ST, Barrett K, Martin JH, Forrester JR, Simon M, Tawil R, Chung SA, Masny PS, Figlewicz DA.
  Source: Neuromuscular Disorders: Nmd. 2003 May; 13(4): 322-33.
  http://www.ncbi.nlm.nih.gov/entrez/query.fcgi?cmd=Retrieve&db=pubmed&dopt=Abstract&list_uids=12868502

- **Facioscapulohumeral muscular dystrophy is uniquely associated with one of the two variants of the 4q subtelomere.**
  Author(s): Lemmers RJ, de Kievit P, Sandkuijl L, Padberg GW, van Ommen GJ, Frants RR, van der Maarel SM.
  Source: Nature Genetics. 2002 October; 32(2): 235-6. Epub 2002 September 23.
  http://www.ncbi.nlm.nih.gov/entrez/query.fcgi?cmd=Retrieve&db=pubmed&dopt=Abstract&list_uids=12355084

- **Facioscapulohumeral muscular dystrophy presenting isolated monomelic lower limb atrophy. Report of two patients with and without 4q35 rearrangement.**
  Author(s): Uncini A, Galluzzi G, Di Muzio A, De Angelis MV, Ricci E, Scoppetta C, Servidei S.
  Source: Neuromuscular Disorders: Nmd. 2002 November; 12(9): 874-7.
  http://www.ncbi.nlm.nih.gov/entrez/query.fcgi?cmd=Retrieve&db=pubmed&dopt=Abstract&list_uids=12398841

- **Facioscapulohumeral muscular dystrophy.**
  Author(s): Tawil R.
  Source: Curr Neurol Neurosci Rep. 2004 January; 4(1): 51-4. Review.
  http://www.ncbi.nlm.nih.gov/entrez/query.fcgi?cmd=Retrieve&db=pubmed&dopt=Abstract&list_uids=14683629

- **Facioscapulohumeral muscular dystrophy. Phenotype-genotype correlation in patients with borderline D4Z4 repeat numbers.**
  Author(s): Butz M, Koch MC, Muller-Felber W, Lemmers RJ, van der Maarel SM, Schreiber H.
  Source: Journal of Neurology. 2003 August; 250(8): 932-7.
  http://www.ncbi.nlm.nih.gov/entrez/query.fcgi?cmd=Retrieve&db=pubmed&dopt=Abstract&list_uids=12928911

- **Familial arachnoid cysts associated with oculopharyngeal muscular dystrophy.**
  Author(s): Jadeja KJ, Grewal RP.
  Source: Journal of Clinical Neuroscience: Official Journal of the Neurosurgical Society of Australasia. 2003 January; 10(1): 125-7.
  http://www.ncbi.nlm.nih.gov/entrez/query.fcgi?cmd=Retrieve&db=pubmed&dopt=Abstract&list_uids=12464544

- **Fetal muscle biopsy as a diagnostic tool in Duchenne muscular dystrophy.**
  Author(s): Nevo Y, Shomrat R, Yaron Y, Orr-Urtreger A, Harel S, Legum C.
  Source: Prenatal Diagnosis. 1999 October; 19(10): 921-6.
  http://www.ncbi.nlm.nih.gov/entrez/query.fcgi?cmd=Retrieve&db=pubmed&dopt=Abstract&list_uids=10521816

- **FKRP (826C>A) frequently causes limb-girdle muscular dystrophy in German patients.**
  Author(s): Walter MC, Petersen JA, Stucka R, Fischer D, Schroder R, Vorgerd M, Schroers A, Schreiber H, Hanemann CO, Knirsch U, Rosenbohm A, Huebner A, Barisic N, Horvath R, Komoly S, Reilich P, Muller-Felber W, Pongratz D, Muller JS, Auerswald EA, Lochmuller H.
  Source: Journal of Medical Genetics. 2004 April; 41(4): E50.
  http://www.ncbi.nlm.nih.gov/entrez/query.fcgi?cmd=Retrieve&db=pubmed&dopt=Abstract&list_uids=15060126

- **FKRP gene mutations cause congenital muscular dystrophy, mental retardation, and cerebellar cysts.**
  Author(s): Topaloglu H, Brockington M, Yuva Y, Talim B, Haliloglu G, Blake D, Torelli S, Brown SC, Muntoni F.
  Source: Neurology. 2003 March 25; 60(6): 988-92.
  http://www.ncbi.nlm.nih.gov/entrez/query.fcgi?cmd=Retrieve&db=pubmed&dopt=Abstract&list_uids=12654965

- **Founder-haplotype analysis in Fukuyama-type congenital muscular dystrophy (FCMD).**
  Author(s): Kobayashi K, Nakahori Y, Mizuno K, Miyake M, Kumagai T, Honma A, Nonaka I, Nakamura Y, Tokunaga K, Toda T.
  Source: Human Genetics. 1998 September; 103(3): 323-7.
  http://www.ncbi.nlm.nih.gov/entrez/query.fcgi?cmd=Retrieve&db=pubmed&dopt=Abstract&list_uids=9799088

- **Four novel plectin gene mutations in Japanese patients with epidermolysis bullosa with muscular dystrophy disclosed by heteroduplex scanning and protein truncation tests.**
  Author(s): Takizawa Y, Shimizu H, Rouan F, Kawai M, Udono M, Pulkkinen L, Nishikawa T, Uitto J.
  Source: The Journal of Investigative Dermatology. 1999 January; 112(1): 109-12.
  http://www.ncbi.nlm.nih.gov/entrez/query.fcgi?cmd=Retrieve&db=pubmed&dopt=Abstract&list_uids=9886273

- **Fracture prevalence in Duchenne muscular dystrophy.**
  Author(s): McDonald DG, Kinali M, Gallagher AC, Mercuri E, Muntoni F, Roper H, Jardine P, Jones DH, Pike MG.
  Source: Developmental Medicine and Child Neurology. 2002 October; 44(10): 695-8.
  http://www.ncbi.nlm.nih.gov/entrez/query.fcgi?cmd=Retrieve&db=pubmed&dopt=Abstract&list_uids=12418795

- **Frequent low penetrance mutations in the Lamin A/C gene, causing Emery Dreifuss muscular dystrophy.**
  Author(s): Vytopil M, Ricci E, Dello Russo A, Hanisch F, Neudecker S, Zierz S, Ricotti R, Demay L, Richard P, Wehnert M, Bonne G, Merlini L, Toniolo D.
  Source: Neuromuscular Disorders: Nmd. 2002 December; 12(10): 958-63.
  http://www.ncbi.nlm.nih.gov/entrez/query.fcgi?cmd=Retrieve&db=pubmed&dopt=Abstract&list_uids=12467752

- **FRG1, a gene in the FSH muscular dystrophy region on human chromosome 4q35, is highly conserved in vertebrates and invertebrates.**
  Author(s): Grewal PK, Todd LC, van der Maarel S, Frants RR, Hewitt JE.
  Source: Gene. 1998 August 17; 216(1): 13-9.
  http://www.ncbi.nlm.nih.gov/entrez/query.fcgi?cmd=Retrieve&db=pubmed&dopt=Abstract&list_uids=9714712

- **Fukutin expression in glial cells and neurons: implication in the brain lesions of Fukuyama congenital muscular dystrophy.**
  Author(s): Yamamoto T, Kato Y, Karita M, Takeiri H, Muramatsu F, Kobayashi M, Saito K, Osawa M.
  Source: Acta Neuropathologica. 2002 September; 104(3): 217-24. Epub 2002 June 21.
  http://www.ncbi.nlm.nih.gov/entrez/query.fcgi?cmd=Retrieve&db=pubmed&dopt=Abstract&list_uids=12172906

- **Fukuyama-type congenital muscular dystrophy (FCMD) and alpha-dystroglycanopathy.**
  Author(s): Toda T, Kobayashi K, Takeda S, Sasaki J, Kurahashi H, Kano H, Tachikawa M, Wang F, Nagai Y, Taniguchi K, Taniguchi M, Sunada Y, Terashima T, Endo T, Matsumura K.
  Source: Congenit Anom (Kyoto). 2003 June; 43(2): 97-104. Review.
  http://www.ncbi.nlm.nih.gov/entrez/query.fcgi?cmd=Retrieve&db=pubmed&dopt=Abstract&list_uids=12893968

- **Fukuyama-type congenital muscular dystrophy: a case report in the Japanese population living in Brazil.**
  Author(s): Zanoteli E, Rocha JC, Narumia LK, Fireman MA, Moura LS, Oliveira AS, Gabbai AA, Fukuda Y, Kinoshita M, Toda T.
  Source: Acta Neurologica Scandinavica. 2002 August; 106(2): 117-21.
  http://www.ncbi.nlm.nih.gov/entrez/query.fcgi?cmd=Retrieve&db=pubmed&dopt=Abstract&list_uids=12100373

- **Functional domains of the nucleus: implications for Emery-Dreifuss muscular dystrophy.**
  Author(s): Maraldi NM, Lattanzi G, Sabatelli P, Ognibene A, Squarzoni S.
  Source: Neuromuscular Disorders: Nmd. 2002 November; 12(9): 815-23. Review.
  http://www.ncbi.nlm.nih.gov/entrez/query.fcgi?cmd=Retrieve&db=pubmed&dopt=Abstract&list_uids=12398831

- **Functional muscle ischemia in neuronal nitric oxide synthase-deficient skeletal muscle of children with Duchenne muscular dystrophy.**
  Author(s): Sander M, Chavoshan B, Harris SA, Iannaccone ST, Stull JT, Thomas GD, Victor RG.
  Source: Proceedings of the National Academy of Sciences of the United States of America. 2000 December 5; 97(25): 13818-23.
  http://www.ncbi.nlm.nih.gov/entrez/query.fcgi?cmd=Retrieve&db=pubmed&dopt=Abstract&list_uids=11087833

- **gamma-sarcoglycan deficiency muscular dystrophy in two adults.**
  Author(s): Lin KL, Wang HS, Chen ST, Ro LS.
  Source: J Formos Med Assoc. 2000 October; 99(10): 789-91.
  http://www.ncbi.nlm.nih.gov/entrez/query.fcgi?cmd=Retrieve&db=pubmed&dopt=Abstract&list_uids=11061077

- **Gastric emptying time in children with progressive muscular dystrophy.**
  Author(s): Okan M, Alper E, Cil E, Eralp O, Agir H.
  Source: Turk J Pediatr. 1997 January-March; 39(1): 69-74.
  http://www.ncbi.nlm.nih.gov/entrez/query.fcgi?cmd=Retrieve&db=pubmed&dopt=Abstract&list_uids=10868196

- **Gastric wall weakening resulting in separate perforations in a patient with Duchenne's muscular dystrophy.**
  Author(s): Dinan D, Levine MS, Gordon AR, Rubesin SE, Rombeau JL.
  Source: Ajr. American Journal of Roentgenology. 2003 September; 181(3): 807-8.
  http://www.ncbi.nlm.nih.gov/entrez/query.fcgi?cmd=Retrieve&db=pubmed&dopt=Abstract&list_uids=12933486

- **GCG repeats and phenotype in oculopharyngeal muscular dystrophy.**
  Author(s): Muller T, Schroder R, Zierz S.
  Source: Muscle & Nerve. 2001 January; 24(1): 120-2.
  http://www.ncbi.nlm.nih.gov/entrez/query.fcgi?cmd=Retrieve&db=pubmed&dopt=Abstract&list_uids=11150975

- **Gene deletion and carrier detection in the family of Becker muscular dystrophy by short tandem repeat sequence polymorphism.**
  Author(s): Cai S, Shen D, Wang J.
  Source: Chinese Medical Journal. 1999 March; 112(3): 242-5.
  http://www.ncbi.nlm.nih.gov/entrez/query.fcgi?cmd=Retrieve&db=pubmed&dopt=Abstract&list_uids=11593558

- **Gene expression comparison of biopsies from Duchenne muscular dystrophy (DMD) and normal skeletal muscle.**
  Author(s): Haslett JN, Sanoudou D, Kho AT, Bennett RR, Greenberg SA, Kohane IS, Beggs AH, Kunkel LM.
  Source: Proceedings of the National Academy of Sciences of the United States of America. 2002 November 12; 99(23): 15000-5. Epub 2002 Nov 01.
  http://www.ncbi.nlm.nih.gov/entrez/query.fcgi?cmd=Retrieve&db=pubmed&dopt=Abstract&list_uids=12415109

- **Gene expression profiling of Duchenne muscular dystrophy skeletal muscle.**
  Author(s): Haslett JN, Sanoudou D, Kho AT, Han M, Bennett RR, Kohane IS, Beggs AH, Kunkel LM.
  Source: Neurogenetics. 2003 August; 4(4): 163-71. Epub 2003 April 16.
  http://www.ncbi.nlm.nih.gov/entrez/query.fcgi?cmd=Retrieve&db=pubmed&dopt=Abstract&list_uids=12698323

- **Gene removes muscular dystrophy symptoms in mouse model.**
  Author(s): Senior K.
  Source: Lancet. 2001 September 22; 358(9286): 990.
  http://www.ncbi.nlm.nih.gov/entrez/query.fcgi?cmd=Retrieve&db=pubmed&dopt=Abstract&list_uids=11583760

- **Gene therapy for muscular dystrophy - a review of promising progress.**
  Author(s): Gregorevic P, Chamberlain JS.
  Source: Expert Opinion on Biological Therapy. 2003 August; 3(5): 803-14. Review.
  http://www.ncbi.nlm.nih.gov/entrez/query.fcgi?cmd=Retrieve&db=pubmed&dopt=Abstract&list_uids=12880380

- **Gene therapy of muscular dystrophy.**
  Author(s): Chamberlain JS.
  Source: Human Molecular Genetics. 2002 October 1; 11(20): 2355-62. Review.
  http://www.ncbi.nlm.nih.gov/entrez/query.fcgi?cmd=Retrieve&db=pubmed&dopt=Abstract&list_uids=12351570

- **Genetic and physical mapping at the limb-girdle muscular dystrophy locus (LGMD2B) on chromosome 2p.**
  Author(s): Bashir R, Keers S, Strachan T, Passos-Bueno R, Zatz M, Weissenbach J, Le Paslier D, Meisler M, Bushby K.
  Source: Genomics. 1996 April 1; 33(1): 46-52.
  http://www.ncbi.nlm.nih.gov/entrez/query.fcgi?cmd=Retrieve&db=pubmed&dopt=Abstract&list_uids=8617508

- **Genetic counseling for childless women at risk for Duchenne muscular dystrophy.**
  Author(s): Eggers S, Pavanello RC, Passos-Bueno MR, Zatz M.
  Source: American Journal of Medical Genetics. 1999 October 29; 86(5): 447-53.
  http://www.ncbi.nlm.nih.gov/entrez/query.fcgi?cmd=Retrieve&db=pubmed&dopt=Abstract&list_uids=10508987

- **Genetic epidemiology of congenital muscular dystrophy in a sample from north-east Italy.**
  Author(s): Mostacciuolo ML, Miorin M, Martinello F, Angelini C, Perini P, Trevisan CP.
  Source: Human Genetics. 1996 March; 97(3): 277-9.
  http://www.ncbi.nlm.nih.gov/entrez/query.fcgi?cmd=Retrieve&db=pubmed&dopt=Abstract&list_uids=8786062

- **Genetic heterogeneity in three Chinese children with Fukuyama congenital muscular dystrophy.**
  Author(s): Jong YJ, Kobayashi K, Toda T, Kondo E, Huang SC, Shen YZ, Nonaka I, Fukuyama Y.
  Source: Neuromuscular Disorders: Nmd. 2000 February; 10(2): 108-12.
  http://www.ncbi.nlm.nih.gov/entrez/query.fcgi?cmd=Retrieve&db=pubmed&dopt=Abstract&list_uids=10714585

- **Genetic polymorphism in muscle biopsies of Duchenne and Becker muscular dystrophy patients.**
  Author(s): Anand A, Prabhakar S, Kaul D.
  Source: Neurology India. 1999 September; 47(3): 218-23.
  http://www.ncbi.nlm.nih.gov/entrez/query.fcgi?cmd=Retrieve&db=pubmed&dopt=Abstract&list_uids=10514583

- **Genomic analysis of facioscapulohumeral muscular dystrophy.**
  Author(s): Clapp J, Bolland DJ, Hewitt JE.
  Source: Brief Funct Genomic Proteomic. 2003 October; 2(3): 213-23. Review.
  http://www.ncbi.nlm.nih.gov/entrez/query.fcgi?cmd=Retrieve&db=pubmed&dopt=Abstract&list_uids=15239924

- **Gentamicin treatment of Duchenne and Becker muscular dystrophy due to nonsense mutations.**
  Author(s): Wagner KR, Hamed S, Hadley DW, Gropman AL, Burstein AH, Escolar DM, Hoffman EP, Fischbeck KH.
  Source: Annals of Neurology. 2001 June; 49(6): 706-11.
  http://www.ncbi.nlm.nih.gov/entrez/query.fcgi?cmd=Retrieve&db=pubmed&dopt=Abstract&list_uids=11409421

- **Glucocorticoid corticosteroids for Duchenne muscular dystrophy.**
  Author(s): Manzur AY, Kuntzer T, Pike M, Swan A.
  Source: Cochrane Database Syst Rev. 2004; (2): Cd003725. Review.
  http://www.ncbi.nlm.nih.gov/entrez/query.fcgi?cmd=Retrieve&db=pubmed&dopt=Abstract&list_uids=15106215

- **Glycosylation defects: a new mechanism for muscular dystrophy?**
  Author(s): Grewal PK, Hewitt JE.
  Source: Human Molecular Genetics. 2003 October 15; 12 Spec No 2: R259-64. Epub 2003 August 12. Review.
  http://www.ncbi.nlm.nih.gov/entrez/query.fcgi?cmd=Retrieve&db=pubmed&dopt=Abstract&list_uids=12925572

- **Glycosylation eases muscular dystrophy.**
  Author(s): Muntoni F, Brockington M, Brown SC.
  Source: Nature Medicine. 2004 July; 10(7): 676-7.
  http://www.ncbi.nlm.nih.gov/entrez/query.fcgi?cmd=Retrieve&db=pubmed&dopt=Abstract&list_uids=15229511

- **Haplotype-phenotype correlation in Fukuyama congenital muscular dystrophy.**
  Author(s): Saito K, Osawa M, Wang ZP, Ikeya K, Fukuyama Y, Kondo-Iida E, Toda T, Ohashi H, Kurosawa K, Wakai S, Kaneko K.
  Source: American Journal of Medical Genetics. 2000 May 29; 92(3): 184-90.
  http://www.ncbi.nlm.nih.gov/entrez/query.fcgi?cmd=Retrieve&db=pubmed&dopt=Abstract&list_uids=10817652

- **Harnessing the potential of dystrophin-related proteins for ameliorating Duchenne's muscular dystrophy.**
  Author(s): Krag TO, Gyrd-Hansen M, Khurana TS.
  Source: Acta Physiologica Scandinavica. 2001 March; 171(3): 349-58. Review.
  http://www.ncbi.nlm.nih.gov/entrez/query.fcgi?cmd=Retrieve&db=pubmed&dopt=Abstract&list_uids=11412148

- **Heart to heart: from nuclear proteins to Emery-Dreifuss muscular dystrophy.**
  Author(s): Morris GE, Manilal S.
  Source: Human Molecular Genetics. 1999; 8(10): 1847-51. Review.
  http://www.ncbi.nlm.nih.gov/entrez/query.fcgi?cmd=Retrieve&db=pubmed&dopt=Abstract&list_uids=10469836

- **Heart-specific localization of emerin: new insights into Emery-Dreifuss muscular dystrophy.**
  Author(s): Cartegni L, di Barletta MR, Barresi R, Squarzoni S, Sabatelli P, Maraldi N, Mora M, Di Blasi C, Cornelio F, Merlini L, Villa A, Cobianchi F, Toniolo D.
  Source: Human Molecular Genetics. 1997 December; 6(13): 2257-64.
  http://www.ncbi.nlm.nih.gov/entrez/query.fcgi?cmd=Retrieve&db=pubmed&dopt=Abstract&list_uids=9361031

- **Heterogeneity in familial dominant Paget disease of bone and muscular dystrophy.**
  Author(s): Waggoner B, Kovach MJ, Winkelman M, Cai D, Khardori R, Gelber D, Kimonis VE.
  Source: American Journal of Medical Genetics. 2002 March 15; 108(3): 187-91.
  http://www.ncbi.nlm.nih.gov/entrez/query.fcgi?cmd=Retrieve&db=pubmed&dopt=Abstract&list_uids=11891683

- **Heterogeneity of classic congenital muscular dystrophy with involvement of the central nervous system: report of five atypical cases.**
  Author(s): Reed UC, Marie SK, Vainzof M, Gobbo LF, Gurgel JE, Carvalho MS, Resende MB, Espindola AA, Zatz M, Diament A.
  Source: Journal of Child Neurology. 2000 March; 15(3): 172-8.
  http://www.ncbi.nlm.nih.gov/entrez/query.fcgi?cmd=Retrieve&db=pubmed&dopt=Abstract&list_uids=10757473

- **Heterozygous myogenic factor 6 mutation associated with myopathy and severe course of Becker muscular dystrophy.**
  Author(s): Kerst B, Mennerich D, Schuelke M, Stoltenburg-Didinger G, von Moers A, Gossrau R, van Landeghem FK, Speer A, Braun T, Hubner C.
  Source: Neuromuscular Disorders: Nmd. 2000 December; 10(8): 572-7.
  http://www.ncbi.nlm.nih.gov/entrez/query.fcgi?cmd=Retrieve&db=pubmed&dopt=Abstract&list_uids=11053684

- **High dose weekly oral prednisone improves strength in boys with Duchenne muscular dystrophy.**
  Author(s): Connolly AM, Schierbecker J, Renna R, Florence J.
  Source: Neuromuscular Disorders: Nmd. 2002 December; 12(10): 917-25.
  http://www.ncbi.nlm.nih.gov/entrez/query.fcgi?cmd=Retrieve&db=pubmed&dopt=Abstract&list_uids=12467746

- **High frequency of de novo deletions in Mexican Duchenne and Becker muscular dystrophy patients. Implications for genetic counseling.**
  Author(s): Alcantara MA, Villarreal MT, Del Castillo V, Gutierrez G, Saldana Y, Maulen I, Lee R, Macias M, Orozco L.
  Source: Clinical Genetics. 1999 May; 55(5): 376-80.
  http://www.ncbi.nlm.nih.gov/entrez/query.fcgi?cmd=Retrieve&db=pubmed&dopt=Abstract&list_uids=10422811

- **High resolution magnetic resonance imaging of the brain in the dy/dy mouse with merosin-deficient congenital muscular dystrophy.**
  Author(s): Dubowitz DJ, Tyszka JM, Sewry CA, Moats RA, Scadeng M, Dubowitz V.
  Source: Neuromuscular Disorders: Nmd. 2000 June; 10(4-5): 292-8.
  http://www.ncbi.nlm.nih.gov/entrez/query.fcgi?cmd=Retrieve&db=pubmed&dopt=Abstract&list_uids=10838257

- **Hip subluxation and dislocation in Duchenne muscular dystrophy.**
  Author(s): Chan KG, Galasko CS, Delaney C.
  Source: Journal of Pediatric Orthopaedics. Part B / European Paediatric Orthopaedic Society, Pediatric Orthopaedic Society of North America. 2001 July; 10(3): 219-25.
  http://www.ncbi.nlm.nih.gov/entrez/query.fcgi?cmd=Retrieve&db=pubmed&dopt=Abstract&list_uids=11497366

- **HnRNP A1 and A/B interaction with PABPN1 in oculopharyngeal muscular dystrophy.**
  Author(s): Fan X, Messaed C, Dion P, Laganiere J, Brais B, Karpati G, Rouleau GA.
  Source: The Canadian Journal of Neurological Sciences. Le Journal Canadien Des Sciences Neurologiques. 2003 August; 30(3): 244-51.
  http://www.ncbi.nlm.nih.gov/entrez/query.fcgi?cmd=Retrieve&db=pubmed&dopt=Abstract&list_uids=12945950

- **Homozygosity for autosomal dominant facioscapulohumeral muscular dystrophy (FSHD) does not result in a more severe phenotype.**
  Author(s): Tonini MM, Pavanello RC, Gurgel-Giannetti J, Lemmers RJ, van der Maarel SM, Frants RR, Zatz M.
  Source: Journal of Medical Genetics. 2004 February; 41(2): E17.
  http://www.ncbi.nlm.nih.gov/entrez/query.fcgi?cmd=Retrieve&db=pu
  bmed&dopt=Abstract&list_uids=14757867

- **Homozygotes for oculopharyngeal muscular dystrophy have a severe form of the disease.**
  Author(s): Blumen SC, Brais B, Korczyn AD, Medinsky S, Chapman J, Asherov A, Nisipeanu P, Codere F, Bouchard JP, Fardeau M, Tome FM, Rouleau GA.
  Source: Annals of Neurology. 1999 July; 46(1): 115-8.
  http://www.ncbi.nlm.nih.gov/entrez/query.fcgi?cmd=Retrieve&db=pu
  bmed&dopt=Abstract&list_uids=10401788

- **Homozygous alpha-sarcoglycan mutation in two siblings: one asymptomatic and one steroid-responsive mild limb-girdle muscular dystrophy patient.**
  Author(s): Angelini C, Fanin M, Menegazzo E, Freda MP, Duggan DJ, Hoffman EP.
  Source: Muscle & Nerve. 1998 June; 21(6): 769-75.
  http://www.ncbi.nlm.nih.gov/entrez/query.fcgi?cmd=Retrieve&db=pu
  bmed&dopt=Abstract&list_uids=9585331

- **How the magnitude of clinical severity and recurrence risk affects reproductive decisions in adult males with different forms of progressive muscular dystrophy.**
  Author(s): Eggers S, Zatz M.
  Source: Journal of Medical Genetics. 1998 March; 35(3): 189-95.
  http://www.ncbi.nlm.nih.gov/entrez/query.fcgi?cmd=Retrieve&db=pu
  bmed&dopt=Abstract&list_uids=9541101

- **Human epsilon-sarcoglycan is highly related to alpha-sarcoglycan (adhalin), the limb girdle muscular dystrophy 2D gene.**
  Author(s): McNally EM, Ly CT, Kunkel LM.
  Source: Febs Letters. 1998 January 23; 422(1): 27-32.
  http://www.ncbi.nlm.nih.gov/entrez/query.fcgi?cmd=Retrieve&db=pu
  bmed&dopt=Abstract&list_uids=9475163

- **Hyperkalaemic cardiac arrest in a manifesting carrier of Duchenne muscular dystrophy following general anaesthesia.**
  Author(s): Kerr TP, Duward A, Hodgson SV, Hughes E, Robb SA.
  Source: European Journal of Pediatrics. 2001 September; 160(9): 579-80.
  http://www.ncbi.nlm.nih.gov/entrez/query.fcgi?cmd=Retrieve&db=pubmed&dopt=Abstract&list_uids=11585084

- **Hyperproliferation of synapses on spinal motor neurons of Duchenne muscular dystrophy and myotonic dystrophy patients.**
  Author(s): Nagao M, Kato S, Hayashi H, Misawa H.
  Source: Acta Neuropathologica. 2003 December; 106(6): 557-60. Epub 2003 August 14.
  http://www.ncbi.nlm.nih.gov/entrez/query.fcgi?cmd=Retrieve&db=pubmed&dopt=Abstract&list_uids=12920538

- **Hypomethylation of D4Z4 in 4q-linked and non-4q-linked facioscapulohumeral muscular dystrophy.**
  Author(s): van Overveld PG, Lemmers RJ, Sandkuijl LA, Enthoven L, Winokur ST, Bakels F, Padberg GW, van Ommen GJ, Frants RR, van der Maarel SM.
  Source: Nature Genetics. 2003 December; 35(4): 315-7. Epub 2003 November 23.
  http://www.ncbi.nlm.nih.gov/entrez/query.fcgi?cmd=Retrieve&db=pubmed&dopt=Abstract&list_uids=14634647

- **Identical de novo mutation at the D4F104S1 locus in monozygotic male twins affected by facioscapulohumeral muscular dystrophy (FSHD) with different clinical expression.**
  Author(s): Tupler R, Barbierato L, Memmi M, Sewry CA, De Grandis D, Maraschio P, Tiepolo L, Ferlini A.
  Source: Journal of Medical Genetics. 1998 September; 35(9): 778-83.
  http://www.ncbi.nlm.nih.gov/entrez/query.fcgi?cmd=Retrieve&db=pubmed&dopt=Abstract&list_uids=9733041

- **Identical dysferlin mutation in limb-girdle muscular dystrophy type 2B and distal myopathy.**
  Author(s): Illarioshkin SN, Ivanova-Smolenskaya IA, Greenberg CR, Nylen E, Sukhorukov VS, Poleshchuk VV, Markova ED, Wrogemann K.
  Source: Neurology. 2000 December 26; 55(12): 1931-3.
  http://www.ncbi.nlm.nih.gov/entrez/query.fcgi?cmd=Retrieve&db=pubmed&dopt=Abstract&list_uids=11134403

- **Identification of a novel truncating mutation (S171X) in the Emerin gene in five members of a Caucasian American family with Emery-Dreifuss muscular dystrophy.**
  Author(s): Menache CC, Brown CA, Donnelly JH, Shapiro F, Darras BT.
  Source: Human Mutation. 2000 July; 16(1): 94.
  http://www.ncbi.nlm.nih.gov/entrez/query.fcgi?cmd=Retrieve&db=pubmed&dopt=Abstract&list_uids=10874323

- **Identification of an HLA-A*0201-restricted epitopic peptide from human dystrophin: application in duchenne muscular dystrophy gene therapy.**
  Author(s): Ginhoux F, Doucet C, Leboeuf M, Lemonnier FA, Danos O, Davoust J, Firat H.
  Source: Molecular Therapy: the Journal of the American Society of Gene Therapy. 2003 August; 8(2): 274-83.
  http://www.ncbi.nlm.nih.gov/entrez/query.fcgi?cmd=Retrieve&db=pubmed&dopt=Abstract&list_uids=12907150

- **Identification of lamin A/C (LMNA) gene mutations in Korean patients with autosomal dominant Emery-Dreifuss muscular dystrophy and limb-girdle muscular dystrophy 1B.**
  Author(s): Ki CS, Hong JS, Jeong GY, Ahn KJ, Choi KM, Kim DK, Kim JW.
  Source: Journal of Human Genetics. 2002; 47(5): 225-8.
  http://www.ncbi.nlm.nih.gov/entrez/query.fcgi?cmd=Retrieve&db=pubmed&dopt=Abstract&list_uids=12032588

- **Identification of transcripts from a subtraction library which might be responsible for the mild phenotype in an intrafamilially variable course of Duchenne muscular dystrophy.**
  Author(s): Sifringer M, Uhlenberg B, Lammel S, Hanke R, Neumann B, von Moers A, Koch I, Speer A.
  Source: Human Genetics. 2004 January; 114(2): 149-56. Epub 2003 November 05.
  http://www.ncbi.nlm.nih.gov/entrez/query.fcgi?cmd=Retrieve&db=pubmed&dopt=Abstract&list_uids=14600829

- **Immune responses to dystropin: implications for gene therapy of Duchenne muscular dystrophy.**
  Author(s): Ferrer A, Wells KE, Wells DJ.
  Source: Gene Therapy. 2000 September; 7(17): 1439-46.
  http://www.ncbi.nlm.nih.gov/entrez/query.fcgi?cmd=Retrieve&db=pubmed&dopt=Abstract&list_uids=11001363

- **Immunocytochemistry of nuclear domains and Emery-Dreifuss muscular dystrophy pathophysiology.**
  Author(s): Maraldi NM, Lattanzi G, Sabatelli P, Ognibene A, Columbaro M, Capanni C, Rutigliano C, Mattioli E, Squarzoni S.
  Source: Eur J Histochem. 2003; 47(1): 3-16. Review.
  http://www.ncbi.nlm.nih.gov/entrez/query.fcgi?cmd=Retrieve&db=pubmed&dopt=Abstract&list_uids=12685553

- **Immunohistochemical staining of dystrophin on formalin-fixed paraffin-embedded sections in Duchenne/Becker muscular dystrophy and manifesting carriers of Duchenne muscular dystrophy.**
  Author(s): Hoshino S, Ohkoshi N, Watanabe M, Shoji S.
  Source: Neuromuscular Disorders: Nmd. 2000 August; 10(6): 425-9.
  http://www.ncbi.nlm.nih.gov/entrez/query.fcgi?cmd=Retrieve&db=pubmed&dopt=Abstract&list_uids=10899449

- **Immunological hurdles in the path to gene therapy for Duchenne muscular dystrophy.**
  Author(s): Wells DJ, Ferrer A, Wells KE.
  Source: Expert Reviews in Molecular Medicine [electronic Resource]. 2002 November 4; 2002: 1-23. Review.
  http://www.ncbi.nlm.nih.gov/entrez/query.fcgi?cmd=Retrieve&db=pubmed&dopt=Abstract&list_uids=14585159

- **Increased expression of IGF-binding protein-5 in Duchenne muscular dystrophy (DMD) fibroblasts correlates with the fibroblast-induced downregulation of DMD myoblast growth: an in vitro analysis.**
  Author(s): Melone MA, Peluso G, Galderisi U, Petillo O, Cotrufo R.
  Source: Journal of Cellular Physiology. 2000 October; 185(1): 143-53.
  http://www.ncbi.nlm.nih.gov/entrez/query.fcgi?cmd=Retrieve&db=pubmed&dopt=Abstract&list_uids=10942528

- **Increased resting energy expenditure in subjects with Emery-Dreifuss muscular dystrophy.**
  Author(s): Vaisman N, Katzenellenbogen S, Nevo Y.
  Source: Neuromuscular Disorders: Nmd. 2004 February; 14(2): 142-6.
  http://www.ncbi.nlm.nih.gov/entrez/query.fcgi?cmd=Retrieve&db=pubmed&dopt=Abstract&list_uids=14733961

- **Increased solubility of lamins and redistribution of lamin C in X-linked Emery-Dreifuss muscular dystrophy fibroblasts.**
  Author(s): Markiewicz E, Venables R, Mauricio-Alvarez-Reyes, Quinlan R, Dorobek M, Hausmanowa-Petrucewicz I, Hutchison C.
  Source: Journal of Structural Biology. 2002 October-December; 140(1-3): 241-53.
  http://www.ncbi.nlm.nih.gov/entrez/query.fcgi?cmd=Retrieve&db=pubmed&dopt=Abstract&list_uids=12490172

- **Indications for a novel muscular dystrophy pathway. gamma-filamin, the muscle-specific filamin isoform, interacts with myotilin.**
  Author(s): van der Ven PF, Wiesner S, Salmikangas P, Auerbach D, Himmel M, Kempa S, Hayess K, Pacholsky D, Taivainen A, Schroder R, Carpen O, Furst DO.
  Source: The Journal of Cell Biology. 2000 October 16; 151(2): 235-48.
  http://www.ncbi.nlm.nih.gov/entrez/query.fcgi?cmd=Retrieve&db=pubmed&dopt=Abstract&list_uids=11038172

- **Inheritance of a 38-kb fragment in apparently sporadic facioscapulohumeral muscular dystrophy.**
  Author(s): Vitelli F, Villanova M, Malandrini A, Bruttini M, Piccini M, Merlini L, Guazzi G, Renieri A.
  Source: Muscle & Nerve. 1999 October; 22(10): 1437-41.
  http://www.ncbi.nlm.nih.gov/entrez/query.fcgi?cmd=Retrieve&db=pubmed&dopt=Abstract&list_uids=10487912

- **Integrin alpha 7 beta 1 in muscular dystrophy/myopathy of unknown etiology.**
  Author(s): Pegoraro E, Cepollaro F, Prandini P, Marin A, Fanin M, Trevisan CP, El-Messlemani AH, Tarone G, Engvall E, Hoffman EP, Angelini C.
  Source: American Journal of Pathology. 2002 June; 160(6): 2135-43.
  http://www.ncbi.nlm.nih.gov/entrez/query.fcgi?cmd=Retrieve&db=pubmed&dopt=Abstract&list_uids=12057917

- **Intranuclear inclusions in oculopharyngeal muscular dystrophy contain poly(A) binding protein 2.**
  Author(s): Becher MW, Kotzuk JA, Davis LE, Bear DG.
  Source: Annals of Neurology. 2000 November; 48(5): 812-5.
  http://www.ncbi.nlm.nih.gov/entrez/query.fcgi?cmd=Retrieve&db=pubmed&dopt=Abstract&list_uids=11079550

- **Involvement of the ubiquitin-proteasome pathway and molecular chaperones in oculopharyngeal muscular dystrophy.**
  Author(s): Abu-Baker A, Messaed C, Laganiere J, Gaspar C, Brais B, Rouleau GA.
  Source: Human Molecular Genetics. 2003 October 15; 12(20): 2609-23. Epub 2003 August 27.
  http://www.ncbi.nlm.nih.gov/entrez/query.fcgi?cmd=Retrieve&db=pubmed&dopt=Abstract&list_uids=12944420

- **Is there selection in favour of heterozygotes in families with merosin-deficient congenital muscular dystrophy?**
  Author(s): D'Alessandro M, Naom I, Ferlini A, Sewry C, Dubowitz V, Muntoni F.
  Source: Human Genetics. 1999 October; 105(4): 308-13.
  http://www.ncbi.nlm.nih.gov/entrez/query.fcgi?cmd=Retrieve&db=pubmed&dopt=Abstract&list_uids=10543397

- **It is bundle branch reentry linked to any kind of muscular dystrophy?**
  Author(s): Merino JL, Peinado R.
  Source: Journal of Cardiovascular Electrophysiology. 1998 December; 9(12): 1397-8.
  http://www.ncbi.nlm.nih.gov/entrez/query.fcgi?cmd=Retrieve&db=pubmed&dopt=Abstract&list_uids=9869540

- **Juvenile limb-girdle muscular dystrophy. Clinical, histopathological and genetic data from a small community living in the Reunion Island.**
  Author(s): Fardeau M, Hillaire D, Mignard C, Feingold N, Feingold J, Mignard D, de Ubeda B, Collin H, Tome FM, Richard I, Beckmann J.
  Source: Brain; a Journal of Neurology. 1996 February; 119 (Pt 1): 295-308.
  http://www.ncbi.nlm.nih.gov/entrez/query.fcgi?cmd=Retrieve&db=pubmed&dopt=Abstract&list_uids=8624690

- **Laminin alpha 2-chain gene mutations in two siblings presenting with limb-girdle muscular dystrophy.**
  Author(s): Naom I, D'Alessandro M, Sewry CA, Philpot J, Manzur AY, Dubowitz V, Muntoni F.
  Source: Neuromuscular Disorders: Nmd. 1998 October; 8(7): 495-501.
  http://www.ncbi.nlm.nih.gov/entrez/query.fcgi?cmd=Retrieve&db=pubmed&dopt=Abstract&list_uids=9829280

- **Late-onset autosomal recessive limb-girdle muscular dystrophy with rimmed vacuoles.**
  Author(s): Nakamura A, Yoshida K, Ikeda S.
  Source: Clinical Neurology and Neurosurgery. 2004 March; 106(2): 122-8.
  http://www.ncbi.nlm.nih.gov/entrez/query.fcgi?cmd=Retrieve&db=pubmed&dopt=Abstract&list_uids=15003303

- **Late-onset distal muscular dystrophy affecting the posterior calves.**
  Author(s): Katz JS, Rando TA, Barohn RJ, Saperstein DS, Jackson CE, Wicklund M, Amato AA.
  Source: Muscle & Nerve. 2003 October; 28(4): 443-8.
  http://www.ncbi.nlm.nih.gov/entrez/query.fcgi?cmd=Retrieve&db=pubmed&dopt=Abstract&list_uids=14506716

- **Life-long course and molecular characterization of the original Dutch family with epidermolysis bullosa simplex with muscular dystrophy due to a homozygous novel plectin point mutation.**
  Author(s): Koss-Harnes D, Hoyheim B, Jonkman MF, de Groot WP, de Weerdt CJ, Nikolic B, Wiche G, Gedde-Dahl T Jr.
  Source: Acta Dermato-Venereologica. 2004; 84(2): 124-31.
  http://www.ncbi.nlm.nih.gov/entrez/query.fcgi?cmd=Retrieve&db=pubmed&dopt=Abstract&list_uids=15206692

- **Limb girdle muscular dystrophy type 2A (CAPN3): mapping using allelic association.**
  Author(s): Lonjou C, Collins A, Beckmann J, Allamand V, Morton N.
  Source: Human Heredity. 1998 November-December; 48(6): 333-7.
  http://www.ncbi.nlm.nih.gov/entrez/query.fcgi?cmd=Retrieve&db=pubmed&dopt=Abstract&list_uids=9813455

- **Limb girdle muscular dystrophy: use of dHPLC and direct sequencing to detect sarcoglycan gene mutations in a New Zealand cohort.**
  Author(s): Love DR.
  Source: Clinical Genetics. 2004 January; 65(1): 55-60.
  http://www.ncbi.nlm.nih.gov/entrez/query.fcgi?cmd=Retrieve&db=pubmed&dopt=Abstract&list_uids=15032976

- **Limb-girdle muscular dystrophy 2I: phenotypic variability within a large consanguineous Bedouin family associated with a novel FKRP mutation.**
  Author(s): Harel T, Goldberg Y, Shalev SA, Chervinski I, Ofir R, Birk OS.
  Source: European Journal of Human Genetics: Ejhg. 2004 January; 12(1): 38-43.
  http://www.ncbi.nlm.nih.gov/entrez/query.fcgi?cmd=Retrieve&db=pubmed&dopt=Abstract&list_uids=14523375

- **Limb-girdle muscular dystrophy in a 71-year-old woman with an R27Q mutation in the CAV3 gene.**
  Author(s): Figarella-Branger D, Pouget J, Bernard R, Krahn M, Fernandez C, Levy N, Pellissier JF.
  Source: Neurology. 2003 August 26; 61(4): 562-4. Review.
  http://www.ncbi.nlm.nih.gov/entrez/query.fcgi?cmd=Retrieve&db=pubmed&dopt=Abstract&list_uids=12939441

- **Limb-girdle muscular dystrophy in Guipuzcoa (Basque Country, Spain).**
  Author(s): Urtasun M, Saenz A, Roudaut C, Poza JJ, Urtizberea JA, Cobo AM, Richard I, Garcia Bragado F, Leturcq F, Kaplan JC, Marti Masso JF, Beckmann JS, Lopez de Munain A.
  Source: Brain; a Journal of Neurology. 1998 September; 121 (Pt 9): 1735-47.
  http://www.ncbi.nlm.nih.gov/entrez/query.fcgi?cmd=Retrieve&db=pubmed&dopt=Abstract&list_uids=9762961

- **Llama-derived phage display antibodies in the dissection of the human disease oculopharyngeal muscular dystrophy.**
  Author(s): van Koningsbruggen S, de Haard H, de Kievit P, Dirks RW, van Remoortere A, Groot AJ, van Engelen BG, den Dunnen JT, Verrips CT, Frants RR, van der Maarel SM.
  Source: Journal of Immunological Methods. 2003 August; 279(1-2): 149-61.
  http://www.ncbi.nlm.nih.gov/entrez/query.fcgi?cmd=Retrieve&db=pubmed&dopt=Abstract&list_uids=12969556

- **Loss of a single amino acid from dystrophin resulting in Duchenne muscular dystrophy with retention of dystrophin protein.**
  Author(s): Becker K, Robb SA, Hatton Z, Yau SC, Abbs S, Roberts RG.
  Source: Human Mutation. 2003 June; 21(6): 651.
  http://www.ncbi.nlm.nih.gov/entrez/query.fcgi?cmd=Retrieve&db=pubmed&dopt=Abstract&list_uids=14961551

- **Malignant hyperthermia-like episode in Becker muscular dystrophy.**
  Author(s): Kleopa KA, Rosenberg H, Heiman-Patterson T.
  Source: Anesthesiology. 2000 December; 93(6): 1535-7.
  http://www.ncbi.nlm.nih.gov/entrez/query.fcgi?cmd=Retrieve&db=pubmed&dopt=Abstract&list_uids=11149452

- **Mechanism and timing of mitotic rearrangements in the subtelomeric D4Z4 repeat involved in facioscapulohumeral muscular dystrophy.**
  Author(s): Lemmers RJ, Van Overveld PG, Sandkuijl LA, Vrieling H, Padberg GW, Frants RR, van der Maarel SM.
  Source: American Journal of Human Genetics. 2004 July; 75(1): 44-53. Epub 2004 May 20.
  http://www.ncbi.nlm.nih.gov/entrez/query.fcgi?cmd=Retrieve&db=pubmed&dopt=Abstract&list_uids=15154112

- **Merosin negative congenital muscular dystrophy: a short report.**
  Author(s): Ralte AM, Sharma MC, Gulati S, Das M, Sarkar C.
  Source: Neurology India. 2003 September; 51(3): 417-9.
  http://www.ncbi.nlm.nih.gov/entrez/query.fcgi?cmd=Retrieve&db=pubmed&dopt=Abstract&list_uids=14652462

- **Mitochondrial abnormalities in genetically assessed oculopharyngeal muscular dystrophy.**
  Author(s): Gambelli S, Malandrini A, Ginanneschi F, Berti G, Cardaioli E, De Stefano R, Franci M, Salvadori C, Mari F, Bruttini M, Rossi A, Federico A, Renieri A.
  Source: European Neurology. 2004; 51(3): 144-7. Epub 2004 February 27.
  http://www.ncbi.nlm.nih.gov/entrez/query.fcgi?cmd=Retrieve&db=pubmed&dopt=Abstract&list_uids=14988608

- **Molecular basis of facioscapulohumeral muscular dystrophy.**
  Author(s): Tupler R, Gabellini D.
  Source: Cellular and Molecular Life Sciences: Cmls. 2004 March; 61(5): 557-66. Review.
  http://www.ncbi.nlm.nih.gov/entrez/query.fcgi?cmd=Retrieve&db=pubmed&dopt=Abstract&list_uids=15004695

- **Motor unit changes in inflammatory myopathy and progressive muscular dystrophy.**
  Author(s): Rowinska-Marcinska K, Szmidt-Salkowska E, Kopec A, Wawro A, Karwanska A.
  Source: Electromyogr Clin Neurophysiol. 2000 October-November; 40(7): 431-9.
  http://www.ncbi.nlm.nih.gov/entrez/query.fcgi?cmd=Retrieve&db=pubmed&dopt=Abstract&list_uids=11142114

- **Muscular dystrophy meets the gene chip: new insights into disease pathogenesis.**
  Author(s): Chamberlain JS.
  Source: The Journal of Cell Biology. 2000 December 11; 151(6): F43-5.
  http://www.ncbi.nlm.nih.gov/entrez/query.fcgi?cmd=Retrieve&db=pubmed&dopt=Abstract&list_uids=11121429

- **Muscular dystrophy overview: genetics and diagnosis.**
  Author(s): Mathews KD.
  Source: Neurologic Clinics. 2003 November; 21(4): 795-816. Review.
  http://www.ncbi.nlm.nih.gov/entrez/query.fcgi?cmd=Retrieve&db=pubmed&dopt=Abstract&list_uids=14743650

- **Myopathy phenotype in transgenic mice expressing mutated PABPN1 as a model of oculopharyngeal muscular dystrophy.**
  Author(s): Hino H, Araki K, Uyama E, Takeya M, Araki M, Yoshinobu K, Miike K, Kawazoe Y, Maeda Y, Uchino M, Yamamura K.
  Source: Human Molecular Genetics. 2004 January 15; 13(2): 181-90. Epub 2003 November 25.
  http://www.ncbi.nlm.nih.gov/entrez/query.fcgi?cmd=Retrieve&db=pubmed&dopt=Abstract&list_uids=14645203

- **Myotilin is mutated in limb girdle muscular dystrophy 1A.**
  Author(s): Hauser MA, Horrigan SK, Salmikangas P, Torian UM, Viles KD, Dancel R, Tim RW, Taivainen A, Bartoloni L, Gilchrist JM, Stajich JM, Gaskell PC, Gilbert JR, Vance JM, Pericak-Vance MA, Carpen O, Westbrook CA, Speer MC.
  Source: Human Molecular Genetics. 2000 September 1; 9(14): 2141-7.
  http://www.ncbi.nlm.nih.gov/entrez/query.fcgi?cmd=Retrieve&db=pubmed&dopt=Abstract&list_uids=10958653

- **New aspects of calcium signaling in skeletal muscle cells: implications in Duchenne muscular dystrophy.**
  Author(s): Gailly P.
  Source: Biochimica Et Biophysica Acta. 2002 November 4; 1600(1-2): 38-44. Review.
  http://www.ncbi.nlm.nih.gov/entrez/query.fcgi?cmd=Retrieve&db=pubmed&dopt=Abstract&list_uids=12445457

- **New FKRP mutations causing congenital muscular dystrophy associated with mental retardation and central nervous system abnormalities. Identification of a founder mutation in Tunisian families.**
  Author(s): Louhichi N, Triki C, Quijano-Roy S, Richard P, Makri S, Meziou M, Estournet B, Mrad S, Romero NB, Ayadi H, Guicheney P, Fakhfakh F.
  Source: Neurogenetics. 2004 February; 5(1): 27-34. Epub 2003 December 02.
  http://www.ncbi.nlm.nih.gov/entrez/query.fcgi?cmd=Retrieve&db=pubmed&dopt=Abstract&list_uids=14652796

- **New molecular mechanism for Ullrich congenital muscular dystrophy: a heterozygous in-frame deletion in the COL6A1 gene causes a severe phenotype.**
  Author(s): Pan TC, Zhang RZ, Sudano DG, Marie SK, Bonnemann CG, Chu ML.
  Source: American Journal of Human Genetics. 2003 August; 73(2): 355-69. Epub 2003 July 01.
  http://www.ncbi.nlm.nih.gov/entrez/query.fcgi?cmd=Retrieve&db=pubmed&dopt=Abstract&list_uids=12840783

- **New treatment alternatives for Duchenne and Becker muscular dystrophy.**
  Author(s): Restrepo S.
  Source: Neurology. 2004 March 23; 62(6): E10.
  http://www.ncbi.nlm.nih.gov/entrez/query.fcgi?cmd=Retrieve&db=pubmed&dopt=Abstract&list_uids=15037729

- **Newborn screening for Duchenne muscular dystrophy.**
  Author(s): Parsons EP, Bradley DM, Clarke AJ.
  Source: Archives of Disease in Childhood. 2003 January; 88(1): 91-2.
  http://www.ncbi.nlm.nih.gov/entrez/query.fcgi?cmd=Retrieve&db=pubmed&dopt=Abstract&list_uids=12495984

- **NO skeletal muscle derived relaxing factor in Duchenne muscular dystrophy.**
  Author(s): Bredt DS.
  Source: Proceedings of the National Academy of Sciences of the United States of America. 1998 December 8; 95(25): 14592-3.
  http://www.ncbi.nlm.nih.gov/entrez/query.fcgi?cmd=Retrieve&db=pubmed&dopt=Abstract&list_uids=9843933

- **NO vascular control in Duchenne muscular dystrophy.**
  Author(s): Crosbie RH.
  Source: Nature Medicine. 2001 January; 7(1): 27-9.
  http://www.ncbi.nlm.nih.gov/entrez/query.fcgi?cmd=Retrieve&db=pubmed&dopt=Abstract&list_uids=11135610

- **Non-operative treatment for perforated gastro-duodenal peptic ulcer in Duchenne muscular dystrophy: a case report.**
  Author(s): Brinkman JM, Oddens JR, Van Royen BJ, Wever J, Olsman JG.
  Source: Bmc Surgery [electronic Resource]. 2004 January 08; 4(1): 1.
  http://www.ncbi.nlm.nih.gov/entrez/query.fcgi?cmd=Retrieve&db=pubmed&dopt=Abstract&list_uids=14713321

- **Nuclear accumulation of expanded PABP2 gene product in oculopharyngeal muscular dystrophy.**
  Author(s): Uyama E, Tsukahara T, Goto K, Kurano Y, Ogawa M, Kim YJ, Uchino M, Arahata K.
  Source: Muscle & Nerve. 2000 October; 23(10): 1549-54.
  http://www.ncbi.nlm.nih.gov/entrez/query.fcgi?cmd=Retrieve&db=pubmed&dopt=Abstract&list_uids=11003790

- **Obstructive sleep apnea syndrome complicating oculopharyngeal muscular dystrophy.**
  Author(s): Dedrick DL, Brown LK.
  Source: Chest. 2004 January; 125(1): 334-6.
  http://www.ncbi.nlm.nih.gov/entrez/query.fcgi?cmd=Retrieve&db=pubmed&dopt=Abstract&list_uids=14718463

- **Occidental-type cerebromuscular dystrophy versus congenital muscular dystrophy with merosin deficiency.**
  Author(s): Castro-Gago M.
  Source: Child's Nervous System: Chns: Official Journal of the International Society for Pediatric Neurosurgery. 1998 October; 14(10): 531.
  http://www.ncbi.nlm.nih.gov/entrez/query.fcgi?cmd=Retrieve&db=pubmed&dopt=Abstract&list_uids=9840374

- **Occipito-temporal polymicrogyria and subclinical muscular dystrophy.**
  Author(s): Zolkipli Z, Hartley L, Brown S, Rutherford M, Cowan F, Mercuri E, Muntoni F.
  Source: Neuropediatrics. 2003 April; 34(2): 92-5.
  http://www.ncbi.nlm.nih.gov/entrez/query.fcgi?cmd=Retrieve&db=pubmed&dopt=Abstract&list_uids=12776231

- **Oculopharyngeal muscular dystrophy (OPMD) due to a small duplication in the PABPN1 gene.**
  Author(s): van der Sluijs BM, van Engelen BG, Hoefsloot LH.
  Source: Human Mutation. 2003 May; 21(5): 553.
  http://www.ncbi.nlm.nih.gov/entrez/query.fcgi?cmd=Retrieve&db=pubmed&dopt=Abstract&list_uids=12673802

- **Oculopharyngeal muscular dystrophy with limb girdle weakness as major complaint.**
  Author(s): Van Der Sluijs BM, Hoefsloot LH, Padberg GW, Van Der Maarel SM, Van Engelen BG.
  Source: Journal of Neurology. 2003 November; 250(11): 1307-12.
  http://www.ncbi.nlm.nih.gov/entrez/query.fcgi?cmd=Retrieve&db=pubmed&dopt=Abstract&list_uids=14648146

- **Oculopharyngeal muscular dystrophy: a late-onset polyalanine disease.**
  Author(s): Brais B.
  Source: Cytogenetic and Genome Research. 2003; 100(1-4): 252-60. Review.
  http://www.ncbi.nlm.nih.gov/entrez/query.fcgi?cmd=Retrieve&db=pubmed&dopt=Abstract&list_uids=14526187

- **Optimization of power wheelchair control for patients with severe Duchenne muscular dystrophy.**
  Author(s): Pellegrini N, Guillon B, Prigent H, Pellegrini M, Orlikovski D, Raphael JC, Lofaso F.
  Source: Neuromuscular Disorders: Nmd. 2004 May; 14(5): 297-300.
  http://www.ncbi.nlm.nih.gov/entrez/query.fcgi?cmd=Retrieve&db=pubmed&dopt=Abstract&list_uids=15099587

- **Origins and early descriptions of "Duchenne muscular dystrophy".**
  Author(s): Tyler KL.
  Source: Muscle & Nerve. 2003 October; 28(4): 402-22.
  http://www.ncbi.nlm.nih.gov/entrez/query.fcgi?cmd=Retrieve&db=pubmed&dopt=Abstract&list_uids=14506712

- **Orthodontic treatment of a case of Becker muscular dystrophy.**
  Author(s): Suda N, Matsuda A, Yoda S, Ishizaki T, Higashibori N, Kim F, Otani-Saito K, Ohyama K.
  Source: Orthodontics & Craniofacial Research. 2004 February; 7(1): 55-62.
  http://www.ncbi.nlm.nih.gov/entrez/query.fcgi?cmd=Retrieve&db=pubmed&dopt=Abstract&list_uids=14989756

- **Oxidative stress in the brain of Fukuyama type congenital muscular dystrophy: immunohistochemical study on astrocytes.**
  Author(s): Yamamoto T, Shibata N, Kobayashi M, Saito K, Osawa M.
  Source: Journal of Child Neurology. 2002 November; 17(11): 793-9.
  http://www.ncbi.nlm.nih.gov/entrez/query.fcgi?cmd=Retrieve&db=pubmed&dopt=Abstract&list_uids=12585716

- **Pathological changes of the myonuclear fibrous lamina and internal nuclear membrane in two cases of autosomal dominant limb-girdle muscular dystrophy with atrioventricular conduction disturbance (LGMD1B).**
  Author(s): Matsubara S, Kitaguchi T.
  Source: Acta Neuropathologica. 2004 February; 107(2): 111-8. Epub 2003 December 11.
  http://www.ncbi.nlm.nih.gov/entrez/query.fcgi?cmd=Retrieve&db=pubmed&dopt=Abstract&list_uids=14673599

- **Persistent hypertransaminasemia as the presenting findings of muscular dystrophy in childhood.**
  Author(s): Lin YC, Lee WT, Huang SF, Young C, Wang PJ, Shen YZ.
  Source: Acta Paediatr Taiwan. 1999 November-December; 40(6): 424-9.
  http://www.ncbi.nlm.nih.gov/entrez/query.fcgi?cmd=Retrieve&db=pubmed&dopt=Abstract&list_uids=10927957

- **Pilot study of myoblast transfer in the treatment of Becker muscular dystrophy.**
  Author(s): Neumeyer AM, Cros D, McKenna-Yasek D, Zawadzka A, Hoffman EP, Pegoraro E, Hunter RG, Munsat TL, Brown RH Jr.
  Source: Neurology. 1998 August; 51(2): 589-92.
  http://www.ncbi.nlm.nih.gov/entrez/query.fcgi?cmd=Retrieve&db=pubmed&dopt=Abstract&list_uids=9710042

- **Pilot trial of albuterol in Duchenne and Becker muscular dystrophy.**
  Author(s): Fowler EG, Graves MC, Wetzel GT, Spencer MJ.
  Source: Neurology. 2004 March 23; 62(6): 1006-8.
  http://www.ncbi.nlm.nih.gov/entrez/query.fcgi?cmd=Retrieve&db=pubmed&dopt=Abstract&list_uids=15037714

- **Pneumothorax associated with long-term non-invasive positive pressure ventilation in Duchenne muscular dystrophy.**
  Author(s): Vianello A, Arcaro G, Gallan F, Ori C, Bevilacqua M.
  Source: Neuromuscular Disorders: Nmd. 2004 June; 14(6): 353-5.
  http://www.ncbi.nlm.nih.gov/entrez/query.fcgi?cmd=Retrieve&db=pubmed&dopt=Abstract&list_uids=15145335

- **Prenatal diagnosis of limb-girdle muscular dystrophy type 2C.**
Author(s): Dincer P, Piccolo F, Leturcq F, Kaplan JC, Jeanpierre M, Topaloglu H.
Source: Prenatal Diagnosis. 1998 December; 18(12): 1300-3.
http://www.ncbi.nlm.nih.gov/entrez/query.fcgi?cmd=Retrieve&db=pubmed&dopt=Abstract&list_uids=9885023

- **Progression of cardiac involvement in patients with myotonic dystrophy, Becker's muscular dystrophy and mitochondrial myopathy during a 2-year follow-up.**
Author(s): Stollberger C, Finsterer J, Keller H, Mamoli B, Slany J.
Source: Cardiology. 1998 December; 90(3): 173-9.
http://www.ncbi.nlm.nih.gov/entrez/query.fcgi?cmd=Retrieve&db=pubmed&dopt=Abstract&list_uids=9892765

- **Progression of scoliosis after spinal fusion in Duchenne's muscular dystrophy.**
Author(s): Gaine WJ, Lim J, Stephenson W, Galasko CS.
Source: The Journal of Bone and Joint Surgery. British Volume. 2004 May; 86(4): 550-5.
http://www.ncbi.nlm.nih.gov/entrez/query.fcgi?cmd=Retrieve&db=pubmed&dopt=Abstract&list_uids=15174552

- **Properties of Ca2+-activated K+ channels in erythrocytes from patients with myotonic muscular dystrophy.**
Author(s): Pellegrino M, Pellegrini M, Bigini P, Scimemi A.
Source: Muscle & Nerve. 1998 November; 21(11): 1465-72.
http://www.ncbi.nlm.nih.gov/entrez/query.fcgi?cmd=Retrieve&db=pubmed&dopt=Abstract&list_uids=9771671

- **Pseudohypertrophy of the temporalis muscle in Xp21 muscular dystrophy.**
Author(s): Richards P, Saywell WR, Heywood P.
Source: Developmental Medicine and Child Neurology. 2000 November; 42(11): 786-7.
http://www.ncbi.nlm.nih.gov/entrez/query.fcgi?cmd=Retrieve&db=pubmed&dopt=Abstract&list_uids=11104355

- **QT dispersion in patients with Duchenne-type progressive muscular dystrophy.**
  Author(s): Yotsukura M, Yamamoto A, Kajiwara T, Nishimura T, Sakata K, Ishihara T, Ishikawa K.
  Source: American Heart Journal. 1999 April; 137(4 Pt 1): 672-7.
  http://www.ncbi.nlm.nih.gov/entrez/query.fcgi?cmd=Retrieve&db=pubmed&dopt=Abstract&list_uids=10097228

- **Quantitative and qualitative alterations of dystrophin are expressed in muscle cell cultures of Xp21 muscular dystrophy patients (Duchenne and Becker type).**
  Author(s): Mongini T, Doriguzzi C, Palmucci L, Chiado-Piat L.
  Source: European Journal of Clinical Investigation. 1996 April; 26(4): 322-4.
  http://www.ncbi.nlm.nih.gov/entrez/query.fcgi?cmd=Retrieve&db=pubmed&dopt=Abstract&list_uids=8732491

- **Quantitative assessment of calf circumference in Duchenne muscular dystrophy patients.**
  Author(s): Beenakker EA, de Vries J, Fock JM, van Tol M, Brouwer OF, Maurits NM, van der Hoeven JH.
  Source: Neuromuscular Disorders: Nmd. 2002 October; 12(7-8): 639-42.
  http://www.ncbi.nlm.nih.gov/entrez/query.fcgi?cmd=Retrieve&db=pubmed&dopt=Abstract&list_uids=12207931

- **Quantitative ELISA for platelet m-calpain: a phenotypic index for detection of carriers of Duchenne muscular dystrophy.**
  Author(s): Hussain T, Kumar DV, Sundaram C, Mohandas S, Anandaraj MP.
  Source: Clinica Chimica Acta; International Journal of Clinical Chemistry. 1998 January 12; 269(1): 13-20.
  http://www.ncbi.nlm.nih.gov/entrez/query.fcgi?cmd=Retrieve&db=pubmed&dopt=Abstract&list_uids=9498100

- **Quantitative MR evaluation of body composition in patients with Duchenne muscular dystrophy.**
  Author(s): Leroy-Willig A.
  Source: European Radiology. 2003 December; 13(12): 2710-1; Author Reply 2712. Epub 2003 March 26.
  http://www.ncbi.nlm.nih.gov/entrez/query.fcgi?cmd=Retrieve&db=pubmed&dopt=Abstract&list_uids=14634784

- **Quantitative MR evaluation of body composition in patients with Duchenne muscular dystrophy.**
  Author(s): Pichiecchio A, Uggetti C, Egitto MG, Berardinelli A, Orcesi S, Gorni KO, Zanardi C, Tagliabue A.
  Source: European Radiology. 2002 November; 12(11): 2704-9. Epub 2002 May 08.
  http://www.ncbi.nlm.nih.gov/entrez/query.fcgi?cmd=Retrieve&db=pubmed&dopt=Abstract&list_uids=12386760

- **Reasons to be cheerful. Genetic diagnosis and therapy are offering hope to people with muscular dystrophy.**
  Author(s): Bird C.
  Source: Nurs Times. 2001 August 2-8; 97(31): 25. No Abstract Available.
  http://www.ncbi.nlm.nih.gov/entrez/query.fcgi?cmd=Retrieve&db=pubmed&dopt=Abstract&list_uids=11957528

- **Recurrent pneumothoraces associated with nocturnal noninvasive ventilation in a patient with muscular dystrophy.**
  Author(s): Choo-Kang LR, Ogunlesi FO, McGrath-Morrow SA, Crawford TO, Marcus CL.
  Source: Pediatric Pulmonology. 2002 July; 34(1): 73-8.
  http://www.ncbi.nlm.nih.gov/entrez/query.fcgi?cmd=Retrieve&db=pubmed&dopt=Abstract&list_uids=12112801

- **Re-evaluation of reading frame-shift hypothesis in Duchenne and Becker muscular dystrophy.**
  Author(s): Pandey GS, Kesari A, Mukherjee M, Mittal RD, Mittal B.
  Source: Neurology India. 2003 September; 51(3): 367-9.
  http://www.ncbi.nlm.nih.gov/entrez/query.fcgi?cmd=Retrieve&db=pubmed&dopt=Abstract&list_uids=14652441

- **Relationship between utrophin and regenerating muscle fibers in duchenne muscular dystrophy.**
  Author(s): Shim JY, Kim TS.
  Source: Yonsei Medical Journal. 2003 February; 44(1): 15-23.
  http://www.ncbi.nlm.nih.gov/entrez/query.fcgi?cmd=Retrieve&db=pubmed&dopt=Abstract&list_uids=12619170

- **Remission of clinical signs in early duchenne muscular dystrophy on intermittent low-dosage prednisolone therapy.**
  Author(s): Dubowitz V, Kinali M, Main M, Mercuri E, Muntoni F.
  Source: European Journal of Paediatric Neurology: Ejpn: Official Journal of the European Paediatric Neurology Society. 2002; 6(3): 153-9.
  http://www.ncbi.nlm.nih.gov/entrez/query.fcgi?cmd=Retrieve&db=pubmed&dopt=Abstract&list_uids=12363102

- **Removal of dystroglycan causes severe muscular dystrophy in zebrafish embryos.**
  Author(s): Parsons MJ, Campos I, Hirst EM, Stemple DL.
  Source: Development (Cambridge, England). 2002 July; 129(14): 3505-12.
  http://www.ncbi.nlm.nih.gov/entrez/query.fcgi?cmd=Retrieve&db=pubmed&dopt=Abstract&list_uids=12091319

- **Restriction map of a YAC and cosmid contig encompassing the oculopharyngeal muscular dystrophy candidate region on chromosome 14q11.2-q13.**
  Author(s): Xie YG, Rochefort D, Brais B, Howard H, Han FY, Gou LP, Maciel P, The BT, Larsson C, Rouleau GA.
  Source: Genomics. 1998 September 1; 52(2): 201-4.
  http://www.ncbi.nlm.nih.gov/entrez/query.fcgi?cmd=Retrieve&db=pubmed&dopt=Abstract&list_uids=9782086

- **Role of apoptosis in Duchenne's muscular dystrophy.**
  Author(s): Serdaroglu A, Gucuyener K, Erdem S, Kose G, Tan E, Okuyaz C.
  Source: Journal of Child Neurology. 2002 January; 17(1): 66-8.
  http://www.ncbi.nlm.nih.gov/entrez/query.fcgi?cmd=Retrieve&db=pubmed&dopt=Abstract&list_uids=11913578

- **Role of dystrophin isoforms and associated proteins in muscular dystrophy (review).**
  Author(s): Culligan KG, Mackey AJ, Finn DM, Maguire PB, Ohlendieck K.
  Source: International Journal of Molecular Medicine. 1998 December; 2(6): 639-48. Review.
  http://www.ncbi.nlm.nih.gov/entrez/query.fcgi?cmd=Retrieve&db=pubmed&dopt=Abstract&list_uids=9850730

- **Sequence specificity of aminoglycoside-induced stop condon readthrough: potential implications for treatment of Duchenne muscular dystrophy.**
  Author(s): Howard MT, Shirts BH, Petros LM, Flanigan KM, Gesteland RF, Atkins JF.
  Source: Annals of Neurology. 2000 August; 48(2): 164-9.
  http://www.ncbi.nlm.nih.gov/entrez/query.fcgi?cmd=Retrieve&db=pubmed&dopt=Abstract&list_uids=10939566

- **Severe classical congenital muscular dystrophy and merosin expression.**
  Author(s): Vajsar J, Chitayat D, Becker LE, Ho M, Ben-Zeev B, Jay V.
  Source: Clinical Genetics. 1998 September; 54(3): 193-8.
  http://www.ncbi.nlm.nih.gov/entrez/query.fcgi?cmd=Retrieve&db=pubmed&dopt=Abstract&list_uids=9788720

- **Severe limb girdle muscular dystrophy in Spanish gypsies: further evidence for a founder mutation in the gamma-sarcoglycan gene.**
  Author(s): Lasa A, Piccolo F, de Diego C, Jeanpierre M, Colomer J, Rodriguez MJ, Urtizberea JA, Baiget M, Kaplan J, Gallano P.
  Source: European Journal of Human Genetics: Ejhg. 1998 July-August; 6(4): 396-9.
  http://www.ncbi.nlm.nih.gov/entrez/query.fcgi?cmd=Retrieve&db=pubmed&dopt=Abstract&list_uids=9781048

- **Severe mucous membrane involvement in epidermolysis bullosa simplex with muscular dystrophy due to a novel plectin gene mutation.**
  Author(s): Schara U, Tucke J, Mortier W, Nusslein T, Rouan F, Pfendner E, Zillikens D, Bruckner-Tuderman L, Uitto J, Wiche G, Schroder R.
  Source: European Journal of Pediatrics. 2004 April; 163(4-5): 218-22. Epub 2004 February 13.
  http://www.ncbi.nlm.nih.gov/entrez/query.fcgi?cmd=Retrieve&db=pubmed&dopt=Abstract&list_uids=14963703

- **Specific cognitive deficits are common in children with Duchenne muscular dystrophy.**
  Author(s): Wicksell RK, Kihlgren M, Melin L, Eeg-Olofsson O.
  Source: Developmental Medicine and Child Neurology. 2004 March; 46(3): 154-9.
  http://www.ncbi.nlm.nih.gov/entrez/query.fcgi?cmd=Retrieve&db=pubmed&dopt=Abstract&list_uids=14995084

- **Steroid treatment and the development of scoliosis in males with duchenne muscular dystrophy.**
  Author(s): Alman BA, Raza SN, Biggar WD.
  Source: The Journal of Bone and Joint Surgery. American Volume. 2004 March; 86-A(3): 519-24.
  http://www.ncbi.nlm.nih.gov/entrez/query.fcgi?cmd=Retrieve&db=pubmed&dopt=Abstract&list_uids=14996877

- **Stiffness of knee extensors in Duchenne muscular dystrophy.**
  Author(s): Cornu C, Goubel F, Fardeau M.
  Source: Muscle & Nerve. 1998 December; 21(12): 1772-4.
  http://www.ncbi.nlm.nih.gov/entrez/query.fcgi?cmd=Retrieve&db=pubmed&dopt=Abstract&list_uids=9843081

- **Subclinical Becker's muscular dystrophy presenting with severe heart failure.**
  Author(s): Yokota R, Shirotani M, Kouchi I, Hirai T, Uemori N, Ohta Y, Mitsui Y, Hattori R.
  Source: Intern Med. 2004 March; 43(3): 204-8.
  http://www.ncbi.nlm.nih.gov/entrez/query.fcgi?cmd=Retrieve&db=pubmed&dopt=Abstract&list_uids=15098601

- **Succinylcholine-induced cardiac arrest in unsuspected becker muscular dystrophy--a case report.**
  Author(s): Wu CC, Tseng CS, Shen CH, Yang TC, Chi KP, Ho WM.
  Source: Acta Anaesthesiol Sin. 1998 September; 36(3): 165-8.
  http://www.ncbi.nlm.nih.gov/entrez/query.fcgi?cmd=Retrieve&db=pubmed&dopt=Abstract&list_uids=9874866

- **The Duchenne muscular dystrophy population in Denmark, 1977-2001: prevalence, incidence and survival in relation to the introduction of ventilator use.**
  Author(s): Jeppesen J, Green A, Steffensen BF, Rahbek J.
  Source: Neuromuscular Disorders: Nmd. 2003 December; 13(10): 804-12.
  http://www.ncbi.nlm.nih.gov/entrez/query.fcgi?cmd=Retrieve&db=pubmed&dopt=Abstract&list_uids=14678803

- **The effects of knee-ankle-foot orthoses in the treatment of Duchenne muscular dystrophy: review of the literature.**
  Author(s): Bakker JP, de Groot IJ, Beckerman H, de Jong BA, Lankhorst GJ.
  Source: Clinical Rehabilitation. 2000 August; 14(4): 343-59. Review.
  http://www.ncbi.nlm.nih.gov/entrez/query.fcgi?cmd=Retrieve&db=pubmed&dopt=Abstract&list_uids=10945419

- **The first European family with tibial muscular dystrophy outside the Finnish population.**
  Author(s): de Seze J, Udd B, Haravuori H, Sablonniere B, Maurage CA, Hurtevent JF, Boutry N, Stojkovic T, Schraen S, Petit H, Vermersch P.
  Source: Neurology. 1998 December; 51(6): 1746-8.
  http://www.ncbi.nlm.nih.gov/entrez/query.fcgi?cmd=Retrieve&db=pubmed&dopt=Abstract&list_uids=9855539

- **The Golden Freeway: a preliminary evaluation of a pilot study advancing information technology as a social intervention for boys with Duchenne muscular dystrophy and their families.**
  Author(s): Soutter J, Hamilton N, Russell P, Russell C, Bushby K, Sloper P, Bartlett K.
  Source: Health & Social Care in the Community. 2004 January; 12(1): 25-33.
  http://www.ncbi.nlm.nih.gov/entrez/query.fcgi?cmd=Retrieve&db=pubmed&dopt=Abstract&list_uids=14675362

- **The sarcoglycan complex in limb-girdle muscular dystrophy.**
  Author(s): Lim LE, Campbell KP.
  Source: Current Opinion in Neurology. 1998 October; 11(5): 443-52. Review.
  http://www.ncbi.nlm.nih.gov/entrez/query.fcgi?cmd=Retrieve&db=pubmed&dopt=Abstract&list_uids=9847993

- **The strength and functional performance in patients with facioscapulohumeral muscular dystrophy.**
  Author(s): Lue YJ, Chen SS.
  Source: Kaohsiung J Med Sci. 2000 May; 16(5): 248-54.
  http://www.ncbi.nlm.nih.gov/entrez/query.fcgi?cmd=Retrieve&db=pubmed&dopt=Abstract&list_uids=10969520

- **Three-tiered noninvasive diagnosis in 96% of patients with Duchenne muscular dystrophy (DMD).**
  Author(s): Yan J, Feng J, Buzin CH, Scaringe W, Liu Q, Mendell JR, den Dunnen J, Sommer SS.
  Source: Human Mutation. 2004 February; 23(2): 203-4.
  http://www.ncbi.nlm.nih.gov/entrez/query.fcgi?cmd=Retrieve&db=pubmed&dopt=Abstract&list_uids=14722924

- **Tracheocoele in a Duchenne muscular dystrophy patient. Case report.**
  Author(s): Piazza C, Bolzoni A, Cavaliere S, Peretti G.
  Source: Acta Otorhinolaryngol Ital. 2003 June; 23(3): 194-8.
  http://www.ncbi.nlm.nih.gov/entrez/query.fcgi?cmd=Retrieve&db=pubmed&dopt=Abstract&list_uids=14677314

- **Transgenic overexpression of dystroglycan does not inhibit muscular dystrophy in mdx mice.**
  Author(s): Hoyte K, Jayasinha V, Xia B, Martin PT.
  Source: American Journal of Pathology. 2004 February; 164(2): 711-8.
  http://www.ncbi.nlm.nih.gov/entrez/query.fcgi?cmd=Retrieve&db=pubmed&dopt=Abstract&list_uids=14742274

- **Two cases of chromosome 4q35-linked early onset facioscapulohumeral muscular dystrophy with mental retardation and epilepsy.**
  Author(s): Miura K, Kumagai T, Matsumoto A, Iriyama E, Watanabe K, Goto K, Arahata K.
  Source: Neuropediatrics. 1998 October; 29(5): 239-41.
  http://www.ncbi.nlm.nih.gov/entrez/query.fcgi?cmd=Retrieve&db=pubmed&dopt=Abstract&list_uids=9810558

- **Ullrich scleroatonic muscular dystrophy is caused by recessive mutations in collagen type VI.**
  Author(s): Camacho Vanegas O, Bertini E, Zhang RZ, Petrini S, Minosse C, Sabatelli P, Giusti B, Chu ML, Pepe G.
  Source: Proceedings of the National Academy of Sciences of the United States of America. 2001 June 19; 98(13): 7516-21. Epub 2001 May 29.
  http://www.ncbi.nlm.nih.gov/entrez/query.fcgi?cmd=Retrieve&db=pubmed&dopt=Abstract&list_uids=11381124

- **Ultrasound tissue characterization detects preclinical myocardial structural changes in children affected by Duchenne muscular dystrophy.**
  Author(s): Giglio V, Pasceri V, Messano L, Mangiola F, Pasquini L, Dello Russo A, Damiani A, Mirabella M, Galluzzi G, Tonali P, Ricci E.
  Source: Journal of the American College of Cardiology. 2003 July 16; 42(2): 309-16.
  http://www.ncbi.nlm.nih.gov/entrez/query.fcgi?cmd=Retrieve&db=pubmed&dopt=Abstract&list_uids=12875769

- **Unequal crossing-over in unique PABP2 mutations in Japanese patients: a possible cause of oculopharyngeal muscular dystrophy.**
  Author(s): Nakamoto M, Nakano S, Kawashima S, Ihara M, Nishimura Y, Shinde A, Kakizuka A.
  Source: Archives of Neurology. 2002 March; 59(3): 474-7.
  http://www.ncbi.nlm.nih.gov/entrez/query.fcgi?cmd=Retrieve&db=pubmed&dopt=Abstract&list_uids=11890856

- **Unique PABP2 mutations in "Cajuns" suggest multiple founders of oculopharyngeal muscular dystrophy in populations with French ancestry.**
  Author(s): Scacheri PC, Garcia C, Hebert R, Hoffman EP.
  Source: American Journal of Medical Genetics. 1999 October 29; 86(5): 477-81.
  http://www.ncbi.nlm.nih.gov/entrez/query.fcgi?cmd=Retrieve&db=pubmed&dopt=Abstract&list_uids=10508991

- **Unusual expression of emerin in a patient with X-linked Emery-Dreifuss muscular dystrophy.**
  Author(s): Di Blasi C, Morandi L, Raffaele di Barletta M, Bione S, Bernasconi P, Cerletti M, Bono R, Blasevich F, Toniolo D, Mora M.
  Source: Neuromuscular Disorders: Nmd. 2000 December; 10(8): 567-71.
  http://www.ncbi.nlm.nih.gov/entrez/query.fcgi?cmd=Retrieve&db=pubmed&dopt=Abstract&list_uids=11053683

- **Unusual laminin alpha2 processing in myoblasts from a patient with a novel variant of congenital muscular dystrophy.**
  Author(s): Lattanzi G, Muntoni F, Sabatelli P, Squarzoni S, Maraldi NM, Cenni V, Villanova M, Columbaro M, Merlini L, Marmiroli S.
  Source: Biochemical and Biophysical Research Communications. 2000 November 2; 277(3): 639-42.
  http://www.ncbi.nlm.nih.gov/entrez/query.fcgi?cmd=Retrieve&db=pubmed&dopt=Abstract&list_uids=11062006

- **Unusual triplet expansion associated with neurogenic changes in a family with oculopharyngeal muscular dystrophy.**
  Author(s): Schober R, Kress W, Grahmann F, Kellermann S, Baum P, Gunzel S, Wagner A.
  Source: Neuropathology: Official Journal of the Japanese Society of Neuropathology. 2001 March; 21(1): 45-52.
  http://www.ncbi.nlm.nih.gov/entrez/query.fcgi?cmd=Retrieve&db=pubmed&dopt=Abstract&list_uids=11304042

- **Use of a CEPH meiotic breakpoint panel to refine the locus of limb-girdle muscular dystrophy type 1A (LGMD1A) to a 2-Mb interval on 5q31.**
  Author(s): Bartoloni L, Horrigan SK, Viles KD, Gilchrist JM, Stajich JM, Vance JM, Yamaoka LH, Pericak-Vance MA, Westbrook CA, Speer MC.
  Source: Genomics. 1998 December 1; 54(2): 250-5.
  http://www.ncbi.nlm.nih.gov/entrez/query.fcgi?cmd=Retrieve&db=pubmed&dopt=Abstract&list_uids=9828127

- **Vaginal delivery in a woman with limb-girdle muscular dystrophy. A case report.**
  Author(s): Ayoubi JM, Meddoun M, Jouk PS, Favier M, Pons JC.
  Source: J Reprod Med. 2000 June; 45(6): 498-500.
  http://www.ncbi.nlm.nih.gov/entrez/query.fcgi?cmd=Retrieve&db=pubmed&dopt=Abstract&list_uids=10900585

- **Validity of the EK scale: a functional assessment of non-ambulatory individuals with Duchenne muscular dystrophy or spinal muscular atrophy.**
  Author(s): Steffensen B, Hyde S, Lyager S, Mattsson E.
  Source: Physiotherapy Research International: the Journal for Researchers and Clinicians in Physical Therapy. 2001; 6(3): 119-34.
  http://www.ncbi.nlm.nih.gov/entrez/query.fcgi?cmd=Retrieve&db=pubmed&dopt=Abstract&list_uids=11725594

- **Valley sign in Becker muscular dystrophy and outliers of Duchenne and Becker muscular dystrophy.**
  Author(s): Pradhan S.
  Source: Neurology India. 2004 June; 52(2): 203-5.
  http://www.ncbi.nlm.nih.gov/entrez/query.fcgi?cmd=Retrieve&db=pubmed&dopt=Abstract&list_uids=15269471

- **Valley sign in duchenne muscular dystrophy: importance in patients with inconspicuous calves.**
  Author(s): Pradhan S.
  Source: Neurology India. 2002 June; 50(2): 184-6.
  http://www.ncbi.nlm.nih.gov/entrez/query.fcgi?cmd=Retrieve&db=pubmed&dopt=Abstract&list_uids=12134184

- **Value of myofibrillar protein catabolic rate in Duchenne muscular dystrophy. A study after lower limb surgery.**
  Author(s): Forst J, Kruger P, Forst R.
  Source: Archives of Orthopaedic and Trauma Surgery. 2000; 120(1-2): 38-41.
  http://www.ncbi.nlm.nih.gov/entrez/query.fcgi?cmd=Retrieve&db=pubmed&dopt=Abstract&list_uids=10653102

- **Vascular tortuosity and Coats'-like retinal changes in facioscapulohumeral muscular dystrophy.**
  Author(s): Tekin NF, Saatci AO, Kavukcu S.
  Source: Ophthalmic Surgery and Lasers. 2000 January-February; 31(1): 82-3.
  http://www.ncbi.nlm.nih.gov/entrez/query.fcgi?cmd=Retrieve&db=pubmed&dopt=Abstract&list_uids=10976570

- **Vertebral compression in Duchenne muscular dystrophy following deflazacort.**
  Author(s): Talim B, Malaguti C, Gnudi S, Politano L, Merlini L.
  Source: Neuromuscular Disorders: Nmd. 2002 March; 12(3): 294-5.
  http://www.ncbi.nlm.nih.gov/entrez/query.fcgi?cmd=Retrieve&db=pubmed&dopt=Abstract&list_uids=11801403

- **Vertebral fractures in boys with Duchenne muscular dystrophy.**
  Author(s): Bothwell JE, Gordon KE, Dooley JM, MacSween J, Cummings EA, Salisbury S.
  Source: Clinical Pediatrics. 2003 May; 42(4): 353-6.
  http://www.ncbi.nlm.nih.gov/entrez/query.fcgi?cmd=Retrieve&db=pubmed&dopt=Abstract&list_uids=12800730

- **Very low penetrance in 85 Japanese families with facioscapulohumeral muscular dystrophy 1A.**
  Author(s): Goto K, Nishino I, Hayashi YK.
  Source: Journal of Medical Genetics. 2004 January; 41(1): E12.
  http://www.ncbi.nlm.nih.gov/entrez/query.fcgi?cmd=Retrieve&db=pubmed&dopt=Abstract&list_uids=14729852

- **Voiding dysfunction in Duchenne muscular dystrophy.**
  Author(s): Robson WL, Leung AK.
  Source: Archives of Disease in Childhood. 2004 January; 89(1): 92.
  http://www.ncbi.nlm.nih.gov/entrez/query.fcgi?cmd=Retrieve&db=pubmed&dopt=Abstract&list_uids=14709529

- **Walker-Warburg syndrome is genetically distinct from Fukuyama type congenital muscular dystrophy.**
  Author(s): Chadani Y, Kondoh T, Kamimura N, Matsumoto T, Matsuzaka T, Kobayashi O, Kondo-Iida E, Kobayashi K, Nonaka I, Toda T.
  Source: Journal of the Neurological Sciences. 2000 August 15; 177(2): 150-3.
  http://www.ncbi.nlm.nih.gov/entrez/query.fcgi?cmd=Retrieve&db=pubmed&dopt=Abstract&list_uids=10980312

- **What is muscular dystrophy? Forty years of progressive ignorance.**
  Author(s): Dubowitz V.
  Source: Journal of the Royal College of Physicians of London. 2000 September-October; 34(5): 464-8.
  http://www.ncbi.nlm.nih.gov/entrez/query.fcgi?cmd=Retrieve&db=pubmed&dopt=Abstract&list_uids=11077661

- **What's in a name? Muscular dystrophy revisited.**
  Author(s): Dubowitz V.
  Source: European Journal of Paediatric Neurology: Ejpn: Official Journal of the European Paediatric Neurology Society. 1998; 2(6): 279-84. Review.
  http://www.ncbi.nlm.nih.gov/entrez/query.fcgi?cmd=Retrieve&db=pubmed&dopt=Abstract&list_uids=10727193

- **What's new in neuromuscular disorders? Nuclear envelope and Emery-Dreifuss muscular dystrophy.**
  Author(s): Mercuri E, Muntoni F.
  Source: European Journal of Paediatric Neurology: Ejpn: Official Journal of the European Paediatric Neurology Society. 2001; 5(1): 3-5.
  http://www.ncbi.nlm.nih.gov/entrez/query.fcgi?cmd=Retrieve&db=pubmed&dopt=Abstract&list_uids=11277362

- **White matter abnormalities in congenital muscular dystrophy.**
  Author(s): Leyten QH, Gabreels FJ, Renier WO, van Engelen BG, ter Laak HJ, Sengers RC, Thijssen HO.
  Source: Journal of the Neurological Sciences. 1995 April; 129(2): 162-9.
  http://www.ncbi.nlm.nih.gov/entrez/query.fcgi?cmd=Retrieve&db=pubmed&dopt=Abstract&list_uids=7608731

- **Why did the heated discussion arise between Erb and Landouzy-Dejerine concerning the priority in describing the facio-scapulo-humeral muscular dystrophy and what is the main reason for this famous discussion?**
  Author(s): Kazakov V.
  Source: Neuromuscular Disorders: Nmd. 2001 May; 11(4): 421.
  http://www.ncbi.nlm.nih.gov/entrez/query.fcgi?cmd=Retrieve&db=pubmed&dopt=Abstract&list_uids=11369197

- **Why is the reproductive performance lower in Becker (BMD) as compared to limb girdle (LGMD) muscular dystrophy male patients?**
  Author(s): Eggers S, Lauriano V, Melo M, Takata RI, Akiyama J, Passos-Bueno MR, Gentil V, Frota-Pessoa O, Zatz M.
  Source: American Journal of Medical Genetics. 1995 February 27; 60(1): 27-32.
  http://www.ncbi.nlm.nih.gov/entrez/query.fcgi?cmd=Retrieve&db=pubmed&dopt=Abstract&list_uids=7485231

- **X-chromosomal (p21) muscular dystrophy and left ventricular diastolic and systolic function.**
  Author(s): Brockmeier K, Schmitz L, von Moers A, Koch H, Vogel M, Bein G.
  Source: Pediatric Cardiology. 1998 March-April; 19(2): 139-44.
  http://www.ncbi.nlm.nih.gov/entrez/query.fcgi?cmd=Retrieve&db=pubmed&dopt=Abstract&list_uids=9565505

- **X-linked Emery-Dreifuss muscular dystrophy can be diagnosed from skin biopsy or blood sample.**
  Author(s): Mora M, Cartegni L, Di Blasi C, Barresi R, Bione S, Raffaele di Barletta M, Morandi L, Merlini L, Nigro V, Politano L, Donati MA, Cornelio F, Cobianchi F, Toniolo D.
  Source: Annals of Neurology. 1997 August; 42(2): 249-53.
  http://www.ncbi.nlm.nih.gov/entrez/query.fcgi?cmd=Retrieve&db=pubmed&dopt=Abstract&list_uids=9266737

- **Xp21 muscular dystrophy due to X chromosome inversion.**
  Author(s): Baxter PS, Maltby EL, Quarrell O.
  Source: Neurology. 1997 July; 49(1): 260.
  http://www.ncbi.nlm.nih.gov/entrez/query.fcgi?cmd=Retrieve&db=pubmed&dopt=Abstract&list_uids=9222202

- **YAC and cosmid contigs encompassing the Fukuyama-type congenital muscular dystrophy (FCMD) candidate region on 9q31.**
  Author(s): Miyake M, Nakahori Y, Matsushita I, Kobayashi K, Mizuno K, Hirai M, Kanazawa I, Nakagome Y, Tokunaga K, Toda T.
  Source: Genomics. 1997 March 1; 40(2): 284-93.
  http://www.ncbi.nlm.nih.gov/entrez/query.fcgi?cmd=Retrieve&db=pubmed&dopt=Abstract&list_uids=9119396

- **You need more than nocturnal NIPPV to manage Duchenne's muscular dystrophy.**
  Author(s): Bach JR.
  Source: Chest. 1995 February; 107(2): 592.
  http://www.ncbi.nlm.nih.gov/entrez/query.fcgi?cmd=Retrieve&db=pubmed&dopt=Abstract&list_uids=7842813

Vocabulary Builder

The following vocabulary builder provides definitions of words used in this chapter that have not been defined in previous chapters:

Ameliorating: A changeable condition which prevents the consequence of a failure or accident from becoming as bad as it otherwise would. [NIH]

Amplification: The production of additional copies of a chromosomal DNA sequence, found as either intrachromosomal or extrachromosomal DNA. [NIH]

Apnea: Cessation of breathing. [NIH]

ATP: ATP an abbreviation for adenosine triphosphate, a compound which serves as a carrier of energy for cells. [NIH]

Attenuated: Strain with weakened or reduced virulence. [NIH]

Avian: A plasmodial infection in birds. [NIH]

Axonal: Condition associated with metabolic derangement of the entire neuron and is manifest by degeneration of the distal portion of the nerve fiber. [NIH]

Bioengineering: The application of engineering principles to the solution of biological problems, for example, remote-handling devices, life-support systems, controls, and displays. [NIH]

Biophysics: The science of physical phenomena and processes in living organisms. [NIH]

Bowen: Intraepithelial epithelioma affecting the skin and sometimes the mucous membranes. [NIH]

Caspase: Enzyme released by the cell at a crucial stage in apoptosis in order to shred all cellular proteins. [NIH]

Cataracts: In medicine, an opacity of the crystalline lens of the eye obstructing partially or totally its transmission of light. [NIH]

CDNA: Synthetic DNA reverse transcribed from a specific RNA through the action of the enzyme reverse transcriptase. DNA synthesized by reverse transcriptase using RNA as a template. [NIH]

Cloning: The production of a number of genetically identical individuals; in genetic engineering, a process for the efficient replication of a great number of identical DNA molecules. [NIH]

CMV: A virus that belongs to the herpes virus group. [NIH]

Complementation: The production of a wild-type phenotype when two different mutations are combined in a diploid or a heterokaryon and tested in trans-configuration. [NIH]

Continuum: An area over which the vegetation or animal population is of constantly changing composition so that homogeneous, separate communities cannot be distinguished. [NIH]

Crawford: Variation of the luminosity of a light stimulus with position of entry of the light pencil through the pupil. [NIH]

Cytotoxicity: Quality of being capable of producing a specific toxic action upon cells of special organs. [NIH]

Deletion: A genetic rearrangement through loss of segments of DNA (chromosomes), bringing sequences, which are normally separated, into close proximity. [NIH]

Density: The logarithm to the base 10 of the opacity of an exposed and processed film. [NIH]

Diaphragm: Contraceptive intra-uterine device. [NIH]

Diploid: Having two sets of chromosomes. [NIH]

Dissection: Cutting up of an organism for study. [NIH]

Dystrophic: Pertaining to toxic habitats low in nutrients. [NIH]

EEG: A graphic recording of the changes in electrical potential associated with the activity of the cerebral cortex made with the electroencephalogram. [NIH]

Effector: It is often an enzyme that converts an inactive precursor molecule into an active second messenger. [NIH]

Egger: Line formed by the attachment of the hyaloideo-capsular ligament to the posterior capsule of the crystalline lens, in a ring of about 9 mm in diameter. [NIH]

ELISA: A sensitive analytical technique in which an enzyme is complexed to an antigen or antibody. A substrate is then added which generates a color proportional to the amount of binding. This method can be adapted to a solid-phase technique. [NIH]

Enzymatic: Phase where enzyme cuts the precursor protein. [NIH]

Eosinophil: A polymorphonuclear leucocyte with large eosinophilic granules in its cytoplasm, which plays a role in hypersensitivity reactions. [NIH]

Epitope: A molecule or portion of a molecule capable of binding to the combining site of an antibody. For every given antigenic determinant, the body can construct a variety of antibody-combining sites, some of which fit almost perfectly, and others which barely fit. [NIH]

Escalation: Progressive use of more harmful drugs. [NIH]

Eukaryote: An organism (or a cell) that carries its genetic material physically constrained within a nuclear membrane, separate from the cytoplasm. [NIH]

Excitability: Property of a cardiac cell whereby, when the cell is depolarized to a critical level (called threshold), the membrane becomes permeable and a regenerative inward current causes an action potential. [NIH]

Excitotoxicity: Excessive exposure to glutamate or related compounds can kill brain neurons, presumably by overstimulating them. [NIH]

Exon: The part of the DNA that encodes the information for the actual amino acid sequence of the protein. In many eucaryotic genes, the coding sequences consist of a series of exons alternating with intron sequences. [NIH]

Extensor: A muscle whose contraction tends to straighten a limb; the antagonist of a flexor. [NIH]

Extraocular: External to or outside of the eye. [NIH]

Frameshift: A type of mutation which causes out-of-phase transcription of the base sequence; such mutations arise from the addition or delection of nucleotide(s) in numbers other than 3 or multiples of 3. [NIH]

Fuchs: A spur of indented, iridic, posterior pigment epithelium into the posterior surface of the sphincter pupillae muscle, about midway along its length, associated with the junction of a few fibers of the dilator pupillae muscle. [NIH]

Genetics: The biological science that deals with the phenomena and mechanisms of heredity. [NIH]

GTPase: Enzyme that hydrolyzes guanosine triphosphate (GTP). [NIH]

Handicap: A handicap occurs as a result of disability, but disability does not always constitute a handicap. A handicap may be said to exist when a disability causes a substantial and continuing reduction in a person's capacity to function socially and vocationally. [NIH]

Heterogeneity: The property of one or more samples or populations which implies that they are not identical in respect of some or all of their parameters, e. g. heterogeneity of variance. [NIH]

Heterozygotes: Having unlike alleles at one or more corresponding loci on homologous chromosomes. [NIH]

Holt: An empirical method for computing compensation for loss of vision, based on the assumption that the total loss of vision of one eye is an 18% loss of the total function of the body. [NIH]

Homodimer: Protein-binding "activation domains" always combine with identical proteins. [NIH]

Hybrid: Cross fertilization between two varieties or, more usually, two species of vines, see also crossing. [NIH]

Infections: The illnesses caused by an organism that usually does not cause disease in a person with a normal immune system. [NIH]

Initiation: Mutation induced by a chemical reactive substance causing cell changes; being a step in a carcinogenic process. [NIH]

Insight: The capacity to understand one's own motives, to be aware of one's own psychodynamics, to appreciate the meaning of symbolic behavior. [NIH]

Koch: It was an early form of tuberculin of low specificity, devised by Robert Koch and made by heat concentration of a broth culture of Mycobacterium tuberculosis. [NIH]

Ligands: A RNA simulation method developed by the MIT. [NIH]

Linkage: The tendency of two or more genes in the same chromosome to remain together from one generation to the next more frequently than expected according to the law of independent assortment. [NIH]

Migration: The systematic movement of genes between populations of the same species, geographic race, or variety. [NIH]

Mitotic: Cell resulting from mitosis. [NIH]

Modeling: A treatment procedure whereby the therapist presents the target behavior which the learner is to imitate and make part of his repertoire. [NIH]

Modification: A change in an organism, or in a process in an organism, that is acquired from its own activity or environment. [NIH]

Monitor: An apparatus which automatically records such physiological signs as respiration, pulse, and blood pressure in an anesthetized patient or one undergoing surgical or other procedures. [NIH]

Monoclonal: An antibody produced by culturing a single type of cell. It therefore consists of a single species of immunoglobulin molecules. [NIH]

MRNA: The RNA molecule that conveys from the DNA the information that is to be translated into the structure of a particular polypeptide molecule. [NIH]

Networks: Pertaining to a nerve or to the nerves, a meshlike structure of interlocking fibers or strands. [NIH]

Nucleus: A body of specialized protoplasm found in nearly all cells and containing the chromosomes. [NIH]

Orbicularis: A thin layer of fibers that originates at the posterior lacrimal crest and passes outward and forward, dividing into two slips which surround the canaliculi. [NIH]

Orderly: A male hospital attendant. [NIH]

Outpatient: A patient who is not an inmate of a hospital but receives diagnosis or treatment in a clinic or dispensary connected with the hospital. [NIH]

Patch: A piece of material used to cover or protect a wound, an injured part, etc.: a patch over the eye. [NIH]

Pathologies: The study of abnormality, especially the study of diseases. [NIH]

Pediatrics: The branch of medical science concerned with children and their diseases. [NIH]

Pharmacodynamic: Is concerned with the response of living tissues to chemical stimuli, that is, the action of drugs on the living organism in the absence of disease. [NIH]

Pharmacokinetic: The mathematical analysis of the time courses of absorption, distribution, and elimination of drugs. [NIH]

Phenotypes: An organism as observed, i. e. as judged by its visually perceptible characters resulting from the interaction of its genotype with the environment. [NIH]

Phosphorylated: Attached to a phosphate group. [NIH]

Photoreceptor: Receptor capable of being activated by light stimuli, as a rod or cone cell of the eye. [NIH]

Physiology: The science that deals with the life processes and functions of organismus, their cells, tissues, and organs. [NIH]

Plasmid: An autonomously replicating, extra-chromosomal DNA molecule found in many bacteria. Plasmids are widely used as carriers of cloned genes. [NIH]

Polymerase: An enzyme which catalyses the synthesis of DNA using a single DNA strand as a template. The polymerase copies the template in the 5'-3'direction provided that sufficient quantities of free nucleotides, dATP and dTTP are present. [NIH]

Polymorphism: The occurrence together of two or more distinct forms in the same population. [NIH]

Postsynaptic: Nerve potential generated by an inhibitory hyperpolarizing stimulation. [NIH]

Potassium: It is essential to the ability of muscle cells to contract. [NIH]

Prion: Small proteinaceous infectious particles that resist inactivation by procedures modifying nucleic acids and contain an abnormal isoform of a cellular protein which is a major and necessary component. [NIH]

Probe: An instrument used in exploring cavities, or in the detection and dilatation of strictures, or in demonstrating the potency of channels; an elongated instrument for exploring or sounding body cavities. [NIH]

Promoter: A chemical substance that increases the activity of a carcinogenic process. [NIH]

Prone: Having the front portion of the body downwards. [NIH]

Protease: Any enzyme that catalyzes hydrolysis of a protein. [NIH]

Protocol: The detailed plan for a clinical trial that states the trial's rationale, purpose, drug or vaccine dosages, length of study, routes of administration, who may participate, and other aspects of trial design. [NIH]

Recombination: The formation of new combinations of genes as a result of segregation in crosses between genetically different parents; also the rearrangement of linked genes due to crossing-over. [NIH]

Reentry: Reexcitation caused by continuous propagation of the same impulse for one or more cycles. [NIH]

Repressor: Any of the specific allosteric protein molecules, products of regulator genes, which bind to the operator of operons and prevent RNA polymerase from proceeding into the operon to transcribe messenger RNA. [NIH]

Sarcomere: The repeating structural unit of a striated muscle fiber. [NIH]

Satellite: Applied to a vein which closely accompanies an artery for some distance; in cytogenetics, a chromosomal agent separated by a secondary constriction from the main body of the chromosome. [NIH]

Schizophrenia: A mental disorder characterized by a special type of disintegration of the personality. [NIH]

Schwann: A neurilemmal cell from the sheath of a peripheral nerve fiber. [NIH]

Scoliosis: A lateral curvature of the spine. [NIH]

Secretory: Secreting; relating to or influencing secretion or the secretions. [NIH]

Senescence: The bodily and mental state associated with advancing age. [NIH]

Senile: Relating or belonging to old age; characteristic of old age; resulting from infirmity of old age. [NIH]

Sequencing: The determination of the order of nucleotides in a DNA or RNA chain. [NIH]

Sequester: A portion of dead bone which has become detached from the healthy bone tissue, as occurs in necrosis. [NIH]

Specificity: Degree of selectivity shown by an antibody with respect to the number and types of antigens with which the antibody combines, as well as with respect to the rates and the extents of these reactions. [NIH]

Spectrometer: An apparatus for determining spectra; measures quantities such as wavelengths and relative amplitudes of components. [NIH]

Spectroscopic: The recognition of elements through their emission spectra. [NIH]

Stomatology: The branch of medical science concerned with the mouth and its diseases. [NIH]

Suppression: A conscious exclusion of disapproved desire contrary with repression, in which the process of exclusion is not conscious. [NIH]

Synapse: The region where the processes of two neurons come into close contiguity, and the nervous impulse passes from one to the other; the fibers of the two are intermeshed, but, according to the general view, there is no direct contiguity. [NIH]

Temporal: One of the two irregular bones forming part of the lateral surfaces and base of the skull, and containing the organs of hearing. [NIH]

Therapeutics: The branch of medicine which is concerned with the treatment of diseases, palliative or curative. [NIH]

Tonus: A state of slight tension usually present in muscles even when they are not undergoing active contraction. [NIH]

Transduction: The transfer of genes from one cell to another by means of a viral (in the case of bacteria, a bacteriophage) vector or a vector which is similar to a virus particle (pseudovirion). [NIH]

Translational: The cleavage of signal sequence that directs the passage of the protein through a cell or organelle membrane. [NIH]

Transmitter: A chemical substance which effects the passage of nerve impulses from one cell to the other at the synapse. [NIH]

Ubiquitin: A highly conserved 76 amino acid-protein found in all eukaryotic cells. [NIH]

Ulcer: A localized necrotic lesion of the skin or a mucous surface. [NIH]

Vacuole: A fluid-filled cavity within the cytoplasm of a cell. [NIH]

Vector: Plasmid or other self-replicating DNA molecule that transfers DNA between cells in nature or in recombinant DNA technology. [NIH]

Venom: That produced by the poison glands of the mouth and injected by the fangs of poisonous snakes. [NIH]

Virion: A complete, mature, infectious virus particle. [NIH]

Vitro: Descriptive of an event or enzyme reaction under experimental investigation occurring outside a living organism. Parts of an organism or microorganism are used together with artificial substrates and/or conditions. [NIH]

CHAPTER 4. PATENTS ON MUSCULAR DYSTROPHY

Overview

You can learn about innovations relating to muscular dystrophy by reading recent patents and patent applications. Patents can be physical innovations (e.g. chemicals, pharmaceuticals, medical equipment) or processes (e.g. treatments or diagnostic procedures). The United States Patent and Trademark Office defines a patent as a grant of a property right to the inventor, issued by the Patent and Trademark Office.[20] Patents, therefore, are intellectual property. For the United States, the term of a new patent is 20 years from the date when the patent application was filed. If the inventor wishes to receive economic benefits, it is likely that the invention will become commercially available to patients with muscular dystrophy within 20 years of the initial filing. It is important to understand, therefore, that an inventor's patent does not indicate that a product or service is or will be commercially available to patients with muscular dystrophy. The patent implies only that the inventor has "the right to exclude others from making, using, offering for sale, or selling" the invention in the United States. While this relates to U.S. patents, similar rules govern foreign patents.

In this chapter, we show you how to locate information on patents and their inventors. If you find a patent that is particularly interesting to you, contact the inventor or the assignee for further information.

---

[20]Adapted from The U. S. Patent and Trademark Office: http://www.uspto.gov/web/offices/pac/doc/general/whatis.htm.

Patents on Muscular Dystrophy

By performing a patent search focusing on muscular dystrophy, you can obtain information such as the title of the invention, the names of the inventor(s), the assignee(s) or the company that owns or controls the patent, a short abstract that summarizes the patent, and a few excerpts from the description of the patent. The abstract of a patent tends to be more technical in nature, while the description is often written for the public. Full patent descriptions contain much more information than is presented here (e.g. claims, references, figures, diagrams, etc.). We will tell you how to obtain this information later in the chapter. The following is an example of the type of information that you can expect to obtain from a patent search on muscular dystrophy:

- **Beta-sarcoglycan nucleic acid sequence, and nucleic acid probes**

  Inventor(s): Beckmann; Jacques S. (Charenton-le-Pont, FR), Broux; Odile (L'Hay-les-Roses, FR), Campbell; Kevin P. (Iowa City, IA), Duclos; Franck (Iowa City, IA), Fardeau; Michel (Sceaux, FR), Jackson; Charles E. (Grosse Pointe, MI), Lim; Leland (Iowa City, IA), Sunada; Yoshihide (Iowa City, IA), Tome; Fernando M. S. (Paris, FR)

  Assignee(s): University of Iowa Research Foundation (Iowa City, IA)

  Patent Number: 5,672,694

  Date filed: October 24, 1995

  Abstract: Disclosed herein is a substantially pure nucleic acid sequence encoding a mammalian 43 kDa non-dystrophin component (beta-sarcoglycan) of the dystrophin-glycoprotein complex. Also disclosed are immunogenic peptides which, when used to immunize a mammal, stimulate the production of antibodies which bind specifically to the beta-sarcoglycan. Mutations in the beta-sarcoglycan gene which are associated with autosomal recessive **limb-girdle muscular dystrophy** are also disclosed. The identification of such mutations enables the design of nucleic acid probes which hybridize specifically to a mutant form of.beta.-sarcoglycan, or the complement thereof, but not to the DNA of the wild-type form of the gene (or the complement thereof), under stringent hybridization conditions. Such probes are useful, for example, in connection with the diagnosis of autosomal recessive **limb-girdle muscular dystrophy.** In addition, the identification of such mutations enables the diagnosis of autosomal recessive **limb-girdle muscular dystrophy** through the use of direct DNA sequencing techniques.

Excerpt(s): The dystrophin-glycoprotein complex (DGC) is a large oligomeric complex of sarcolemmal proteins and glycoproteins. It consists of dystrophin, a large, F-actin binding intracellular protein; syntrophin, a 59 kDa intracellular protein triplet; adhalin, a 50 kDa transmembrane glycoprotein; a 43 kDa transmembrane glycoprotein doublet (.beta.-dystroglycan and A3b); a 35 kDa transmembrane glycoprotein; a 25 kDa transmembrane protein; and.alpha.-dystroglycan, a large extracellular laminin-binding glycoprotein. Together, the dystrophin-glycoprotein complex is believed to act as a structural link between the cytoskeleton and the extracellular matrix, thereby conferring stability to the sarcolemma and protecting muscle cells from contraction-induced damage and necrosis.... The DGC has been implicated in several forms of **muscular dystrophy.** In Duchenne **muscular dystrophy** (DMD), mutations in the dystrophin gene cause the complete absence of dystrophin and a dramatic reduction of its associated glycoproteins at the sarcolemma resulting in a severe dystrophic phenotype. In the milder Becker **muscular dystrophy,** mutations in dystrophin result in the production of a dysfunctional protein. More recently, severe childhood autosomal recessive **muscular dystrophy** (SCARMD2 or LGMD2D) was shown to be caused by missense mutations in the adhalin gene, which result in the reduction of adhalin at the sarcolemma. Non-Fukuyama congenital **muscular dystrophy** (CMD) has recently been linked close to the merosin locus on chromosome 6q which is likely to be responsible for this disease. Thus, in these muscular dystrophies, mutations in one component of the DGC cause the disruption of the complex and consequently lead to the dystrophic process.... The limb girdle muscular dystrophies (LGMDs) represent a clinically heterogeneous group of diseases which are characterized by progressive weakness of the pelvic and shoulder girdle muscles. These disorders may be inherited in an autosomal dominant or recessive fashion, the latter being more common with an estimated prevalence of 10.sup.-5. Several genes have been implicated in the etiology of these disorders. The autosomal dominant form, LGMD1A, was mapped to 5q22-q3425 (Speer et al., Am. J. Hum. Genet. 50:1211 (1992)), while four genes involved in the autosomal recessive forms were mapped to chromosomes 2p13--p16 (LGMD2B, Bashir et al., Hum. Mol. Genet. 3:455 (1994)), 13q12 (LGMD2C, Ben Othmane et al., Nature Genet. 2:315 (1992); Azibi et al., Hum. Mol. Genet. 2:1423 (1993)), 15q15.1 (LGMD2A, Beckmann et al., C. R. Acad. Sci. Paris 312, 141 (1991)) and 17q12-q21.33 (LGMD2D, Roberds et al. Cell 78: 625 (1994)). The genes responsible for LGMD2D and LGMD2A have been identified: the 50 kDa adhalin glycoprotein (Roberds et al., Cell 78:625 (1994)) and muscle-specific calpain (Richard et al. Cell 87:27 1995)), respectively.

Web site: http://www.delphion.com/details?pn=US05672694__

- **Antibodies to dystrophin and uses therefor**

Inventor(s): Hoffman; Eric P. (Newton, MA), Koenig; Michel (Boston, MA), Kunkel; Louis M. (Hyde Park, MA), Monaco; Anthony (Boston, MA)

Assignee(s): The Children's Medical Center Corporation (Boston, MA)

Patent Number: 5,541,074

Date filed: November 21, 1994

Abstract: The invention relates to a **muscular dystrophy** (MD) probe comprising a substantially purified single-stranded nucleic acid sequence capable of hybridizing to a region of DNA on a human X chromosome between the deletion break point at Xp21.3 and the translocation break point at X;11. The invention also relates to a 14 kb cDNA corresponding to the complete MD gene and probes produced therefrom useful in genetic methods of diagnosis of MD. Furthermore, the invention relates to the polypeptide, dystrophin, which corresponds to the MD gene product, and antibodies thereto that are useful in a variety of methods for immunodiagnosis of MD.

Excerpt(s): This invention relates to the detection and treatment of hereditary disease, and in particular to the detection and diagnosis of Duchenne, Becker and Outlier muscular dystrophies (MD) by various methods.... Duchenne **muscular dystrophy** (DMD) is an X-linked recessive genetic disorder which affects about 1 in 3,300 males. Traits associated with DMD (DMD) phenotype) are well known and may include elevated creatine phosphokinase levels in serum (at least 10.times. the normal level), delayed development of motor function, and muscle weakness characterized by the replacement of muscle fiber with adipose and fibrose tissue accompanied by a marked variation in muscle size. Until recently, carrier identification in DMD families generally was accomplished by detecting elevated levels of creatine phosphokinase in serum.... Becker **muscular dystrophy** (BMD) is also an X-linked recessive genetic disorder, but occurs at only 10% of the frequency of DMD. BMD is a more benign form of **muscular dystrophy** which follows a less rapid clinical course than DMD. Both DMD and BMD are caused by mutations in the DMD gene located in the Xp21 region of the short arm of the human X chromosome.

Web site: http://www.delphion.com/details?pn=US05541074__

- **Apparatus and method for aiding transmission**

Inventor(s): Hayashi; Hideki (Tokyo, JP), Ichiyoshi; Hiroyuki (Kawasaki, JP), Kadota; Toshihiko (Kawasaki, JP), Koizumi; Hiroyuki (Tokyo, JP)

Assignee(s): Canon Kabushiki Kaisha (Tokyo, JP)

Patent Number: 5,967,996

Date filed: March 12, 1997

Abstract: An apparatus and a method for aiding the transmission of intent enables a severely physically-handicapped person, who has lost muscular energy due to amyotrophic lateral sclerosis (ALS), **muscular dystrophy** or the like, to transmit his/her intent through an electroencephalogram wave. A mechanical switch and an electroencephalogram wave switch are used in combination to allow the transmission of intent over the entire period of such a disease.

Excerpt(s): The present invention relates to an apparatus and a method for aiding the transmission of intent, which enable a severely physically-handicapped person, who has lost muscular energy due to amyotrophic lateral sclerosis (ALS), **muscular dystrophy** or the like, to transmit his/her intent through an electroencephalogram wave.... The number of physically-handicapped persons, who lose motor functions while retaining their brain function, is expected to increase in the coming aged society. In the case of such diseases as ALS or **muscular dystrophy,** which are known as incurable diseases, patients' losing the means for transmitting their intent in medical care environments is leading to a significant increase in the medical care cost for medical treatment, medical attendance, and nursing. Further, there is strong demand for mutual transmission of intent between patients, who still retain human intelligence and senses, and people who attend on the patients over a long period.... A disease such as ALS and **muscular dystrophy** causes the muscular function of a human body to be lost slowly and no aiding apparatus is available for transmitting intent, which can be used over the entire period of the progressive disease of a patient.

Web site: http://www.delphion.com/details?pn=US05967996__

- **Changes in laminin subunit composition are diagnostic of Fukuyama congenital muscular dystrophy**

Inventor(s): Arahata; Kiichi (Tokyo, JP), Engvall; Eva (Rancho Santa Fe, CA)

Assignee(s): La Jolla Cancer Research Foundation (La Jolla, CA)

Patent Number: 5,780,244

Date filed: February 14, 1994

Abstract: The present invention relates to a method for detecting altered expression or localization of a cytoskeleton/basal lamina protein in a tissue sample obtained from an individual, wherein the altered expression or localization are associated with a **muscular dystrophy** such as Fukuyama congenital **muscular dystrophy** (FCMD). The invention provides an immunohistochemical method for detecting the expression and localization in a tissue, such as muscle, of laminin M (merosin), which is a protein component of the basal lamina, wherein certain defined changes are diagnostic of individuals predisposed to FCMD. The invention also provides a prenatal diagnostic screening procedure, using a tissue such as placenta, wherein the screening procedure can identify an individual predisposed to FCMD. The invention further provides methods for identifying an individual predisposed to other muscular dystrophies such as Walker-Warburg Syndrome (WWS) and muscle-eye-brain disease of the Finnish type (MEB).

Excerpt(s): This invention relates generally to the field of medicine and more specifically to methods for detecting changes in the expression of laminin M protein and of M chain mRNA that are diagnostic of Fukuyama congenital **muscular dystrophy** (FCMD). The invention further relates to methods of identifying agents that can reduce or prevent the symptoms associated with FCMD and to methods of treating an FCMD patient.... The basal lamina of muscle fibers is a specialized extracellular matrix that has a static structure that contributes to the proper migration, proliferation and regeneration of myogenic cells during development or after injury or tissue grafting (Alberts et al., Molecular Biology of the Cell (Garland Publ., Inc. 1989); Sanes et al., Myology (McGraw-Hill Book Co., NY, 1986); Martin, G. R., Ann. Rev. Cell Biol. 3:37-85 (1987); Alameddine et al., Neuromusc. Dis. 1:143-152 (1991)). The components of the basal lamina include laminin, type IV collagen, fibronectin and heparan-sulfate proteoglycan. The large laminin protein, which has a molecular weight of approximately 850 kilodaltons (kdal), is a heterotrimer consisting of two smaller chains (B1, S or B2) and one larger chain (A or M) which are arranged in the shape of a cross. Thus, laminin trimers have various structures such as A-B1-B2, M-B1-B2, A-S-

B2 and M-S-B2. Other laminins such as kalinin and K-laminin contain an A chain homolog, designated K (Marinkovich et al., J. Cell Biol. 119:695-703 (1992)).... Laminin is found adjacent to the plasma membrane of muscle fibers, where its multiple functional domains bind type IV collagen, proteoglycans and laminin receptor proteins, such as integrins (Hynes and Lander, Cell 68:303-322 (1992)) and the 156 kdal dystrophin-associated glycoprotein (DAG) (Ibraghimov-Beskrovnaya et al., Nature 355:696-702 (1992)), which are present on the plasma membrane of the muscle fibers. The various laminin isoforms can be either ubiquitously expressed or tissue-specific (Leivo and Engvall, Proc. Natl. Acad. Sci. USA 85:1544-1548 (1988); Ehrig et al., Proc. Natl. Acad. Sci. USA 87:3264-3268 (1990); Sanes et al., J. Cell Biol. 111:1685-1699 (1990)). For example, laminin M (merosin) contains an M chain subunit that is specific for striated muscle, Schwann cells and trophoblast, where it replaces the "A" subunit in the ubiquitous non-muscle laminin polyprotein (Leivo and Engvall (1988); Wewer et al., Lab. Invest. 66:378-389 (1992)).

Web site: http://www.delphion.com/details?pn=US05780244__

- **Diagnosis of myotonic muscular dystrophy**

Inventor(s): Caskey; C. Thomas (West University, TX), Fenwick; Raymond G. (Sugarland, TX), Friedman; David L. (Houston, TX), Fu; Ying-Hui (Columbus, OH), Pizzuti; Antonio (Milan, IT)

Assignee(s): Baylor College of Medicine (Houston, TX)

Patent Number: 5,552,282

Date filed: June 6, 1993

Abstract: The present invention includes a DNA clone from the **myotonic muscular dystrophy** gene, a cosmid probe to the myotonic dystrophy site, as well as methods of detecting **myotonic muscular dystrophy** using RFLP. The method involves the steps of digesting DNA from an individual to be tested with a restriction endonuclease and detecting the restriction fragment length polymorphism with hybridization to probes within the myotonic muscular locus and southern blot analysis. Alternatively, the **myotonic muscular dystrophy** gene can be measured by determining the amount of mRNA or measuring the amount of protein with an antibody. Further, the **myotonic muscular dystrophy** gene defect can be detected using either fluorescence in situ hybridization or pulsed field gel electrophoresis using the probes described herein.

Excerpt(s): This invention relates to the field of molecular diagnosis of **myotonic muscular dystrophy**.... The **myotonic muscular dystrophy** (DM) disease is the most common adult **muscular dystrophy** in man with a prevalence of 1 in 10,000. The disorder is inherited in an autosomal dominant manner with variable expression of symptoms from individual to individual within a given family. Furthermore, the phenomenon of anticipation (increasing disease severity over generations) is well documented for DM. This is particularly evident when an affected mother transmits the gene for the disease to her offspring. These offspring have a high incidence of mental retardation and profound infantile myotonia. Adult patients with DM manifest a pleiotropic set of symptoms including myotonia, cardiac arrhythmias, cataracts, frontal baldness, hypogonadism, and other endocrine dysfunctions. There is no evidence that **myotonic muscular dystrophy** may be caused by defects in more than one gene.... A **myotonic muscular dystrophy** gene has been mapped to human chromosome position 19q13.3. Both a genetic and physical map of the region was developed by a group of investigators acting as a voluntary consortium under sponsorship of the **Muscular Dystrophy** Association. The genetic linkage studies identified two RFLP alleles, D10 and X75, which are polymerase chain reaction (PCR)-based dinucleotide polymorphisms and are tightly linked to DM.

Web site: http://www.delphion.com/details?pn=US05552282__

- **Gene replacement therapy for muscular dystrophy**

  Inventor(s): Campbell; Kevin P. (Iowa City, IA), Davidson; Beverly (Iowa City, IA), Duclos; Franck (Iowa City, IA), Holt; Kathleen H. (Corlville, IA), Lim; Leland E. (Iowa City, IA), Straub; Volker (Essen, IA), Williamson; Roger (Iowa City, IA)

  Assignee(s): University of Iowa Research Foundation (Iowa City, IA)

  Patent Number: 6,262,035

  Date filed: October 1, 1998

  Abstract: Disclosed is a method for treating a patient suffering from the disease sarcoglycan-deficient **limb-girdle muscular dystrophy** by gene replacement therapy. Sarcoglycan gene replacement therapy produces extensive long-term expression of the sarcoglycan species which restores the entire sarcoglycan complex, results in the stable association of alph.alpha.-dystroglycan with the sarcolemma, and eliminates the morphological markers of **limb-girdle muscular dystrophy.** In another aspect, the invention relates to a method for determining a specific defective sarcoglycan species in the tissue of a patient. The method involves culture of muscle cells obtained from the patient, and the independent introduction of expression vectors encoding each of the sarcoglycan species,.alpha.,.beta.,.gamma., and.delta., into the cultured cells with subsequent assaying for restoration of the dystrophin-glycoprotein complex. In another aspect, the invention relates to a mouse, and cells derived therefrom, homozygous for a disrupted.alpha.-sarcoglycan gene. The disruption prevents the synthesis of functional.alpha.-sarcoglycan in cells of the mouse and results in the mutant mouse having no detectable sarcospan,.beta.-,.gamma.-,.delta.-sarcoglycan, and reduced.alpha.-dystroglycan in the sarcolemma of skeletal and cardiac muscles, and a reduction of dystrophin in skeletal muscle, when compared to tissue of a mouse lacking a disrupted.alpha.-sarcoglycan gene. In another aspect, the invention relates to methods for screening for therapeutic agents useful in the treatment of sarcoglycan-deficient **limb-girdle muscular dystrophy.** The methods involve administering a candidate therapeutic agent to a mouse, or cells derived therefrom, and assaying for therapeutic effects on the mouse or cells, with the determination of therapeutic effects being a reduction or reversal in disease progression, or a restoration of the dystroglycan complex.

Excerpt(s): The term **muscular dystrophy** describes a group of diseases characterized by hereditary progressive muscle weakness and degeneration. Several muscular dystrophies are caused by mutations in genes that encode sarcolemmal proteins, including certain types of **limb-girdle muscular dystrophy** (LGMD). LGMD is genetically and clinically heterogeneous; it may be inherited in an autosomal dominant or recessive manner, and may have different rates of progression and severity. A unifying theme among the LGMDs is the initial involvement of the shoulder and pelvic girdle muscles, with relative sparing of most other muscle groups (Jackson et al., Pediatrics 41, 495-501 (1968); Bushby, K. M., Neuromusc Disord 5, 71-74 (1995)).... The pace of discovery in the field of **muscular dystrophy** research has been rapid since the discovery of the Duchenne and Becker **muscular dystrophy** (DMD) gene in 1986 (Monaco et al., Nature 323, 646-650 (1986)). The DMD gene encodes dystrophin, a large cytoskeletal protein that together with other molecular components makes up the dystrophin-glycoprotein complex (DGC). The dystrophin-glycoprotein complex (DGC) is a large oligomeric complex of sarcolemmal proteins and glycoproteins in skeletal and cardiac muscle (Campbell, K. P. Cell 80, 675-679 (1995); Ozawa et al., Hum. Mol. Genet. 4, 1711-1716 (1995)). This complex consists of dystrophin, a large cytoskeletal protein which binds F-actin;.alpha.- and.beta.-dystroglycan, which bind laminin and the cysteine-rich region of dystrophin, respectively;.alpha.-,.beta.-,.gamma.-, and.delta.-sarcoglycan (.delta.-SG), which form a distinct subcomplex; and sarcospan, a 25 kDa protein predicted to span the membrane four times (Crosbie et al., J. Biol. Chem. 272, 31221-31224 (1997). The DGC spans the sarcolemma and is believed to play an essential role in maintaining the normal architecture of the muscle sarcolemma by constituting a link between the subsarcolemmal cytoskeleton and the extracellular matrix. This structural linkage is thought to protect muscle fibers from the mechanical stress of contraction.... Mutations in different components of the DGC lead to similar dystrophic features, suggesting that the function of the DGC as a whole is dependent on intact molecular interactions between its individual subunits. The loss of one component destroys the link, and leads to muscle fiber degeneration. Several components of the DGC have been implicated in several human muscular dystrophies (Straub et al., Curr. Opin. Neurol. 10, 168-175 (1997)). Mutations in dystrophin cause Duchenne and Becker **muscular dystrophy** (DMD) (Hoffman et al., Cell 51, 919-928 (1987)). Two forms of congenital **muscular dystrophy** are caused by mutations in the extracellular matrix protein laminin 2 (Helbling-Leclerc et al., Nature Genet. 11, 216-218 (1995); Allamand et al., Hum. Mol. Genet. 6, 747-752 (1997)). Mutations in each of.alpha.-,.beta.-,.gamma.-, and.delta.-SG cause autosomal recessive LGMD types 2D, 2E, 2C, and 2F, respectively (Roberds et al., Cell 78, 625-633 (1994); Piccolo et al., Nature Genet. 10, 243-245 (1995); Lim et al., Nature Genet. 11, 257-265 (1995); Bonneman et al., Nature Genet. 11, 266-273 (1995); Noguchi et al., Science 270, 819-822 (1995); Passos-Bueno et al., Hum. Mol. Genet. 5, 815-820 (1996); Nigro et al., Hum. Mol. Genet. 5, 1179-1186 (1996); Nigro et al., Nature Genet. 14, 195-198 (1996)).

Web site: http://www.delphion.com/details?pn=US06262035__

- **Merosin deficiency-type congenital muscular dystrophy**

Inventor(s): Campbell; Kevin P. (Iowa City, IA), Fardeau; Michel (Sceaux, FR), Sunada; Yoshihide (Iowa City, IA), Tome; Fernando M. S. (Paris, FR)

Assignee(s): University of Iowa Research Foundation (Iowa City, IA)

Patent Number: 5,863,743

Date filed: August 12, 1994

Abstract: Disclosed is a method for aiding in the diagnosis of merosin deficiency-type congenital **muscular dystrophy** (CMD). The method is based on the discovery of a previously unidentified form of CMD which is characterized by a substantial reduction in the levels of merosin in skeletal muscle tissue containing normal levels of dystrophin and dystrophin-associated proteins.

Excerpt(s): Congenital **muscular dystrophy** (CMD), a very disabling muscle disease of early clinical onset, is the most frequent cause of severe neonatal hypotonia. Its manifestations are noticed at birth or in the first months of life and consist of muscle hypotonia, often associated with delayed motor milestones, severe and early contractures and joint deformities. Serum creatine kinase is raised, up to 30 times the normal values, in the early stage of the disease, and then rapidly decreases. The histological changes in the muscle biopsies consist of large variation in the size of muscle fibers, a few necrotic and regenerating fibers, marked increase in endomysial collagen tissue, and no specific ultrastructural features. The diagnosis of CMD has been based on the clinical picture and the morphological changes in the muscle biopsy, but it cannot be made with certainty, as other muscle disorders may present with similar clinico-pathological features.... Within the group of diseases classified as CMD, various forms have been individualized. The two more common forms are the occidental and the Japanese, the latter being associated with severe mental disturbances, and usually referred to as Fukuyama congenital **muscular dystrophy** (FCMD). The genetic lesion responsible for FCMD has recently been mapped to chromosome 9. It is unknown whether or not the rare cases of CMD associated with mental retardation or central nervous system abnormalities observed in occidental countries belong to the same disease entity. The determination of the gene (or genes) responsible for the various forms of CMD is required in order to clearly delineate specific members of the currently ill-defined genus.... The present invention is based on the identification of a novel disease etiology which is responsible for a previously undefined member of the congenital **muscular dystrophy** family. The novel etiology, referred to herein as merosin deficiency-type congenital **muscular dystrophy,** was identified through the study of levels of specific proteins in mammalian muscle tissue.

Web site: http://www.delphion.com/details?pn=US05863743__

- **Method for aiding in the diagnosis of in-frame deletion type congenital muscular dystrophy**

Inventor(s): Allamand; Valerie (Iowa City, IA), Campbell; Kevin P. (Iowa City, IA), Salih; Mustafa (Riyadh, SA), Straub; Volker (Iowa City, IA), Sunada; Yoshihide (Kawaguchi, JP)

Assignee(s): University of Iowa Research Foundation (Iowa City, IA)

Patent Number: 6,136,546

Date filed: April 9, 1998

Abstract: Disclosed are compositions and methods for aiding in the diagnosis of congenital **muscular dystrophy** associated with in-frame deletion in the laminin-2.alpha.2 polypeptide chain in an individual. In a preferred diagnostic method embodiment, an experimental muscle tissue sample is provided from the individual and treated if necessary to render components available for antibody binding. The components of the sample are then separated on the basis of molecular weight. The separated protein components are then transferred to a solid support while maintaining the relative positions established in separation step. The transferred components are then stained with an affinity reagent which is known to bind to a C-terminal domain of the laminin-2.alpha.2 polypeptide chain. Individual afflicted with congenital **muscular dystrophy** associated with in-frame deletion in the laminin-2.alpha.2 polypeptide chain on the basis of positive staining in combination with reduced molecular weight of the laminin-2.alpha.2 polypeptide chain relative to the wild-type laminin-2.alpha.2 polypeptide chain. A preferred composition is a nucleic acid probe for the detection of merosin deletion-type congenital **muscular dystrophy.** The preferred nucleic acid probe is characterized by the ability to bind specifically to a mutant merosin nucleic acid sequence, the mutant merosin nucleic acid sequence comprising a T to C substitution at position 3973 +2 of the consensus donor splice site of exon 25.

Excerpt(s): Laminins are a family of large extracellular glycoproteins which display a complex and still unclear repertoire of biological functions. Laminin-2, the isoform involved in congenital **muscular dystrophy** (CMD), is specifically expressed in the basal lamina of striated muscle and peripheral nerve. As are all members of the laminin family, it is composed of three chains: one heavy (.alpha.2) and two light chains (.beta.1 and.gamma.1) that assemble in a cross-shaped molecule with three short arms and one long arm. The C-terminal ends of each chain interact to form the triple stranded long arm of the molecule, stabilized by disulfide bonds, with a large globular (G) domain contributed to by the.alpha.2-chain. The.alpha.2-chain of laminin consists of 6 domains: I and II are part of the long arm; IIIa, IIIb and V contain cystein-rich EGF-like repeats and are predicted to have rigid rod-like structures; and IVa, IVb and VI are predicted to form globular structures. Laminin.alpha.2-chain has been shown to be a native ligand for.alpha.-dystroglycan, an extracellular component of the dystrophin-associated glycoprotein complex (DGC). This complex constitutes a link between the subsarcolemmal skeleton and the extracellular matrix. A number of components of the DGC have now been shown to be involved in muscular dystrophies suggesting a crucial role of laminin-2 and the components of the DGC in maintaining the integrity of muscle cell function.... Congenital **muscular dystrophy** (CMD) is a clinically and genetically heterogeneous group of autosomal recessive neuromuscular disorders of early onset. In the classic form of CMD, clinical manifestations are limited to skeletal muscle with no clinical involvement of the central nervous system (CNS) although changes in the white matter have been detected by MRI. The histological changes in muscle biopsies consist of connective tissue proliferation, large variation in the size of the muscle fibers as well as some necrotic and regenerating fibers.... Two groups of classical-type CMD cases can be distinguished according to the status of the.alpha.2-chain of laminin-2 (also referred to as merosin) with about half of the cases displaying a deficiency of this protein. However, even these merosin-deficient CMD cases represent a heterogeneous subgroup since some patients display a total deficiency of the.alpha.2-chain of laminin-2 whereas this protein is expressed in others, though at a reduced level. Linkage analyses and homozygosity mapping studies have led to the localization of the CMD locus to chromosome 6q2 (Hillaire et al., Hum. Mol. Genet. 3: 1657-1661 (1994); and Helbling-Leclerc et al., C. R. Acad. Sci. Paris 318: 1245-1252 (1995)), in the region containing the gene encoding the.alpha.2-chain of laminin (LAMA-2) (Vuolteenaho et al., J. Cell Biol. 124: 381-394 (1994)). Recently, mutations affecting this gene have been identified in CMD patients (Helbling-Leclerc et al., Nat. Genet. 11: 216-218 (1995); and Nissinen et al., Am. J. Hum. Genet. 58: 1177-1184 (1996).

Web site: http://www.delphion.com/details?pn=US06136546__

- **Method of in vitro preconditioning healthy donor's myoblasts before transplantation thereof in compatible patients suffering of recessive myopathies like muscular dystrophy, for improving transplantation success**

Inventor(s): Tremblay; Jacques P. (Bernieres, CA)

Assignee(s): Universite Laval (Quebec, CA)

Patent Number: 5,833,978

Date filed: March 16, 1995

Abstract: A method of pretreating healthy donor's myoblast cultures with growth or trophic factors like basic fibroblast growth factor (bFGF) on transplantation to subjects suffering of recessive myopathy like **muscular dystrophy** is disclosed and claimed. Recipient muscles show a higher percentage of functional cells, demonstrated by the higher incidence of dystrophin-positive fibers, and does not require previous preconditioning of recipient muscles by irradiation or toxin administration. Donor mouse myoblasts expressing the reporter gene.beta.- galactosidase were grown with 100 ng/ml bFGF during the last two days before injecting them in the left tibialis anterior (TA) muscles of recipient MHC-compatible mdx mice, an experimental animal model of **muscular dystrophy.** Myoblasts from the same primary cultures were also grown without bFGF and injected in the right TA muscles as control. The recipient mice were immunosuppressed with FK 506. Twenty-eight days after myoblast transplantation, the percentage of.beta.- galactosidase-positive fibers was significantly higher (more than a 4 fold increase) following culture with bFGF than without bFGF. Almost all.beta.-galactosidase-positive-fibers were also dystrophin positive.

Excerpt(s): The present invention is a method for preconditioning healthy donor's myoblasts in vitro before transplantation thereof in compatible patients suffering of recessive myopathies, particularly of **muscular dystrophy.** This in vitro preconditioning improves the success of the transplantation while not requiring an in vivo preconditioning of the patient's muscle by irradiation or by administering muscular toxin.... Duchenne **muscular dystrophy** (DMD) is a progressive disease characterized by the lack of dystrophin under the sarcolemmal membrane.sup.6,19,28,37. One possible way to introduce dystrophin in the muscle fibers of the patients to limit the degeneration is to transplant myoblasts obtained from normal subjects.sup.30,34,35. Several groups have tried myoblast transplantations to DMD patients but poor graft success was observed.sup.17,22,24,38. Even in experimental myoblast transplantation using mdx mice, an animal model of DMD.sup.10,25,29, large amount of dystrophin-positive fibers were observed only when nude mdx mice were previously irradiated to prevent regeneration of the muscle fibers by host myoblasts.sup.32,43. High percentage of dystrophin-positive fibers was also observed in mdx mice immunosuppressed with FK 506 and in SCID mice, in both cases muscles were previously damaged by notexin injection and irradiated.sup.23,27. These results indicate that to obtain successful myoblast transplantation, it is necessary to have not only an immunodeficient mouse or a mouse adequately immunosuppressed but also a host muscle which has been adequately preconditioned. It is, however, impossible in clinical studies to use damaging treatments such as marcaine, notexin and irradiation. If good myoblast transplantation results can be obtained without using such techniques, this would be very helpful for myoblast transplantation in humans.... Recently there has been an increasing interest on the effects of basic fibroblast growth factor (bFGF) and other growth factors on myoblast cultures and myoblast cell lines.sup.1,4,5. Basic FGF has been reported to both stimulate proliferation and inhibit differentiation of skeletal myoblasts in vitro.sup.15,16. Other growth or trophic factors like insulin growth factor I, transferrin, platelet-derived growth factor, epidermal growth factor, adrenocorticotrophin and macrophage colony-stimulating factor as well as C kinase proteins activators or agonists by which the effect of bFGF is mediated.sup.20 may also have similar or even better effects than bFGF on the success of myoblast transplantation. The use of these stimulating properties to enhance the success of transplantation by in vitro preconditioning of donor's cells and to replace at least partially the use of previously known methods of in vivo preconditioning of recipients' cells has never been suggested before.

Web site: http://www.delphion.com/details?pn=US05833978__

- **Method of treating fibrosis in skeletal muscle tissue**

  Inventor(s): Funanage; Vicky L. (Wilmington, DE)

  Assignee(s): The Nemours Foundation (Wilmington, DE)

  Patent Number: 5,604,199

  Date filed: October 16, 1995

  Abstract: A method of treating skeletal muscle fibrosis in mammals. The novel method is effective for reducing the extent of skeletal muscle fibrosis in an individual who suffers from a disorder which targets skeletal muscle tissue, such as Duchenne's and Becker's **muscular dystrophy** and denervation atrophy induced by either trauma or neuromuscular disease. The treatment includes administering to the individual an effective amount of a metalloporphyrin compound, especially hemin, heme arginate, cobalt protoporphyrin IX chloride and cobalt protoporphyrin IX arginate.

  Excerpt(s): This invention relates to a method of treating skeletal muscle disease. More specifically, the invention provides a method of reducing skeletal muscle fibrosis by administering a therapeutic amount of a metalloporphyrin compound.... Skeletal muscle fibrosis is a phenomenon which frequently occurs in diseased or damaged muscle. It is characterized by the excessive growth of fibrous tissue which usually results from the body's attempt to recover from injury. Fibrosis impairs muscle function and causes weakness. The amount of muscle function loss generally increases with the extent of fibrosis. Often fibrosis is progressive and can contribute to the patient's inability to carry out ordinary tasks of independent living, such as grasping objects or walking.... Victims of muscular dystrophies, particularly Becker **muscular dystrophy** (BMD) and the more severely penetrating allelic manifestation, Duchenne **muscular dystrophy** (DMD), frequently suffer from increasing skeletal muscle fibrosis as the disease progresses. BMD patients usually exhibit progressive muscle weakness and wasting. The advance of fibrosis often causes ever greater loss of mobility and a reduced life expectancy. At some point, the patient may become too weak to walk and takes to a wheelchair. Victims of DMD typically lose the ability to walk by their early teen years and experience tragically premature death before the age of twenty. DMD patients typically succumb to cardio-pulmonary complications which may be partly attributable to strain associated with fibrosis-induced muscle function loss and weakness.

Web site: http://www.delphion.com/details?pn=US05604199__

- **Method of treatment for muscular dystrophy**

Inventor(s): Antoku; Yasunobu (Kurume, JP), Koike; Fumihiko (Saga, JP), Sakai; Tetsuo (Yame, JP), Tanaka; Kaoru (Fukuoka, JP), Tsukamoto; Kosuke (Kurume, JP)

Assignee(s): MinoPhagen Pharmaceutical Company (Tokyo, JP)

Patent Number: 5,434,142

Date filed: August 24, 1993

Abstract: Administering to a patient of **muscular dystrophy** a pharmaceutical agent containing glycyrrhizin and/or a pharmaceutically acceptable salt thereof as effective components is effective against **muscular dystrophy**, particularly, Duchenne or Becker **muscular dystrophy** and is highly safe with less side effect.

Excerpt(s): This invention relates to a method of treatment for **muscular dystrophy** and, more particularly, to a method of treatment for **muscular dystrophy** such as Duchenne **muscular dystrophy**, Becker **muscular dystrophy** and the like.... The Duchenne **muscular dystrophy** is a sex-linked recessive disease occuring in childhood, in which muscle weakness and muscular wasting in the proximal parts of extremities and trunk are progressed, resulting in a death at about twenty. The Becker **muscular dystrophy** is also a sex-linked recessive disease showing the same symptoms, although its onset age is older and tile progression is slower, compared with the Duchenne type.... Other muscular dystrophies include **limb-girdle muscular dystrophy**, facioscapulohumeral (FSH) **muscular dystrophy**, congenital **muscular dystrophy**, and the like.

Web site: http://www.delphion.com/details?pn=US05434142__

- **Oligonucleotides for dysferlin, a gene mutated in distal myopathy and limb girdle muscular dystrophy**

Inventor(s): Aoki; Masashi (Sendai, JP), Brown, Jr.; Robert H. (Needham, MA), Ho; Meng F. (Singapore, SG), Liu; Jing (Outremont, CA), Matsuda-Asada; Chie (Brookline, MA)

Assignee(s): The General Hospital Corporation (Boston, MA)

Patent Number: 6,673,909

Date filed: August 25, 1999

Abstract: A novel gene and the protein encoded therein, i.e., dysferlin, are disclosed. This gene and its expression products are associated with **muscular dystrophy,** e.g., Miyoshi myopathy and limb girdle musclular dystrophy 2B.

Excerpt(s): The invention relates to genes involved in the onset of **muscular dystrophy**.... Muscular dystrophies constitute a heterogeneous group of disorders. Most are characterized by weakness and atrophy of the proximal muscles, although in rare myopathies such as "Miyoshi myopathy" symptoms may first arise in distal muscles. Of the various hereditary types of **muscular dystrophy,** several are caused by mutations or deletions in genes encoding individual components of the dystrophin-associated protein (DAP) complex. It is this DAP complex that links the cytoskeletal protein dystrophin to the extracellular matrix protein, laminin-2.... Muscular dystrophies may be classified according to the gene mutations that are associated with specific clinical syndromes. For example, mutations in the gene encoding the cytoskeletal protein dystrophin result in either **Duchenne's Muscular Dystrophy** or Becker's **Muscular Dystrophy,** whereas mutations in the gene encoding the extracellular matrix protein merosin produce Congenital **Muscular Dystrophy.** Muscular dystrophies with an autosomal recessive mode of inheritance include "Miyoshi myopathy" and the several limb-girdle muscular dystrophies (LGMD2). Of the limb-girdle muscular dystrophies, the deficiencies resulting in LGMD2C, D, E, and F result from mutations in genes encoding the membrane-associated sarcoglycan components of the DAP complex.

Web site: http://www.delphion.com/details?pn=US06673909__

- **Purified, native dystrophin**

Inventor(s): Campbell; Kevin P. (Iowa City, IA), Ervasti; James M. (Iowa City, IA), Kahl; Steven D. (Iowa City, IA)

Assignee(s): University of Iowa Research Foundation (Iowa City, IA)

Patent Number: 5,430,129

Date filed: January 16, 1991

Abstract: The invention pertains to pure, native dystrophin of mammalian skeletal muscle and a method of purifying dystrophin from mammalian skeletal muscle. The invention further pertains to a method of diagnosing **muscular dystrophy** by detecting the loss or abnormal structure of pure, native dystrophin from mammalian skeletal muscle. The detection of a loss of dystrophin or an abnormal structure of dystrophin is indicative of **muscular dystrophy.**

Excerpt(s): Muscular dystrophy refers to a group of genetically determined myopathies characterized by progressive atrophy or degeneration of increasing numbers of individual muscle cells. The structural changes observed histologically are essentially the same in the various types of muscular dystrophies. This may, perhaps, suggest a common etiology. However, the distribution of the affected muscles is quite distinctive. This, along with the mode of inheritance, forms the basis of the classification of these diseases. The muscular dystrophies are traditionally subdivided by the patterns of initial muscle involvement, which in turn correlates fairly well with the type of genetic transmission. The three major forms of **muscular dystrophy** are as follows: 1) Duchennes **Muscular Dystrophy** which affects most skeletal muscle groups and is transmitted by an X-linked recessive gene; 2) Limb Girdle **Muscular Dystrophy,** affecting principally the pelvic and shoulder girdle muscles and is transmitted by an autosomal recessive gene; and 3) Facioscapulohumeral **muscular dystrophy,** involves the muscles of the face and shoulder girdle and is transmitted by an autosomal dominant gene.... Recently, the defective gene responsible for Duchenne **muscular dystrophy** (DMD) has been located on the X chromosome. The DMD gene encodes for a large molecular weight protein product called dystrophin. This protein is localized in the sacrolemmal membrane of normal skeletal muscle, but is absent from the skeletal muscle of people with DMD, as well as, dogs and mice with dystrophic muscle. A more benign form of this X-linked recessive disease is Becker's **Muscular Dystrophy** which is caused by an abnormal DMD gene which encodes an abnormal dystrophin protein. The exact function of dystrophin and the reasons why its absence or abnormal structure results in necrosis of dystrophic muscle fibers has not been determined. However, the amino acid sequence of dystrophin suggests that it is a membrane cytoskeletal protein.... The present technology for initial detection and diagnosis of Duchenne or Becker's **Muscular Dystrophy** relies on the use of an immunological probe to identify the presence of dystrophin, the absence of dystrophin, or the abnormal molecular weight or content of dystrophin in human muscle biopsies. Immunological assays, however, are indirect and often plagued by non-specific binding and/or cross-reactivity of the immunological probes (antibodies) with other proteins. Both of these problems can lead to false positive determinations. Conversely, other factors can cause interference with the binding of immunological probes with their target proteins (in this case, dystrophin). This type of problem can cause false negative determinations.

Web site: http://www.delphion.com/details?pn=US05430129__

- **Utrophin gene expression**

Inventor(s): Davies; Kay E. (Oxford, GB), Tinsley; Jonathon M. (Oxford, GB)

Assignee(s): Medical Research Council (London, GB)

Patent Number: 6,518,413

Date filed: July 14, 1998

Abstract: Nucleic acid from which a polypeptide with utrophin function can be expressed, especially mini-genes and chimaeric constructs. Expression significantly decreases the severity of the dystrophic muscle phenotype in an animal model, indicating usefulness in treatment of **muscular dystrophy.** The nucleic acid and encoded polypeptides are also useful in screening for substances to modulate utrophin binding to actin and/or the dystrophin protein complex.

Excerpt(s): The present invention generally relates to the provision of nucleic acid from which a polypeptide with utrophin function can be expressed, especially mini-genes and chimaeric constructs. Expression of a utrophin transgene significantly decreases the severity of the dystrophic muscle phenotype in an animal model.... The severe muscle wasting disorders, Duchenne **muscular dystrophy** (DMD) and the less debilitating Becker **muscular dystrophy** (BMD) are due to mutations in the dystrophin gene. Dystrophin is a large cytoskeletal protein which in muscle is located at the cytoplasmic surface of the sarcolemma, the neuromuscular junction (NMJ) and myotendinous junction (MTJ). The protein is composed of four domains: an actin-binding domain (shown in vitro to bind actin), a rod domain containing triple helical repeats, a cysteine rich (CR) domain and a carboxy-terminal (CT) domain. The majority of the CRCT binds to a complex of proteins and glycoproteins (called the dystrophin protein complex, DPC) spanning the sarcolemma. This complex consists of cytoskeletal syntrophins and dystrobrevin, transmembrane,.beta.-dystroglycan,.alpha.-,.beta.-.delta.-,.gamma.-sarcoglycans and extracellular.alpha.-dystroglycan. The DPC links to laminin-.alpha.2 (merosin) in the extracellular matrix and to the actin cytoskeleton via dystrophin within the cell. The breakdown of the integrity of the DPC due to the loss of, or impairment of dystrophin function, leads to muscle degeneration and the DMD phenotype. The structure of dystrophin and protein interactions within the DPC have been recently reviewed [1,2,3].... There are various approaches which can be adopted for the gene therapy of DMD. These include myoblast transfer, retroviral infection, adenoviral infection and direct injection of plasmid DNA. In most cases the dystrophin gene used in the experiments generates a truncated protein approximately half the size of the full size protein. This dystrophin minigene was modelled on a natural mutation identified in a very mild Becker patient [4]. The cloned version of this truncated minigene is able to reverse the pathological phenotype in the dystrophin deficient mdx mouse [5,6,7] and has had limited success when delivered to mdx muscle by viral vectors [8,9,10]. Although some progress is being made in each of these areas using the mdx mouse as a model system, there are problems related to the number of muscle cells that can be made dystrophin positive, the levels of expression of the gene and the duration of expression [11]. Another problem to be addressed is the rejection of cells expressing dystrophin because of immunological intolerance i.e. dystrophin within these cells will appear foreign to the host immune system given that most DMD patients will never have expressed dystrophin [12,13].

Web site: http://www.delphion.com/details?pn=US06518413__

- **Utrophin gene promotor**

  Inventor(s): Davies; Kay Elizabeth (Oxford, GB), Dennis; Carina (New York, NY), Tinsley; Jonathon Mark (Oxford, GB)

  Assignee(s): Medical Research Council (London, GB)

  Patent Number: 5,972,609

  Date filed: October 22, 1997

  Abstract: Mouse and human utrophin gene promoters are provided. The promoters or fragments and derivatives may be used to control transcription of heterologous sequences, including coding sequences of reporter genes. Expression systems such as host cells containing nucleic acid constructs which comprise a promoter as provided operably linked to a heterologous sequence may be used to screen substances for ability to modulate activity of the utrophin promoter. Substances with such ability may be manufactured and/or used in the preparation of compositions such as medicaments. Up-regulation of utrophin expression may compensate for dystrophin loss in **muscular dystrophy** patients.

Excerpt(s): The present invention is based on cloning of a genomic promoter region of the human utrophin gene and of the mouse utrophin gene.... The severe muscle wasting disorders Duchenne **muscular dystrophy** (DMD) and the less debilitating Becker **muscular dystrophy** (BMD) are due to mutations in the dystrophin gene resulting in a lack of dystrophin or abnormal expression of truncated forms of dystrophin, respectively. Dystrophin is a large cytoskeletal protein (427 kDa with a length of 125 nm) which in muscle is located at the cytoplasmic surface of the sarcolemma, the neuromuscular junction (NMJ) and myotendinous junction (MTJ). It binds to a complex of proteins and glycoproteins spanning the sarcolemma called the dystrophin associated glycoprotein complex (DGC). The breakdown of the integrity of this complex due to loss of, or impairment of dystrophin function, leads to muscle degeneration and the DMD phenotype.... The dystrophin gene is the largest gene so far identified in man, covering over 2.7 megabases and containing 79 exons. The corresponding 14 kb dystrophin mRNA is expressed predominantly in skeletal, cardiac and smooth muscle with lower levels in brain. Transcription of dystrophin in different tissues is regulated from either the brain promoter (predominantly active in neuronal cells) or muscle promoter (differentiated myogenic cells, and primary glial cells) giving rise to differing first exons. A third promoter between the muscle promoter and the second exon of dystrophin regulates expression in cerebellar Purkinje neurons. Recently reviewed in [1,2,3].

Web site: http://www.delphion.com/details?pn=US05972609__

Patent Applications on Muscular Dystrophy

As of December 2000, U.S. patent applications are open to public viewing.[21] Applications are patent requests which have yet to be granted (the process to achieve a patent can take several years). The following patent applications have been filed since December 2000 relating to muscular dystrophy:

---

[21] This has been a common practice outside the United States prior to December 2000.

- **Biglycan and related therapeutics and methods of use**

Inventor(s): Bowe, Mark A.; (Derwood, MD), Creely, Hilliary; (Providence, RI), Fallon, Justin R.; (Harvard, MA), Ferri, Raymond; (Providence, RI), McKechnie, Beth; (Franklin, MA), Rafii, Michael; (Riverside, RI)

Correspondence: ROPES & GRAY LLP; ONE INTERNATIONAL PLACE; BOSTON; MA; 02110-2624; US

Patent Application Number: 20040063627

Date filed: February 20, 2002

Abstract: The invention provides compositions and methods for treating, preventing, and diagnosing diseases or conditions associated with an abnormal level or activity of biglycan; disorders associated with an unstable cytoplasmic membrane, due, e.g., to an unstable dystrophin associated protein complex (DAPC); disorders associated with abnormal synapses or neuromuscular junctions, including those resulting from an abnormal MuSK activation or acetylcholine receptor (AChR) aggregation. Example of diseases include muscular dystrophies, such as **Duchenne's Muscular Dystrophy,** Becker's **Muscular Dystrophy,** neuromuscular disorders and neurological disorders.

Excerpt(s): This application is a continuation-in-part of U.S. Ser. No. 09/715,836 filed 17 Nov. 2000, which claims the benefit of U.S. Provisional Application No. 60/166,253, filed 18 Nov. 1999. This application also claims the benefit of U.S. Provisional Application No. 60/270,053, filed.degree.Feb. 2001. The specifications of each application are specifically incorporated herein.... The dystrophin-associated protein complex (DAPC) links the cytoskeleton to the extracellular matrix and is necessary for maintaining the integrity of the muscle cell.backslash.plasma membrane. The core DAPC consists of the cytoskeletal scaffolding molecule dystrophin and the dystroglycan and sarcoglycan transmembrane subcomplexes. The DAPC also serves to localize key signaling molecules to the cell surface, at least in part through its associated syntrophins (Brenman, et al. (1996) Cell. 84: 757-767; Bredt, et al. (1998), Proc Natl Acad Sci USA. 95: 14592). Mutations in either dystrophin or any of the sarcoglycans result in muscular dystrophies characterized by breakdown of the muscle cell membrane, loss of myofibers, and fibrosis (Hoffman, et al. 1987. Cell. 51: 919; Straub, and Campbell (1997) Curr Opin Neurol. 10: 168). Moreover, mutations in the extracellular matrix protein laminin-.alpha.2, which associates with the DAPC on the cell surface, is the basis of a major congenital **muscular dystrophy** (Helbling-Leclerc, et al. (1995) Nat Genet. 11: 216).... The.alpha.-/.beta.-dystroglycan subcomplex forms a critical structural link in the DAPC. The transmembrane.beta.-dystroglycan and the wholly extracellular.alpha.-dystroglycan arise by proteolytic cleavage of a common precursor (Ibraghimov, et al. (1992) Nature 355: 696; Bowe, et al. (1994) Neuron 12: 1173). The cytoplasmic tail of.beta.-dystroglycan binds dystrophin, while the highly glycosylated, mucin-like.alpha.-dystroglycan binds to several ECM elements including agrin, laminin, and perlecan (Ervasti and Campbell, (1993) J Cell Biol. 122: 809; Bowe, et al. (1994) Neuron. 12: 1173; Gee, et al. (1994) Cell 77: 675; Hemler, (1999) Cell 97: 543). This binding to matrix proteins appears to be essential for assembly of basal lamina, since mice deficient in dystroglycan fail to form these structures and die very early in development (Henry, M. D. and K. P. Campbell. 1998. Cell. 95: 859)..beta.-Dystroglycan can bind the signaling adapter molecule Grb2 and associates indirectly with p125FAK (Yang, et al. (1995) J. Biol. Chem. 270: 11711; Cavaldesi, et al. (1999), J. Neurochem. 72: 01648). Although the significance of these associations remains unknown, these binding properties suggest that dystroglycan may also serve to localize signaling molecules to the cell surface.

Web site: http://appft1.uspto.gov/netahtml/PTO/search-bool.html

- **Diagnostics, assay methods and amelioration of muscular dystrophy symptoms**

Inventor(s): Kaufman, Stephen J.; (Urbana, IL)

Correspondence: GREENLEE WINNER AND SULLIVAN P C; 5370 MANHATTAN CIRCLE; SUITE 201; BOULDER; CO; 80303; US

Patent Application Number: 20020192710

Date filed: February 20, 2002

Abstract: The present disclosure provides compositions and sequences for the diagnosis, genetic therapy of certain muscular dystrophies, especially **muscular dystrophy** resulting from a deficiency in dystrophin protein or a combined deficiency in dystrophin and utrophin, and methods and compositions for the identification of compounds which increase expression of the.alpha.7 integrin. Expression of the integrin.alpha.BX2 polypeptide in muscle cells results in better physical condition in a patient or an animal lacking normal levels of dystrophin or dystrophin and utrophin. The present disclosure further provides immunological and nucleic acid based methods for the diagnosis of scapuloperoneal **muscular dystrophy,** where there is a reduction in or absence of.alpha.7A integrin expression in muscle tissue samples and normal levels of laminin-{fraction (2/4)} in those same samples. The present disclosure further provides methods for identifying compositions which increase the expression of.alpha.7 integrin protein in muscle cells of dystrophy patients.

Excerpt(s): This application claims priority from U.S. Provisional Application 60/270,645 filed Feb. 20, 2001 and from U.S. Provisional Application 60/286,890 filed Apr. 27, 2001, both of which are incorporated herein.... The field of the present invention is the area of medical treatment and diagnosis using molecular technology. In particular, the present invention utilizes gene therapy and drug induced gene expression to ameliorate the physical condition of **muscular dystrophy** patients, especially those lacking dystrophin or lacking dystrophin and utrophin or those with lower than normal levels of.alpha.7 integrin, and in another aspect, this invention relates to the use of nucleic acid probes or primers or immunological probes for detecting the reduction of or lack of expression of the.alpha.7.beta.1 integrin in scapuloperoneal **muscular dystrophy** (SPMD) as well as to the use of assays to identify compounds which induce increased expression via.alpha.7.beta.1 integrin transcriptional regulatory sequences.... Scapuloperoneal (SP) **muscular dystrophy** is one of a heterogenous group of scapuloperoneal syndromes affecting the muscles of the shoulder girdle and peroneal. SP syndromes were formerly grouped as one genetic disease, but clinical analysis and genetic mapping have revealed that this syndrome includes at least two distinct diseases with different underlying genetic defects. SPMD is an autosomal dominant disorder characterized by myopathy and progressive muscle weakening in the shoulder girdle and peroneal muscles. The disease has late onset, with affected individuals first displaying symptoms in their late teens or early twenties and up to the late fifties. This disease affects the legs and feet (with foot drop and hammer toes) and the proximal and/or distal arms. Patients have scapular winging and asymmetry. There is intolerance to exercise. Other symptoms include contractures, hearing loss, twitching, muscle cramps, facial weakness and cardiac disorders. Death results from cardiac or respiratory failure. Although the underlying genetic defect has not been identified previously, SPMD has been mapped by genetic linkage analysis to human chromosome 12q13.3-q15.

Web site: http://appft1.uspto.gov/netahtml/PTO/search-bool.html

- **DNA sequences encoding dystrophin minigenes and methods of use thereof**

Inventor(s): Xiao, Xiao; (Wexford, PA)

Correspondence: David A. Einhorn, Esq.; Anderson Kill & Olick, P.C.; 1251 Avenue of the Americas; New York; NY; 10020; US

Patent Application Number: 20030171312

Date filed: April 30, 2001

Abstract: The present invention provides a series of novel dystrophin minigenes that retain the essential biological functions. The expression of the dystrophin minigenes may be controlled by a regulatory element along with a small polyadenylation signal. The entire gene expression cassettes may be readily packaged into a viral vector, preferably an AAV vector. The present invention further defines the minimal functional domains of dystrophin and provides ways to optimize and create new versions of dystrophin minigenes. Finally, the present invention provides a method of treatment for Duchenne **muscular dystrophy** (DMD) and Becker **muscular dystrophy** (BMD).

Excerpt(s): The present invention relates to novel dystrophin minigenes that retain the essential biological functions of a full length dystrophin gene, and methods of treatment for Duchenne **muscular dystrophy** (DMD) and Becker **muscular dystrophy** (BMD) in a mammalian subject using the dystrophin minigenes.... Duchenne **muscular dystrophy** (DMD) is an X-linked genetic muscle disease affecting 1 of every 3,500 newborn males (Kunkel et al. Nature (London) 322,73-77 [1986]). The progressive muscle degeneration and weakness usually confine the patients to wheelchairs by their early teens, and lead to death by their early twenties. DMD is caused by recessive mutations in the dystrophin gene, the largest gene known to date, which spans nearly 3 million base-pairs on the X-chromosome with 79 exons, a coding sequence of about 11 kb, and a high rate of de novo mutations. (Koenig et al. Cell 50, 509-517 [1987]).... Dystrophin is an enormous rod-like protein of 3,685 amino acids (aa) localized beneath the inner surface of muscle cell membrane (Watkins, S. C. et al. Nature 333, 863-866 [1988]). It functions through four major structural domains: a N-terminal domain (1-756 aa), a central rod domain (757-3122 aa), a cysteine rich (CR) domain (3123-3409aa), and a distal C-terminal domain (3410-3685 aa). The N-terminal domain binds to the F-actin of cytoskeletal structures, while the CR domain along with the distal C-terminal domain anchors to the cell membrane via dystrophin-associated protein (DAP) complexes, thus, dystrophin crosslinks and stabilizes the muscle cell membrane and cytoskeleton. The central rod domain contains 24 triple-helix rod repeats (R1-R24) and 4 hinges (H1-

H4). Each repeat is approximately 109 aa long. (Koenig et al. J Biol Chem 265, 4560-4566 [1990]). The central rod domain presumably functions as a "shock absorber" during muscle contraction. Dystrophin crosslinks and stabilizes the muscle cell membrane and cytoskeleton. The absence of a functional dystrophin results in the loss of DAP complexes and causes instability of myofiber plasma membrane. These deficiencies in turn lead to chronic muscle damage and degenerative pathology.

Web site: http://appft1.uspto.gov/netahtml/PTO/search-bool.html

- **Method and composition for treating obesity by targeting cathepsin**

Inventor(s): Chen, Jingming; (Fremont, CA), Shi, Guo-Ping; (Palo Alto, CA), Yong, Hamilton H.; (Castro Valley, CA)

Correspondence: WILSON SONSINI GOODRICH & ROSATI; 650 PAGE MILL ROAD; PALO ALTO; CA; 943041050

Patent Application Number: 20040009891

Date filed: June 12, 2003

Abstract: Methods and compositions are provided for modulating fat storage of animals by targeting the gene and gene products of cathepsins, particularly cathepsins L, K, and S, and especially cathepsin L. The method comprises: administering to the animal an agent that reduces an in vivo level of cathepsin L activity such that fat storage by the animal is reduced. The methods of the present invention can be used to diagnose obesity, diabetes and related diseases such as hyperinsulinmia, hyperglycermia, hypertension, cardiovascular diseases, **muscular dystrophy** and infertility, as well as to screen for agents that can be used therapeutics for these diseases.

Excerpt(s): This application is a continuation of U.S. application Ser. No. 09/784,642, filed Feb. 14, 2001 and is hereby incorporated herein by reference.... This invention relates to treatment of obesity and related diseases, such as hyperinsulinmia, hyperglycermia, hypertension, cardiovascular diseases, **muscular dystrophy** and infertility. More particularly, the invention relates to methods of treating obesity and non-insulin-dependent (type II) diabetes mellitus (NIDDM) by specifically targeting the genes and gene products of cathepsins.... Obesity is the most important nutritional disorder in the western world, with the estimates of its prevalence ranging from 30% to 50% within the middle-aged population. Obesity is usually defined as a body weight more than 20% in excess of the ideal body weight. Severe obesity can be a chronic disease that affects an increasingly large number of people and requires long-term treatment to promote and sustain weight loss.

Web site: http://appft1.uspto.gov/netahtml/PTO/search-bool.html

- ## METHOD FOR IN VITRO PRECONDITIONING OF MYOBLASTS BEFORE TRANSPLANTATION

Inventor(s): TREMBLAY, JACQUES P.; (QUEBEC, CA)

Correspondence: BIRCH STEWART KOLASCH & BIRCH; PO BOX 747; FALLS CHURCH; VA; 22040-0747; US

Patent Application Number: 20020012657

Date filed: June 9, 1999

Abstract: A method of pretreating healthy donor's myoblast cultures with growth or trophic factors like basic fibroblast growth factor (bFGF) and with concanavalin A on transplantation to subjects suffering of myopathy like **muscular dystrophy** is disclosed and claimed. Recipient muscles show a higher percentage of functional cells, a four-fold increase, demonstrated by the higher incidence of dystrophin-positive fibers, and does not require previous preconditioning of recipient muscles by irradiation or toxin administration. The recipient subjects were immunosuppressed with FK 506. When growing myoblasts with 20.mu.g/ml concanavalin A or 100 ng/ml TPA for two to four days, migration of donor cells in recipient tissue was increased by 3-4 fold. This suggests that, when using primary cultures, metalloproteases are secreted by fibroblasts, resulting in a greater degradation of the extracellular matrix. Both metalloproteases and bFGF appear beneficial for the success of the transplantation. The use of recombinant myoblast expressing metalloproteases is also contemplated.

Excerpt(s): The present invention is a method for preconditioning healthy donor's myoblasts in vitro before transplantation thereof in compatible patients suffering of recessive myopathies, particularly of **muscular dystrophy.** This in vitro preconditioning improves the success of the transplantation while not requiring an in vivo preconditioning of the patient's muscle by irradiation or by administering muscular toxin.... Duchenne **muscular dystrophy** (DMD) is a progressive disease characterized by the lack of dystrophin under the sarcolemmal membrane.sup.6,19,28,37. One possible way to introduce dystrophin in the muscle fibers of the patients to limit the degeneration is to transplant myoblasts obtained from normal subjects.sup.30,34,35. Several groups have tried myoblast transplantations to DMD patients but poor graft success was observed.sup.17,22,24,38. Even in experimental myoblast transplantation using mdx mice, an animal model of DMD.sup.10,25,29, large amount of dystrophin-positive fibers were observed only when nude mdx mice were previously irradiated to prevent regeneration of the muscle fibers by host myoblasts.sup.32,43. High percentage of dystrophin-positive fibers was also observed in mdx mice immunosuppressed with FK 506 and in SCID mice, in both cases muscles were previously damaged by notexin injection and irradiated.sup.23,27. These results indicate that to obtain successful myoblast transplantation, it is necessary to have not only an immunodeficient mouse or a mouse adequately immunosuppressed but also a host muscle which has been adequately preconditioned. It is, however, impossible in clinical studies to use damaging treatments such as marcaine, notexin and irradiation. If good myoblast transplantation results can be obtained without using such techniques, this would be very helpful for myoblast transplantation in humans.... Recently there has been an increasing interest on the effects of basic fibroblast growth factor (bFGF) and other growth factors on myoblast cultures and myoblast cell lines.sup.1,4,5. Basic FGF has been reported to both stimulate proliferation and inhibit differentiation of skeletal myoblasts in vitro.sup.15,16. Other growth or trophic factors like insulin growth factor I, transferrin, platelet-derived growth factor, epidermal growth factor, adrenocorticotrophin and macrophage colony-stimulating factor as well as C kinase proteins activators or agonists by which the effect of bFGF is mediated.sup.20 may also have similar or even better effects than bFGF on the success of myoblast transplantation.sup.7. The use of these stimulating properties to enhance the success of transplantation by in vitro preconditioning of donor's cells and to replace at least partially the use of previously known methods of in vivo preconditioning of recipients' cells has never been suggested before.

Web site: http://appft1.uspto.gov/netahtml/PTO/search-bool.html

- **Method of early detection of duchenne muscular dystrophy and other neuromuscular disease**

Inventor(s): Hampton, Thomas G.; (Framingham, MA)

Correspondence: LAHIVE & COCKFIELD; 28 STATE STREET; BOSTON; MA; 02109; US

Patent Application Number: 20030003052

Date filed: June 19, 2002

Abstract: The mdx mouse is a model of Duchenne **muscular dystrophy.** The present invention describes that mdx mice exhibited clinically relevant cardiac phenotypes. A non-invasive method of recording electrocardiograms (ECGs) was used to a study mdx mice (n=15) and control mice (n=15). The mdx mice had significant tachycardia, consistent with observations in patients with **muscular dystrophy.** Heart-rate was nearly 15% faster in mdx mice than control mice (P<0.01). ECGs revealed significant shortening of the rate-corrected QT interval duration (QTc) in mdx mice compared to control mice (P<0.05). PR interval duration were shorter at baseline in mdx compared to control mice (P<0.05). The muscarinic antagonist atropine significantly increased heart-rate and decreased PR interval duration in C57 mice. Paradoxically, atropine significantly decreased heart-rate and increased PR interval duration in all mdx mice. Pharmacological autonomic blockade and baroreflex sensitivity testing demonstrated an imbalance in autonomic nervous system modulation of heart-rate, with decreased parasympathetic activity and increased sympathetic activity in mdx mice. These electrocardiographic findings in dystrophin-deficient mice provide new bases for diagnosing, understanding, and treating patients with Duchenne **muscular dystrophy.**

Excerpt(s): This application claims priority to U.S. provisional patent application serial No. 60/299,302, filed Jun. 19, 2001, and to U.S. provisional patent application serial No. 60/338,821, filed Nov. 17, 2001. The contents of these provisional patent applications are incorporated herein by reference in their entirety.... Dysfunction of the autonomic nervous system is an under-recognized but important aspect of the etiological and clinical manifestation of neuromuscular disorder such as Duchenne **muscular dystrophy** (DMD). DMD is an X-linked inherited disorder that affects over nearly 30 out of every 100,000 boys born in the United States. The disorder results from a defect in the gene for an enormous protein called dystrophin, which forms part of the scaffold in muscle fibers. Although the disorder is present from the initial stages of fetal development, there is no physical indication at birth that the baby is abnormal. Rarely is there physical diagnosis in the first year of life. Problems are usually not evident until 18 months to 4 years of age. Usually diagnosis is not made until the child is five. Nearly 50% of affected boys do not walk until 18 months of age or later. Duchenne children have difficulty climbing and getting up from the floor. Parents often comment that their child falls frequently. By the age 3 to 5 years, generalized muscle weakness becomes more obvious. Parents may be falsely encouraged by a seeming improvement at school age, but this may be due to natural growth and development. Weakness progresses rapidly after age 8 or 9, resulting in the inability to walk or stand unassisted. Leg braces may make walking possible for a year or two, but by early adolescence walking becomes impossible. There are some boys with Duchenne **muscular dystrophy** who have problems with delay in mental or language development. Eventually all the major muscles are affected.

Lung capacity may decrease, resulting in an increased susceptibility to respiratory infections. Cardiac and respiratory failure are common in Duchenne patients.... Autonomic nervous system abnormalities have now been frequently reported in patients. The cardiac phenotype includes decreased parasympathetic nervous activity and increased sympathetic nervous activity. Currently there is no reliable mode of prenatal diagnosis or cure. For a series of reasons, diagnosis of Duchenne patients using DNA markers from amniocytes is error ridden and deletion mutants are detectable in only 65% of cases. Therefore, early detection of the disease before locomotor or autonomic disturbances reduce quality of life or irreversibly affect outcome of the disease could significantly improve life-quality prospects and longevity in those afflicted with dystrophin-deficiency related diseases.

Web site: http://appft1.uspto.gov/netahtml/PTO/search-bool.html

- **Methods for treating muscular dystrophy**

Inventor(s): Gussoni, Emanuela; (Winchester, MA), Kunkel, Louis M.; (Westwood, MA), Mulligan, Richard C.; (Lincoln, MA), Soneoka, Yuko; (Washington, DC)

Correspondence: HAMILTON, BROOK, SMITH & REYNOLDS, P.C.; 530 VIRGINIA ROAD; P.O. BOX 9133; CONCORD; MA; 01742-9133; US

Patent Application Number: 20020182192

Date filed: March 14, 2002

Abstract: Methods for treating muscle diseases via bone marrow transplantation of either allogeneic cells or autologous cells engineered to express dystrophin or other gene products affected in muscle diseases are disclosed. Bone marrow cells and bone marrow SP cells (a highly purified population of hematopoietic stem cells) can be used in the methods. Muscle diseases include muscular dystrophies, such as Duchenne **muscular dystrophy,** Becker **muscular dystrophy** and limb-girdle muscular dystrophies.

Excerpt(s): This application is a continuation of International Application No. PCT/US00/25128, filed Sep. 14, 2000, which claims the benefit of U.S. Provisional Application No. 60/153,821, filed Sep. 14, 1999. The teachings of the above applications are incorporated herein by reference in their entirety.... There are probably about 3,000 muscle proteins, each encoded by a different gene. Some muscle proteins are part of the structure of muscle fibers, while others influence chemical reactions in the fibers. A defect in a muscle protein gene can lead to a muscle disease. The precise defect in a muscle protein gene can influence the nature and severity of a muscle disease.... Muscular dystrophies are caused by defects in muscle protein genes and are typically progressive disorders mainly of striated muscle that lead to breakdown of muscle integrity, often resulting in death. The histologic picture shows variation in fiber size, muscle cell necrosis and regeneration, and often proliferation of connective and adipose tissue. The precise defect in a muscle protein gene determines the nature and severity of a **muscular dystrophy.** For example, two major types of **muscular dystrophy,** Duchenne **muscular dystrophy** (DMD) and Becker **muscular dystrophy** (BMD), are allelic, lethal degenerative muscle diseases. DMD results from mutations in the dystrophin gene on the X-chromosome (Hoffinan et al., N. Engl. J. Med., 318:1363-1368 (1988)), which usually result in the absence of dystrophin, a cytoskeletal protein in skeletal and cardiac muscle. BMD is the result of mutations in the same gene (Hoffinan et al., N. Engl. J. Med., 318:1363-1368 (1988)), but dystrophin is usually expressed in muscle but at a reduced level and/or as a shorter, internally deleted form, resulting in a milder phenotype.

Web site: http://appft1.uspto.gov/netahtml/PTO/search-bool.html

- **Methods for treating muscular dystrophy**

  Inventor(s): Oron, Amir; (Tel-Aviv, IL), Streeter, Jackson; (Reno, NV)

  Correspondence: KNOBBE MARTENS OLSON & BEAR LLP; 2040 MAIN STREET; FOURTEENTH FLOOR; IRVINE; CA; 92614; US

  Patent Application Number: 20040153130

  Date filed: May 29, 2003

  Abstract: Therapeutic methods for treating or inhibiting a neuromuscular disease or condition, including **muscular dystrophy,** in a subject in need thereof are described, the methods including applying to muscle tissue of the subject a **muscular dystrophy** effective amount of electromagnetic energy having a wavelength in the visible to near-infrared wavelength. In a preferred embodiment, the **muscular dystrophy** effective amount of energy comprises predetermined power density (mW/cm.sup.2) of the electromagnetic energy of at least 1 mW/cm.sup.2, which is provided from a laser or other light energy source.

  Excerpt(s): This application claims priority under 35 U.S.C..sctn. 119(e) to U.S. Provisional Application Serial No. 60/384,050, filed May 29, 2002 and is a continuation-in-part of U.S. patent application Ser. No. 10/287,432, filed Nov. 1, 2002, the disclosures of which are hereby incorporated by reference in their entireties.... The present invention relates in general to therapeutic methods for the treatment of **muscular dystrophy,** and more particularly to methods for treating **muscular**

dystrophy by applying electromagnetic energy.... Muscular dystrophy (MD) encompasses a group of genetically determined muscular disorders that are characterized by progressive wasting and weakness of the skeletal muscle, and often also of the cardiac and smooth muscles or other tissues. See, e.g., K. Arhata, NEUROPATHOLOGY 20:34-41 (2000); C. Angelini and D. M. Bonifati, Neurol. Sci. 21: 919-24 (2002).

Web site: http://appft1.uspto.gov/netahtml/PTO/search-bool.html

- **Pathogenesis of cardiomyopathy**

Inventor(s): Campbell, Kevin P.; (Iowa City, IA), Cohn, Ronald; (Iowa City, IA), Coral, Ramon; (Iowa City, IA), Durbeej, Madeleine; (Iowa City, IA), Williamson, Roger; (Iowa City, IA)

Correspondence: Farrell & Associates, P.C.; P.O. Box 999; York Harbor; ME; 03911; US

Patent Application Number: 20010016952

Date filed: January 4, 2001

Abstract: Disclosed within is a mouse, and cells derived therefrom, which are homozygous for a disrupted.delta.-sarcoglycan gene, the disruption in said gene having been introduced into the mouse or an ancestor of the mouse at an embryonic stage. Said disruption prevents the synthesis of functional.delta.-sarcoglycan in cells of the mouse and results in the mouse having a reduced amount of.beta.- and.epsilon.-sarcoglycan and sarcospan, and a disruption of the sarcoglycan-sarcospan complex in smooth muscle of the mouse. Said disruption also results in a reduced amount of sarcospan,.alpha.-,.beta.-,.gamma.-, and.epsilon.-sarcoglycan in the sarcolemma of skeletal and cardiac muscles of the mouse, compared to the amounts of said components in a mouse lacking disrupted.delta.-sarcoglycan genes. Preferred specific disruptions of the.delta.-sarcoglycan gene are listed. Also disclosed is a mouse, and cells derived therefrom, which are homozygous for a disrupted.beta.-sarcoglycan gene, the disruption in said gene having been introduced into the mouse or an ancestor of the mouse at an embryonic stage. The disruption prevents the synthesis of functional.beta.-sarcoglycan in cells of the mouse and results in the mouse having a reduced amount of.delta.- and.epsilon.-sarcoglycan and sarcospan and.alpha.-dystroglycan in smooth muscle of the mouse. The disruption also results in a disruption of the sarcoglycan-sarcospan complex in smooth muscle of the mouse, and a reduced amount of sarcospan,.alpha.,.gamma.,.delta.- and.epsilon.-sarcoglycan in the sarcolemma of skeletal and cardiac muscles of the mouse, compared to the amounts of the components in a mouse lacking disrupted.beta.-sarcoglycan genes. Preferred specific disruptions of the.beta.-sarcoglycan gene are listed. A method for treating mammalian autosomal recessive **limb-girdle muscular dystrophy** type 2F in an individual is also disclosed. The method comprises, providing an expression vector which encodes a wild-type form of.delta.-sarcoglycan, and introducing the expression vector into skeletal and smooth muscle tissue of the individual under conditions appropriate for expression of the wild-type form of.delta.-sarcoglycan in said tissues. Examples of expression vectors for use in this method are adenovirus expression vector, a gutted adenovirus expression vector, and an adeno-associated expression vector. Also disclosed are methods for treating mammalian autosomal recessive **limb-girdle muscular dystrophy** type 2E, and type 2F, in an individual. The methods comprise, providing an expression vector which encodes a wild-type form of.beta.-sarcoglycan, or.delta.-sarcoglycan, respectively, and introducing the expression vector into skeletal and smooth muscle tissue of the individual under conditions appropriate for expression of the wild-type form of the sarcoglycan gene in said tissues. The.delta.-sarcoglycan deficient, and.beta.-sarcoglycan deficient mice of the present invention are useful in identifying therapeutic compounds for treatment of an individual diagnosed with.delta.-sarcoglycan-deficient **limb-girdle muscular dystrophy,** and beta-sarcoglycan-deficient **limb-girdle muscular dystrophy,** respectively. A therapeutic method for treating ischemic heart disease caused by reduced expression of the sarcoglycan-sarcospan complex in vascular smooth muscle cells of an individual is also provided. The method comprises contacting the vascular smooth muscle cells of the individual with a vascular smooth muscle relaxant, such as Nicorandil. This method is also useful for preventing ischemic injury in skeletal and cardiac muscle of an individual caused by reduced expression of the sarcoglycan-sarcospan complex in the vascular smooth muscle cells of the individual. The method is also useful for treating mammalian autosomal recessive **limb-girdle muscular dystrophy** type 2F or type 2E in an individual. Other methods provided include a method for identifying a therapeutic compound for the treatment of ischemic heart disease in an individual caused by reduced expression of the sarcoglycan-sarcospan complex in the vascular smooth muscle cells of the individual, and also a method for identifying a therapeutic compound for the prevention of ischemic injury in skeletal and cardiac muscle of an individual which is caused by reduced expression of the sarcoglycan-sarcospan complex in vascular smooth muscle cells of the individual.

Excerpt(s): The sarcoglycan complex is a group of single pass transmembrane proteins (.alpha.,.beta.,.delta.and.gamma.-sarcoglycan) which is tightly associated with sarcospan to form a subcomplex within the dystrophin-glycoprotein complex (DGC) in skeletal and cardiac muscle (Campbell et al., Nature 338: 259-362 (1989); Yoshida et al., J. Biochem. 108: 748-752 (1990); Crosbie et al., J. Cell Biol. 145: 153-165 (1999)). The DGC is further comprised of dystrophin, the dystroglycan complex and the syntrophins (Hoffman et al., Cell 51: 919-928 (1987); Froehner et al., Soc. Gen. Physiol. Ser. 52: 197-207 (1997); Durbeej et al., Curr. Opin. Cell. Biol. 10: 594-601 (1998)). The expression of the sarcoglycan-sarcospan complex is necessary to target dystroglycan to the sarcolemma (Duclos et al., J. Cell Biol. 142: 1461-1471 (1998); Duclos et al., Neuromusc. Disord. 8: 30-38 (1998); Holt et al., Mol. Cell 1: 841-848 (1998); Straub et al., Am. J. Path. 153: 1623-1630 (1998)) which in turn confers a link between the extracellular matrix and the F-actin cytoskeleton (Ervasti et al., J. Cell Biol. 122: 809-823 (1993)). Thus, the DGC is thought to protect muscle cells from contraction-induced damage (Petrof et al., Proc. Natl. Acad. Sci. USA 90: 3710-3714 (1993)). In agreement with this hypothesis, mutations in the genes for the sarcoglycans, dystrophin and laminin.alpha.2 chain are responsible for **limb-girdle muscular dystrophy,** Duchenne/Becker **muscular dystrophy** and congenital **muscular dystrophy** respectively (Straub et al., Curr. Opin. Neurol. 10: 168-175 (1997); Lim et al., Curr. Opin. Neurol. 11: 443-452 (1998)). Clinical evidence of cardiomyopathy is variably present in these muscular dystrophies (Towbin, J. A., Curr. Opin. Cell Biol. 10: 131-139 (1998)) but a correlation between the primary mutation of the sarcoglycan genes and cardiomyopathy is yet to be established (Melacini et al., Muscle & Nerve 22: 473-479 (1999)).... Dilated cardiomyopathy is a multifactorial disease that includes both inherited and acquired forms of cardiomyopathy. Inherited cardiomyopathy in humans can be associated with genetic defects occurring in components of the dystrophin-glycoprotein complex (DGC) (Towbin, J. A., Curr. Opin. Cell Biol. 10: 131-139 (1998)). Mutations in the dystrophin gene lead to a high incidence of cardiomyopathy in Duchenne and Becker **muscular dystrophy** patients (DMD/BMD) and can cause X-linked dilated cardiomyopathy (Towbin, J. A., Curr. Opin. Cell Biol. 10: 131-139 (1998)). In addition to these primary genetic causes of cardiomyopathy, recent data suggest that disruption of the DGC underlie the cardiomyopathy associated with enteroviral infection (Badorff et al., Nat. Med. 5: 320-326 (1999)). Consequently, evidence is accumulating that the DGC plays a critical role in the pathogenesis of some forms of inherited and acquired cardiomyopathy. Several components of the DGC are also expressed in smooth muscle (Houzelstein et al., J. Cell Biol. 119: 811-821 (1992); North et al., J. Cell Biol. 120: 1159-1167 (1993); Ozawa, et al., Hum. Mol. Gen. 4: 1711-1716 (1995); Durbeej et al., Curr. Opin. Cell. Biol. 10: 594-601 (1998)). Interestingly, potential smooth muscle dysfunction has been described in patients with Duchenne **muscular dystrophy** (Bahron et al., N. Engl. J. Med. 319: 15-18 (1998); Jaffe et al., Arch. Phys. Med. Rehabil. 71: 742-744 (1990)). However, no smooth muscle dysfunction has been reported in patients with **limb-girdle muscular dystrophy**.... Recently, a fifth sarcoglycan,.epsilon.-sarcoglycan, was cloned and shown to be highly homologous to.alpha.-sarcoglycan (Ettinger et al., J. Biol. Chem. 272: 32534-32538 (1997); McNally et al., FEBS Lett. 422: 27-32 (1998))..epsilon.-sarcoglycan is expressed in skeletal and cardiac muscle, but also in several non-muscle tissues. Whether.epsilon.-sarcoglycan is associated with the other sarcoglycans in striated muscle is yet to be determined. At the immunofluorescence level, however, it has been shown that.epsilon.-sarcoglycan is still present in skeletal muscle of.alpha.-sarcoglycan deficient (Sgca-null mice) mice although the other sarcoglycans are greatly reduced (Duclos et al., J. Cell Biol. 142: 1461-1471 (1998)). This indicates that.epsilon.-sarcoglycan is not an additional member of the known tetrameric complex of.alpha.-,.beta.-,.gamma.- and.delta.-sarcoglycan in skeletal muscle but may be part of a distinct complex at the sarcolemma.

Web site: http://appft1.uspto.gov/netahtml/PTO/search-bool.html

- **Pharmaceutical composition for treatment of duchenne muscular dystrophy**

Inventor(s): Matsuo, Masafumi; (Kobe-shi, JP)

Correspondence: GREENBLUM & BERNSTEIN, P.L.C.; 1941 ROLAND CLARKE PLACE; RESTON; VA; 20191; US

Patent Application Number: 20010056077

Date filed: July 31, 2001

Abstract: A therapeutic pharmaceutical composition for patients of Duchenne **muscular dystrophy** with entire loss of exon 20 in dystrophin mature mRNA is provided. The composition comprise as an active principle an antisense oligonucleotide consisting of a 20 to 50-nucleotide sequence against exon 19 of the dystrophin pre-mRNA.

Excerpt(s): This application is a continuation application of U.S. application Ser. No. 09/563,260 filed May 1, 2000, and which claims priority of Japanese Application No. 140930/99, filed May 21, 1999. The entire disclosure of U.S. application Ser. No. 09/563,260 is considered as being part of the disclosure of this application, and the entire disclosure of U.S. application Ser. No. 09/563,260 is expressly incorporated by reference herein in its entirety.... The present invention relates to the use of an antisense oligonucleotide for the manufacture of a therapeutic pharmaceutical composition for a certain hereditary disease, and more specifically to a therapeutic pharmaceutical composition for Duchenne **muscular dystrophy** intended to induce an exon skipping in the pre-mRNA of a certain abnormal dystrophin gene.... Antisense oligonucleotide strategy has been widely studied for the purpose of inhibiting expression of oncogenes or viral genes. Antisense oligonucleotides have been known to efficiently inhibit de novo synthesis of their respective targeted proteins. For example, it is known that an antisense oligonucleotide against the mRNA encoding IGF-I (Insulin-like Growth Factor-I) inhibits proliferation of rat glioblastoma cells [Askari, F. K., and McDonnell, W. M., N. Engl. J. Med, 334: 316-318 (1996); Trojan, et al., Science, 259: 94-97 (1993), Trojan, et al., Proc. Natl Acad. Sci. U.S.A., 89: 4874-4878 (1992)].

Web site: http://appft1.uspto.gov/netahtml/PTO/search-bool.html

- **Pharmaceutical composition for treatment of Duchenne muscular dystrophy**

Inventor(s): Kamei, Shoichiro; (Kobe-shi, JP), Matsuo, Masafumi; (Kobe-shi, JP)

Correspondence: GREENBLUM & BERNSTEIN, P.L.C.; 1941 ROLAND CLARKE PLACE; RESTON; VA; 20191; US

Patent Application Number: 20020055481

Date filed: August 16, 2001

Abstract: The invention provides an isolated and purified DNA set forth as SEQ ID NO:15 in the Sequence Listing and an antisense oligonucleotide complementary to the DNA. The DNA represents the splicing enhancer sequence (SES) in exon 45 of human dystrophin gene, and serves as a template in preparation of the antisense oligonucleotide, which is used to induce exon 45 skipping in certain group of patient with Duchenne **muscular dystrophy** to restore the reading frame of dystrophin mRNA.

Excerpt(s): The present invention relates to pharmaceutical compositions for treatment of Duchenne **muscular dystrophy,** which pharmaceutical compositions are designed to correct an existing shift of the amino acid reading frame in dystrophin pre-mRNA, by inducing in a predetermined manner an exon skipping in the pre-mRNA having the shifted reading frame as a result of abnormalities in dystrophin gene. More specifically, the present invention relates to a splicing enhancer sequence (SES) in dystrophin gene which can be utilized for the preparation of pharmaceutical compositions for treatment of a specific type of Duchenne

muscular dystrophy, as well as to antisense oligonucleotides against the splicing enhancer sequence, and therapeutic pharmaceutical compositions comprising such oligonucleotides.... Diagnosis has become available today for hereditary diseases caused by abnormal splicing of pre-mRNA molecules. A so far intractable disease, **muscular dystrophy,** has thus come to draw particular attention. **Muscular dystrophy** is divided into two groups: Duchenne **muscular dystrophy** (DMD) and Becker **muscular dystrophy** (BMD). DMD is a hereditary muscular disease of the highest incidence, occurring in one in 3,500 live male births. Patients of DMD at first exhibit a lowered muscular power in their infancy, then suffer a constant progression of muscular atrophy thereafter, and eventually die at around the age of 20. It is in contrast to BMD, in which the onset of the disease is relatively late, somewhere in the adulthood, and though a mild loss of muscular power is observed after the onset of the disease, patients can live nearly a normal life. No drug is so far available for effective treatment of DMD, and therefore development of a drug for its treatment has been longed for by the patients across the world. In 1987, dystrophin gene, the causative gene of DMD, was found by means of retrospective genetics, and BMD also was found to result from abnormality in the same dystrophin gene [Koenig, M. et al., Cell, 50:509-517(1987)].... Dystrophin gene is located in the subregion 21 of the short arm of the X-chromosome. The size of the gene is 3.0 Mb, the largest known human gene. Despite that large size, only 14 kb regions in total of the dystrophin gene do encode the whole dystrophin protein, and those encoding regions are divided into no less than 79 exons which are distributed throughout the gene [Roberts, R G., et al., Genomics, 16:536-538(1993)]. The transcript of dystrophin gene, i.e. pre-mRNA, is spliced into the mature 14 kb mRNA. The gene has eight distinct promoter regions also distributed within the gene and they are responsible for production of distinct mRNAs, respectively [Nishio, H., et al., J. Clin. Invest., 94:1073-1042(1994), Ann, A H. and Kunkel, L M., Nature Genet., 3:283-291(1993), D'Souza, V N. et al., Hum. Mol. Genet., 4:837-842(1995)]. Thus, dystrophin gene and its transcript are structurally very complex.

Web site: http://appft1.uspto.gov/netahtml/PTO/search-bool.html

- **Treatment of congenital muscular dystrophies**

Inventor(s): Ruegg, Markus A.; (Riehen, CH)

Correspondence: LEYDIG VOIT & MAYER, LTD; TWO PRUDENTIAL PLAZA, SUITE 4900; 180 NORTH STETSON AVENUE; CHICAGO; IL; 60601-6780; US

Patent Application Number: 20030224981

Date filed: June 3, 2002

Abstract: Methods of treating congenital **muscular dystrophy** in a mammal, one of which comprises administering to the mammal a therapeutically effective amount of a protein comprising at least one binding domain for a laminin and at least one binding domain for.alpha.-dystroglycan, and the other of which comprises administering to the mammal a therapeutically effective amount of a substance that upregulates endogenous agrin, an isolated and purified non-naturally occurring protein or polypeptide comprising at least one binding domain for a laminin and at least one binding domain for.alpha.-dystroglycan, an isolated and purified nucleic acid encoding the protein or polypeptide, optionally in the form of a recombinant vector, a composition comprising (i) the aforementioned protein or polypeptide or nucleic acid and (ii) a pharmaceutically acceptable carrier, a nonhuman transgenic animal, which expresses the aforementioned protein or polypeptide or comprises and expresses the aforementioned nucleic acid, and a method of identifying a substance that upregulates endogenous agrin in a mammal, which method comprises (i) contacting a mammalian muscle or cells or tissue thereof with a substance, and (ii) comparing the amount of agrin in the mammalian muscle or cells or tissue thereof in the presence of the substance with (a) the amount of agrin in the mammalian muscle or cells or tissue thereof before contact with the substance or (b) the amount of agrin in a mammalian muscle or cells or tissue thereof in the absence of the substance.

Excerpt(s): The present invention relates to a method of treating congenital **muscular dystrophy** in a mammal involving the administration of a protein comprising at least one binding domain for a laminin and at least one binding domain for.alpha.-dystroglycan or a substance that upregulates endogenous agrin, proteins and nucleic acids for use in the method, a composition comprising the protein or nucleic acid, a nonhuman transgenic animal expressing the protein, and a method of identifying a substance that upregulates endogenous agrin in a mammal.... A large number of medical disorders are due to genetic defects that result in the expression of mutated and malfunctioning proteins or even total absence of that protein. Diseases, such as dystrophinopathies (e.g., Duchenne and Becker muscular dystrophies), sarcoglycanopathies, and laminin or collagen deficiencies, affect the body muscle mass and can be considered disorders, for which replacement of the malfunctioning or absent protein could effect treatment.... Congenital **muscular dystrophy** is a specific example of these genetically based disorders. It is a heterogeneous and severe, progressive muscle-wasting disease that frequently leads to death in early childhood (Tome et al., in Neuromuscular Disorders: Clinical and Molecular Genetics (ed., Emery), pp. 21-57 (John Wiley & Sons, West Sussex (1998)); and Miyagoe-Suzuki et al., Microsc. Res Tech. 48: 181-191 (2000)). Most cases of congenital **muscular dystrophy** are caused by mutations in LAMA2, the gene encoding the.alpha.2 chain of the main laminin isoforms expressed by muscle fibers. Muscle fiber deterioration in this disease is thought to be caused by failure to form the primary laminin scaffold, which is necessary for basement membrane structure (Colognato et al., Dev. Dyn. 218: 213-234 (2000)), and the missing interaction between muscle basement membrane and the dystrophin-glycoprotein complex (DGC) (Campbell, Cell 80: 675-679 (1995)) or the integrins (Mayer et al., Nature Genet. 17: 318-323 (1997)).

Web site: http://appft1.uspto.gov/netahtml/PTO/search-bool.html

- **TREATMENT OF HEREDITARY DISEASES WITH GENTAMICIN**

Inventor(s): TREMBLAY, JACQUES P.; (BERNIERES, CA)

Correspondence: DENISE HUBERDEAU; STOCK EXCHANGE TOWER; SUITE 3400; 800 PLACE VICTORIA P O BOX 242; MONTREAL; H4Z1E9; CA

Patent Application Number: 20010051607

Date filed: December 22, 1999

Abstract: This invention relates to a method of treating an inherited disease due to a point mutation producing a stop codon by administering an effective dose of an aminoglycoside antibiotic or a derivative thereof. Mdx mouse, which is an animal model for Duchenne **muscular dystrophy,** has been successfully treated with intramuscularly administered 1 and 5 mg gentamicin, which had for effect to suppress the premature stop mutation by inserting an amino acid at the stop codon. Dystrophin positive muscle fibers not different in number from those of normal mouse were detected at the dose of 5 mg gentamicin.

Excerpt(s): Duchenne **Muscular Dystrophy** (DMD) is due to the mutation of a gene in the X chromosome coding for a protein called dystrophin (Koenig et al. 1987; Hoffman et al. 1987; Bodrug et al. 1987, Arahata et al.

1988; Sugita et al. al 1988). The mutations of the dystrophin vary from one family of patients to another but always lead to the absence of a functional dystrophin protein under the membrane on the muscle fiber (Hoffman et al. 1987; Chelly et al. 1990; Chamberlain et al. 1991; Anderson et al 1992; Kilimann et al. 1992; Roberts et al 1992). The absence of dystrophin leads to an increase vulnerability of the muscle fibers during contraction (Menke 1995). Repeated cycles of damages and repairs produce a progressive reduction of the number of muscle fibers and to loss of strength which confine the patients to a wheel chair by the age of ten and to premature death in their early twenties.... Roughly 70% of the mutations of the dystrophin gene are large deletion of one of several exons (Anderson et al 1992; Kilimann et al. 1992). The other mutations are small point mutations due either to a small deletion of a few base pairs leading to a shift of the reading frame or changes of only one base pair producing a missense or a stop codon (Bullman et al 1991: Chamberlain et al. 1994; Roberts et al. 1992; Clemens et al 1992; Nicholson et al. 1993). Around 5% of all DMD mutations may be due to stop codons.... Cystic fibrosis (CF) is due to a mutation of a gene coding for the CF transmembrane conductance regulator (CFTR) protein. Howard et al. (1996) made experiments with a bronchial epithelial cell line obtained from a CF patient having a premature stop mutation in the CFTR gene. This mutation resulted in a premature end of the synthesis of the CFTR protein and thus in a non-functional protein. They incubated this cell line with aminoglycoside antibiotics G-418 (100 mg/mL) or with gentamicin (200 mg/mL) during 18 to 24 hours. This incubation with gentamicin permitted to suppress the premature stop mutation by inserting an amino acid at the stop codon. A full-length CFTR protein was thus obtained. The suppression of the premature stop codon by gentamicin is mediated by mis-pairing between the stop codon and a near-cognate aminoacyl tRNA. Bedwell et al. (1997) recently demonstrated that this full length CFTR protein resulting from the incubation with the aminoglycoside antibiotics was present in the cell membrane and functional.

Web site: http://appft1.uspto.gov/netahtml/PTO/search-bool.html

- **Treatment of muscular dystrophy with cord blood cells**

Inventor(s): Brown, Robert H. JR.; (Needham, MA), Finklestein, Seth P.; (Needham, MA)

Correspondence: CLARK & ELBING LLP; 101 FEDERAL STREET; BOSTON; MA; 02110; US

Patent Application Number: 20030118565

Date filed: July 23, 2002

Abstract: The invention features methods for treating a patient suffering from **muscular dystrophy** by administration of umbilical cord blood cells, e.g., by IV infusion.

Excerpt(s): This application claims the benefit of the filing date of U.S. provisional patent application No. 60/307,227, filed Jul. 23, 2001.... Muscular dystrophy represents a family of inherited diseases of the muscles. Some forms affect children (e.g., Duchenne dystrophy) and are lethal within two to three decades. Other forms present in adult life and are more slowly progressive. The genes for several dystrophies have been identified, including Duchenne dystrophy (caused by mutations in the dystrophin gene) and the teenage and adult onset Miyoshi dystrophy or its variant, limb girdle dystrophy 2B or LGMD-2B (caused by mutations in the dysferlin gene). These are "loss of function" mutations that prevent expression of the relevant protein in muscle and thereby cause muscle dysfunction. Mouse models for these mutations exist, either arising spontaneously in nature or generated by inactivation or deletion of the relevant genes. These models are useful for testing therapies that might replace the missing protein in muscle and restore normal muscle function.... Differentiated muscle is composed of multi-nucleated cells or myofibers that have an extraordinary capacity to regenerate. This regenerative capacity exists because muscle possesses primitive muscle precursor cells (muscle stem cells and somewhat more mature cells known as "satellite cells"). These cells lie dormant in muscle and can be activated to make new mononucleated muscle cells (myoblasts) that can adhere to one another and fuse to make new, multi-nucleated myotubes, as well as the more mature muscle cells (that are again multinucleated). Because myofibers arise from the fusion of individual myoblasts, a protein made by one muscle cell is readily accessible to be shared with neighboring muscle cells lacking that protein if the two cells fuse into the same myotube.

Web site: http://appft1.uspto.gov/netahtml/PTO/search-bool.html

- **Use of chimeric mutational vectors to change endogenous nucleotide sequences in solid tissues**

Inventor(s): Bartlett, Richard J.; (Weston, FL), Rando, Thomas A.; (Stanford, CA)

Correspondence: PILLSBURY WINTHROP, LLP; P.O. BOX 10500; MCLEAN; VA; 22102; US

Patent Application Number: 20020137717

Date filed: February 20, 2002

Abstract: This invention relates to the field of **muscular dystrophy** and methods for its treatment in humans. This invention also concerns art-recognized animal models of Duchenne **muscular dystrophy** in dogs (GRMD) and mice (mdx). Another aspect concerns chimeric mutational vectors capable of inducing reversion of genetic mutations (i.e., gene repair) causing genetic disease by direct injection into affected tissue. Thus, more generally, the invention envisions direct injection of chimeric mutational vectors into affected tissues to effect gene repair therein.

Excerpt(s): This is a continuation application which claims priority benefit to U.S. patent application Ser. No. 09/576,081, filed May 20, 2000, which claims priority benefit to provisional U.S. Appln. No. 60/135,139, filed May 21, 1999, and provisional U.S. Appln. No. 60/174,388, filed Jan. 5, 2000, all of which are incorporated by reference herein.... The invention concerns methods of treating genetic diseases or other pathologic conditions by making one or more specific changes in endogenous nucleotide sequences of solid tissues. These specific changes are mediated by oligonucleobases called chimeric mutational vectors (CMV). The CMV can be administered directly to the subject in vivo; in particular, the CMV can be injected into a solid tissue in which expression of the mutated gene occurs. Such gene repair can reverse the disease or other pathologic condition caused by the mutation or, alternatively, can introduce a second change that compensates for the disease or condition causing mutation.... The inclusion of a reference in this section is not to be understood as an admission that its teachings were publicly available prior to our invention of the subject matter disclosed herein or that they resulted from someone other than the inventors.

Web site: http://appft1.uspto.gov/netahtml/PTO/search-bool.html

Keeping Current

In order to stay informed about patents and patent applications dealing with muscular dystrophy, you can access the U.S. Patent Office archive via the Internet at **http://www.uspto.gov/patft/index.html**. You will see two broad options: (1) Issued Patent, and (2) Published Applications. To see a list of issued patents, perform the following steps: Under "Issued Patents," click "Quick Search." Then, type "muscular dystrophy" (or synonyms) into the "Term 1" box. After clicking on the search button, scroll down to see the various patents which have been granted to date on muscular dystrophy.

You can also use this procedure to view pending patent applications concerning muscular dystrophy. Simply go back to the following Web address: **http://www.uspto.gov/patft/index.html**. Select "Quick Search" under "Published Applications." Then proceed with the steps listed above.

Vocabulary Builder

The following vocabulary builder provides definitions of words used in this chapter that have not been defined in previous chapters:

Blot: To transfer DNA, RNA, or proteins to an immobilizing matrix such as nitrocellulose. [NIH]

Brace: Any form of splint or appliance used to support the limbs or trunk. [NIH]

Codons: Any triplet of nucleotides (coding unit) in DNA or RNA (if RNA is the carrier of primary genetic information as in some viruses) that codes for particular amino acid or signals the beginning or end of the message. [NIH]

Enhancer: Transcriptional element in the virus genome. [NIH]

Fibronectin: An adhesive glycoprotein. One form circulates in plasma, acting as an opsonin; another is a cell-surface protein which mediates cellular adhesive interactions. [NIH]

Grafting: The operation of transfer of tissue from one site to another. [NIH]

Hammer: The largest of the three ossicles of the ear. [NIH]

Hereditary: Of, relating to, or denoting factors that can be transmitted genetically from one generation to another. [NIH]

Immunofluorescence: A technique for identifying molecules present on the surfaces of cells or in tissues using a highly fluorescent substance coupled to a specific antibody. [NIH]

Morphological: Relating to the configuration or the structure of live organs. [NIH]

Noguchi: A medium composed of fresh rabbit kidney tissue in sterile ascitic fluid under vaseline in narrow tubes. [NIH]

Promotor: In an operon, a nucleotide sequence located at the operator end which contains all the signals for the correct initiation of genetic transcription by the RNA polymerase holoenzyme and determines the maximal rate of RNA synthesis. [NIH]

Purifying: Respiratory equipment whose function is to remove contaminants from otherwise wholesome air. [NIH]

Reversion: A return to the original condition, e. g. the reappearance of the normal or wild type in previously mutated cells, tissues, or organisms. [NIH]

Sendai: A virus that causes an important and widespread infection of laboratory mice; it belongs to the parainfluenza group of mixoviruses. The virus is widely used in cell fusion studies. [NIH]

Translocation: The movement of material in solution inside the body of the plant. [NIH]

CHAPTER 5. BOOKS ON MUSCULAR DYSTROPHY

Overview

This chapter provides bibliographic book references relating to muscular dystrophy. You have many options to locate books on muscular dystrophy. The simplest method is to go to your local bookseller and inquire about titles that they have in stock or can special order for you. Some patients, however, feel uncomfortable approaching their local booksellers and prefer online sources (e.g. **www.amazon.com** and **www.bn.com**). In addition to online booksellers, excellent sources for book titles on muscular dystrophy include the Combined Health Information Database and the National Library of Medicine. Once you have found a title that interests you, visit your local public or medical library to see if it is available for loan.

Book Summaries: Federal Agencies

The Combined Health Information Database collects various book abstracts from a variety of healthcare institutions and federal agencies. To access these summaries, go to **http://chid.nih.gov/detail/detail.html**. You will need to use the "Detailed Search" option. To find book summaries, use the drop boxes at the bottom of the search page where "You may refine your search by." Select the dates and language you prefer. For the format option, select "Monograph/Book." Now type "muscular dystrophy" (or synonyms) into the "For these words:" box. You will only receive results on books. You should check back periodically with this database which is updated every 3 months. The following is a typical result when searching for books on muscular dystrophy:

- **A-Z Reference Book of Syndromes and Inherited Disorders**

Source: London, England: Chapman and Hall. 1996. 394 p.

Contact: Available from Singular Publishing Group, Inc. 401 West 'A' Street, Suite 325, San Diego, CA 92101-7904. (800) 521-8545 or (619) 238-6777. Fax (800) 774-8398 or (619) 238-6789. E-mail: singpub@singpub.com. Website: www.singpub.com. PRICE: $42.95 plus shipping and handling. ISBN: 0412641208.

Summary: This book provides a practical reference for both caregivers and those with a syndrome or inherited disorder. The author describes the disorders and problems of both children and adults, and considers the day-to-day management of conditions. The book is written in nontechnical language while still providing enough detail for medical, nursing, and midwifery professionals. The syndromes and disorders are listed alphabetically by name. Those specifically related to deafness, communication, and speech and language include achondroplasia, Alport's syndrome, Apert's syndrome, Asperger's syndrome, Batten's disease, Beckwith-Wiedeman syndrome, CHARGE syndrome, Cockayne syndrome, Cornelia de Lange syndrome, Crouzon's syndrome, Down's syndrome, Duchenne **muscular dystrophy,** Edward's syndrome, Ehlers-Danlos syndrome, Fabry disease, fetal alcohol syndrome, Fragile X syndrome, Gilles de la Tourette syndrome, Goldenhar syndrome, Hunter's syndrome, Hurler's syndrome, Klinefelter's syndrome, LEOPARD syndrome, Moebius syndrome, Morquio's syndrome, neurofibromatosis, Niemann-Pick disease, Noonan's syndrome, osteogenesis imperfecta, Pierre-Robin syndrome, Prader-Willi syndrome, Rett's syndrome, Reye's syndrome, San Filippo syndrome, Smith-Magenis syndrome, Stickler syndrome, Tay-Sachs disease, Treacher Collins syndrome, Turner's syndrome, Usher's syndrome, Waardenburg's syndrome, and William's syndrome. For each syndrome, the author lists alternative names, incidence, causation (etiology), characteristics or symptoms, management implications (treatment options), prognosis, and self-help groups to contact. Most groups listed are in England. The book concludes with three appendices that provide a discussion of genetics, a listing of regional genetics centers (in England), and a glossary of terms. A subject index is also included. (AA-M).

Chapters on Muscular Dystrophy

Frequently, muscular dystrophy will be discussed within a book, perhaps within a specific chapter. In order to find chapters that are specifically dealing with muscular dystrophy, an excellent source of abstracts is the

Combined Health Information Database. You will need to limit your search to book chapters and muscular dystrophy using the "Detailed Search" option. Go to the following hyperlink: **http://chid.nih.gov/detail/detail.html**. To find book chapters, use the drop boxes at the bottom of the search page where "You may refine your search by." Select the dates and language you prefer, and the format option "Book Chapter." By making these selections and typing in "muscular dystrophy" (or synonyms) into the "For these words:" box, you will only receive results on chapters in books. The following is a typical result when searching for book chapters on muscular dystrophy:

- **Muscular Dystrophy: Duchenne Muscular Dystrophy, Becker Muscular Dystrophy**

  Source: in Plumridge, D., et al., eds. Student with a Genetic Disorder: Educational Implications for Special Education Teachers and for Physical Therapists, Occupational Therapists, and Speech Pathologists. Springfield, IL: Charles C Thomas Publisher. 1993. p. 180-185.

  Contact: Available from Charles C Thomas Publisher. 2600 South First Street, Springfield, IL 62794-9265. (212) 789-8980. Fax (217) 789-9130. PRICE: $75.95 plus shipping and handling (cloth); $39.95 plus shipping and handling (paper). ISBN: 0398058393.

  Summary: Both Duchenne and Becker **muscular dystrophy** are progressive muscle wasting conditions that primarily affect boys. This chapter on **muscular dystrophy** is from a text for special education teachers, physical therapists, occupational therapists, and speech pathologists on the educational implications of genetic disorders. Topics covered include the physical and characteristic features of the disorder, the genetics of the disorder, the cognitive and behavior profiles, the educational implications, physical therapy, occupational therapy, hearing and speech considerations, psychosocial issues, and prognosis. 5 references.

- **Myotonic Dystrophy: Steinert Muscular Dystrophy, Dytrophia Myotonica**

  Source: in Plumridge, D., et al., eds. Student with a Genetic Disorder: Educational Implications for Special Education Teachers and for Physical Therapists, Occupational Therapists, and Speech Pathologists. Springfield, IL: Charles C Thomas Publisher. 1993. p. 186-191.

  Contact: Available from Charles C Thomas Publisher. 2600 South First Street, Springfield, IL 62794-9265. (217) 789-8980. Fax (217) 789-9130.

PRICE: $75.95 plus shipping and handling (cloth); $39.95 plus shipping and handling (paper). ISBN: 0398058393.

Summary: Myotonic dystrophy is a type of **muscular dystrophy** that affects other parts of the body in addition to muscles. This chapter on myotonic dystrophy is from a text for special education teachers, physical therapists, occupational therapists, and speech pathologists on the educational implications of genetic disorders. Topics covered include the physical and characteristic features of the disorder, the genetics of the disorder, the cognitive and behavior profiles, the educational implications, physical therapy, occupational therapy, hearing and speech considerations, psychosocial issues, and prognosis. 6 references.

General Home References

In addition to references for muscular dystrophy, you may want a general home medical guide that spans all aspects of home healthcare. The following list is a recent sample of such guides (sorted alphabetically by title; hyperlinks provide rankings, information, and reviews at Amazon.com):

- **American College of Physicians Complete Home Medical Guide (with Interactive Human Anatomy CD-ROM)** by David R. Goldmann (Editor), American College of Physicians; Hardcover - 1104 pages, Book & CD-Rom edition (1999), DK Publishing; ISBN: 0789444127; http://www.amazon.com/exec/obidos/ASIN/0789444127/icongroupinterna

- **The American Medical Association Guide to Home Caregiving** by the American Medical Association (Editor); Paperback - 256 pages 1 edition (2001), John Wiley & Sons; ISBN: 0471414093; http://www.amazon.com/exec/obidos/ASIN/0471414093/icongroupinterna

- **Anatomica: The Complete Home Medical Reference** by Peter Forrestal (Editor); Hardcover (2000), Book Sales; ISBN: 1740480309; http://www.amazon.com/exec/obidos/ASIN/1740480309/icongroupinterna

- **The HarperCollins Illustrated Medical Dictionary: The Complete Home Medical Dictionary** by Ida G. Dox, et al; Paperback - 656 pages 4th edition (2001), Harper Resource; ISBN: 0062736469; http://www.amazon.com/exec/obidos/ASIN/0062736469/icongroupinterna

- **Mayo Clinic Guide to Self-Care: Answers for Everyday Health Problems** by Philip Hagen, M.D. (Editor), et al; Paperback - 279 pages, 2nd edition (December 15, 1999), Kensington Publishing Corp.; ISBN: 0962786578; http://www.amazon.com/exec/obidos/ASIN/0962786578/icongroupinterna

- **The Merck Manual of Medical Information: Home Edition (Merck Manual of Medical Information Home Edition (Trade Paper)** by Robert Berkow (Editor), Mark H. Beers, M.D. (Editor); Paperback - 1536 pages (2000), Pocket Books; ISBN: 0671027263; http://www.amazon.com/exec/obidos/ASIN/0671027263/icongroupinterna

Chapter 6. Periodicals and News on Muscular Dystrophy

Overview

Keeping up on the news relating to muscular dystrophy can be challenging. Subscribing to targeted periodicals can be an effective way to stay abreast of recent developments on muscular dystrophy. Periodicals include newsletters, magazines, and academic journals.

In this chapter, we suggest a number of news sources and present various periodicals that cover muscular dystrophy beyond and including those which are published by patient associations mentioned earlier. We will first focus on news services, and then on periodicals. News services, press releases, and newsletters generally use more accessible language, so if you do chose to subscribe to one of the more technical periodicals, make sure that it uses language you can easily follow.

News Services and Press Releases

Well before articles show up in newsletters or the popular press, they may appear in the form of a press release or a public relations announcement. One of the simplest ways of tracking press releases on muscular dystrophy is to search the news wires. News wires are used by professional journalists, and have existed since the invention of the telegraph. Today, there are several major "wires" that are used by companies, universities, and other organizations to announce new medical breakthroughs. In the following sample of sources, we will briefly describe how to access each service. These services only post recent news intended for public viewing.

PR Newswire

Perhaps the broadest of the wires is PR Newswire Association, Inc. To access this archive, simply go to **http://www.prnewswire.com**. Below the search box, select the option "The last 30 days." In the search box, type "muscular dystrophy" or synonyms. The search results are shown by order of relevance. When reading these press releases, do not forget that the sponsor of the release may be a company or organization that is trying to sell a particular product or therapy. Their views, therefore, may be biased. The following is typical of press releases that can be found on PR Newswire:

- **PTC Therapeutics Awarded Grant From the Parent Project Muscular Dystrophy for Drug Discovery Research**

   Summary: SOUTH PLAINFIELD, N.J., Sept. 2 /PRNewswire/ -- PTC Therapeutics, Inc.

   (PTC), a biopharmaceutical company focused on the discovery, development, and commercialization of small molecule drugs targeting post-transcriptional control mechanisms, announced today that it has been awarded a grant of $1 million from the Parent Project **Muscular Dystrophy** (PPMD) to discover novel agents to treat Duchenne **muscular dystrophy** (DMD). PTC and PPMD have jointly selected target genes of potential therapeutic relevance to DMD. PTC will apply its proprietary GEMS (Gene Expression Modulation by Small-molecules) technology to identify small molecule compounds that can be developed into novel drugs for the treatment of DMD.

   (Logo: http://www.newscom.com/cgi-bin/prnh/20010919/PTCLOGO)
   "This is the first award PPMD has granted to a biopharmaceutical company and we are proud to have PTC on our team to fight this debilitating disorder," said Pat Furlong, Executive Director, PPMD. "We look forward to working with PTC as they advance their research and hope that this project will lead to potential new treatments for DMD."
   DMD is a disease characterized by muscle weakness and progressive loss of muscle function that results in serious disability and shortened life expectancy. DMD is perhaps the most prevalent of the muscular dystrophies and is the most common genetic disorder diagnosed during childhood today. It is estimated that approximately 20,000 boys worldwide are born with DMD annually.

   "We are extremely pleased to have the strong support of PPMD. This collaboration allows us to investigate potential therapies for DMD beyond the scope of our clinical compound, PTC124, which targets nonsense mutations that cause genetic disorders such as DMD," said Stuart Peltz, Ph.D., President and CEO of PTC Therapeutics. "PTC is committed to finding new treatments for diseases like DMD in which there is a high unmet medical need."

About PTC Therapeutics, Inc.
PTC Therapeutics, Inc. is a biopharmaceutical company focused on the discovery, development, and commercialization of small molecule drugs targeting post-transcriptional control mechanisms. PTC's compounds regulate gene expression by selectively modulating how RNA is used to produce proteins.

Post-transcriptional control processes are the sequence of events in the cell that ultimately regulate how much, and when, each particular protein is produced. By applying this approach, PTC has advanced its drug discovery programs rapidly from targets to preclinical and clinical drug candidates, building a robust pipeline across genetic disorders, oncology, and infectious diseases. For more information please visit http://www.ptcbio.com.

About GEMS
GEMS is PTC's proprietary technology that exploits the regulatory mechanisms found in the untranslated regions of messenger RNA for the rapid identification of small molecule drugs that can treat diseases by selectively increasing or decreasing the expression of key proteins. GEMS is broadly applicable to targets across multiple therapeutic areas including newly identified or previously intractable targets. The ability to identify orally bioavailable molecules that modulate the expression of specific proteins in cells also allows PTC to pursue targets currently only addressed by protein drugs. PTC's preclinical programs in infectious diseases and oncology have validated the applicability of GEMS to identify orally bioavailable compounds that selectively modulate protein expression.

About Parent Project Muscular Dystrophy
Parent Project **Muscular Dystrophy** (PPMD) is a national not-for-profit organization founded in 1994 by parents of children with Duchenne and Becker **muscular dystrophy.** Duchenne **muscular dystrophy** is the most common lethal genetic disorder diagnosed during early childhood, affecting approximately 1 out of every 3,500 boys and 20,000 babies born each year. The organization's mission is to improve the treatment, quality

of life and long-term outlook for all individuals affected by Duchenne **muscular dystrophy** through research, education, advocacy and compassion. PPMD is the largest grassroots organization in the U.S. entirely focused on Duchenne **muscular dystrophy.** It is headquartered in Middletown, Ohio with offices in Fort Lee, New Jersey.

For more information please visit http://www.parentprojectmd.org.

Reuters Health

The Reuters' Medical News and Health eLine databases can be very useful in exploring news archives relating to muscular dystrophy. While some of the listed articles are free to view, others can be purchased for a nominal fee. To access this archive, go to **http://www.reutershealth.com/en/index.html** and search by "muscular dystrophy" (or synonyms). The following was recently listed in this archive for muscular dystrophy:

- **Plasmid-based gene therapy for muscular dystrophy succeeds in preclinical study**
  Source: Reuters Medical News
  Date: October 20, 2003

- **New approach repairs genetic defect in Duchenne muscular dystrophy mouse model**
  Source: Reuters Medical News
  Date: July 07, 2003

- **Researchers fix muscular dystrophy damage in mice**
  Source: Reuters Health eLine
  Date: September 16, 2002

- **Gene problem in muscular dystrophy identified**
  Source: Reuters Health eLine
  Date: August 08, 2002

- **Clues to muscular dystrophy revealed**
  Source: Reuters Health eLine
  Date: July 25, 2002

- **Axcell, Mount Sinai in Alzheimer's, muscular dystrophy protein research pact**
  Source: Reuters Industry Breifing
  Date: November 15, 2001

- **House approves muscular dystrophy research push**
  Source: Reuters Medical News
  Date: September 25, 2001

- **House approves muscular dystrophy funding bill**
  Source: Reuters Industry Breifing
  Date: September 25, 2001

- **Gene therapy fights muscular dystrophy in mice**
  Source: Reuters Health eLine
  Date: September 19, 2001

- **FDA pulls fast track status from muscular dystrophy study**
  Source: Reuters Industry Breifing
  Date: May 01, 2001

- **Key signaling mechanism could point to muscular dystrophy treatment**
  Source: Reuters Medical News
  Date: April 27, 2001

- **Gene therapy for muscular dystrophy promising**
  Source: Reuters Health eLine
  Date: November 30, 2000

- **Repeats in muscular dystrophy gene responsible for disease in mice**
  Source: Reuters Industry Breifing
  Date: September 11, 2000

- **Stem cell transplantation restores dystrophin in mouse muscular dystrophy model**
  Source: Reuters Medical News
  Date: September 23, 1999

- **Sarcoglycan protein deficiency causes muscular dystrophy in mouse model**
  Source: Reuters Medical News
  Date: December 17, 1998

- **Full-length utrophin expression needed to prevent muscular dystrophy in mice**
  Source: Reuters Medical News
  Date: December 14, 1998

- **Gene associated with two types of muscular dystrophy identified**
  Source: Reuters Medical News
  Date: September 03, 1998

- **Utrophin Transgene Corrects Clinical Signs Of Muscular Dystrophy In Mouse Model Of The Disease**
  Source: Reuters Medical News
  Date: April 28, 1998

- **Upregulation Of Utrophin Relieves Muscular Dystrophy In Mice**
  Source: Reuters Medical News
  Date: November 28, 1996

- **Genetic Basis Of Autosomal Recessive Muscular Dystrophy Identified**
  Source: Reuters Medical News
  Date: November 03, 1995

- **Initial Results Of Gene Therapy For Cystic Fibrosis and Duchenne's Muscular Dystrophy Disappointing**
  Source: Reuters Medical News
  Date: September 28, 1995

The NIH

Within MEDLINEplus, the NIH has made an agreement with the New York Times Syndicate, the AP News Service, and Reuters to deliver news that can be browsed by the public. Search news releases at **http://www.nlm.nih.gov/medlineplus/alphanews_a.html.** MEDLINEplus allows you to browse across an alphabetical index. Or you can search by date at **http://www.nlm.nih.gov/medlineplus/newsbydate.html.** Often, news items are indexed by MEDLINEplus within their search engine.

Business Wire

Business Wire is similar to PR Newswire. To access this archive, simply go to **http://www.businesswire.com.** You can scan the news by industry category or company name.

Market Wire

Market Wire is more focused on technology than the other wires. To browse the latest press releases by topic, such as alternative medicine, biotechnology, fitness, healthcare, legal, nutrition, and pharmaceuticals, log on to Market Wire's Medical/Health channel at the following hyperlink **http://www.marketwire.com/mw/release_index?channel=MedicalHealth.** Market Wire's home page is **http://www.marketwire.com/mw/home.** From here, type "muscular dystrophy" (or synonyms) into the search box, and click on "Search News." As this service is technology oriented, you may wish to use it when searching for press releases covering diagnostic procedures or tests.

Search Engines

Free-to-view news can also be found in the news section of your favorite search engines (see the health news page at Yahoo: **http://dir.yahoo.com/Health/News_and_Media/,** or use this Web site's general news search page **http://news.yahoo.com/.** Type in "muscular dystrophy" (or synonyms). If you know the name of a company that is relevant to muscular dystrophy, you can go to any stock trading Web site (such as **www.etrade.com**) and search for the company name there. News items across various news sources are reported on indicated hyperlinks.

BBC

Covering news from a more European perspective, the British Broadcasting Corporation (BBC) allows the public free access to their news archive located at **http://www.bbc.co.uk/.** Search by "muscular dystrophy" (or synonyms).

Academic Periodicals covering Muscular Dystrophy

Academic periodicals can be a highly technical yet valuable source of information on muscular dystrophy. We have compiled the following list of periodicals known to publish articles relating to muscular dystrophy and which are currently indexed within the National Library of Medicine's PubMed database (follow hyperlinks to view more information, summaries, etc., for each). In addition to these sources, to keep current on articles written on muscular dystrophy published by any of the periodicals listed below, you can simply follow the hyperlink indicated or go to **www.ncbi.nlm.nih.gov/pubmed**. Type the periodical's name into the search box to find the latest studies published.

If you want complete details about the historical contents of a periodical, you can also visit **http://www.ncbi.nlm.nih.gov/entrez/jrbrowser.cgi**. Here, type in the name of the journal or its abbreviation, and you will receive an index of published articles. At **http://locatorplus.gov/** you can retrieve more indexing information on medical periodicals (e.g. the name of the publisher). Select the button "Search LOCATORplus." Then type in the name of the journal and select the advanced search option "Journal Title Search." The following is a sample of periodicals which publish articles on muscular dystrophy:

- **AJNR. American Journal of Neuroradiology. (AJNR Am J Neuroradiol)**
  http://www.ncbi.nlm.nih.gov/entrez/jrbrowser.cgi?field=0&regexp=Aj
  nr.+American+Journal+of+Neuroradiology&dispmax=20&dispstart=0

- **AJR. American Journal of Roentgenology. (AJR Am J Roentgenol)**
  http://www.ncbi.nlm.nih.gov/entrez/jrbrowser.cgi?field=0&regexp=Ajr
  .+American+Journal+of+Roentgenology&dispmax=20&dispstart=0

- **American Heart Journal. (Am Heart J)**
  http://www.ncbi.nlm.nih.gov/entrez/jrbrowser.cgi?field=0&regexp=A
  merican+Heart+Journal&dispmax=20&dispstart=0

- **American Journal of Human Genetics. (Am J Hum Genet)**
  http://www.ncbi.nlm.nih.gov/entrez/jrbrowser.cgi?field=0&regexp=A
  merican+Journal+of+Human+Genetics&dispmax=20&dispstart=0

- **American Journal of Medical Genetics. (Am J Med Genet)**
  http://www.ncbi.nlm.nih.gov/entrez/jrbrowser.cgi?field=0&regexp=A
  merican+Journal+of+Medical+Genetics&dispmax=20&dispstart=0

- **American Journal of Pathology. (Am J Pathol)**
  http://www.ncbi.nlm.nih.gov/entrez/jrbrowser.cgi?field=0&regexp=A
  merican+Journal+of+Pathology&dispmax=20&dispstart=0

- **Annals of Neurology. (Ann Neurol)**
  http://www.ncbi.nlm.nih.gov/entrez/jrbrowser.cgi?field=0&regexp=An
  nals+of+Neurology&dispmax=20&dispstart=0

- **Archives of Disease in Childhood. (Arch Dis Child)**
  http://www.ncbi.nlm.nih.gov/entrez/jrbrowser.cgi?field=0&regexp=Ar
  chives+of+Disease+in+Childhood&dispmax=20&dispstart=0

- **Archives of Neurology. (Arch Neurol)**
  http://www.ncbi.nlm.nih.gov/entrez/jrbrowser.cgi?field=0&regexp=Ar
  chives+of+Neurology&dispmax=20&dispstart=0

- **Archives of Orthopaedic and Trauma Surgery. (Arch Orthop Trauma Surg)**
  http://www.ncbi.nlm.nih.gov/entrez/jrbrowser.cgi?field=0&regexp=Ar
  chives+of+Orthopaedic+and+Trauma+Surgery&dispmax=20&dispstart=
  0

- **Arquivos De Neuro-Psiquiatria. (Arq Neuropsiquiatr)**
  http://www.ncbi.nlm.nih.gov/entrez/jrbrowser.cgi?field=0&regexp=Ar
  quivos+De+Neuro-Psiquiatria&dispmax=20&dispstart=0

- **Biochemical and Biophysical Research Communications. (Biochem Biophys Res Commun)**
  http://www.ncbi.nlm.nih.gov/entrez/jrbrowser.cgi?field=0&regexp=Bi
  ochemical+and+Biophysical+Research+Communications&dispmax=20&
  dispstart=0

- **Biochimica Et Biophysica Acta. (Biochim Biophys Acta)**
  http://www.ncbi.nlm.nih.gov/entrez/jrbrowser.cgi?field=0&regexp=Bi
  ochimica+Et+Biophysica+Acta&dispmax=20&dispstart=0

- **Bmc Cell Biology [electronic Resource]. (BMC Cell Biol)**
  http://www.ncbi.nlm.nih.gov/entrez/jrbrowser.cgi?field=0&regexp=B
  mc+Cell+Biology+[electronic+Resource]&dispmax=20&dispstart=0

- **Bmc Surgery [electronic Resource]. (BMC Surg)**
  http://www.ncbi.nlm.nih.gov/entrez/jrbrowser.cgi?field=0&regexp=B
  mc+Surgery+[electronic+Resource]&dispmax=20&dispstart=0

- **Brain; a Journal of Neurology. (Brain)**
  http://www.ncbi.nlm.nih.gov/entrez/jrbrowser.cgi?field=0&regexp=Br
  ain;+a+Journal+of+Neurology&dispmax=20&dispstart=0

- **British Journal of Anaesthesia. (Br J Anaesth)**
  http://www.ncbi.nlm.nih.gov/entrez/jrbrowser.cgi?field=0&regexp=Bri
  tish+Journal+of+Anaesthesia&dispmax=20&dispstart=0

- **Cellular and Molecular Life Sciences: Cmls. (Cell Mol Life Sci)**
  http://www.ncbi.nlm.nih.gov/entrez/jrbrowser.cgi?field=0&regexp=Ce
  llular+and+Molecular+Life+Sciences+:+Cmls&dispmax=20&dispstart=0

- **Child's Nervous System: Chns: Official Journal of the International Society for Pediatric Neurosurgery. (Childs Nerv Syst)**
  http://www.ncbi.nlm.nih.gov/entrez/jrbrowser.cgi?field=0&regexp=Ch
  ild's+Nervous+System+:+Chns+:+Official+Journal+of+the+International
  +Society+for+Pediatric+Neurosurgery&dispmax=20&dispstart=0

- **Chinese Medical Journal. (Chin Med J (Engl))**
  http://www.ncbi.nlm.nih.gov/entrez/jrbrowser.cgi?field=0&regexp=Chinese+Medical+Journal&dispmax=20&dispstart=0

- **Clinica Chimica Acta; International Journal of Clinical Chemistry. (Clin Chim Acta)**
  http://www.ncbi.nlm.nih.gov/entrez/jrbrowser.cgi?field=0&regexp=Clinica+Chimica+Acta;+International+Journal+of+Clinical+Chemistry&dispmax=20&dispstart=0

- **Clinical Biochemistry. (Clin Biochem)**
  http://www.ncbi.nlm.nih.gov/entrez/jrbrowser.cgi?field=0&regexp=Clinical+Biochemistry&dispmax=20&dispstart=0

- **Clinical Chemistry. (Clin Chem)**
  http://www.ncbi.nlm.nih.gov/entrez/jrbrowser.cgi?field=0&regexp=Clinical+Chemistry&dispmax=20&dispstart=0

- **Clinical Genetics. (Clin Genet)**
  http://www.ncbi.nlm.nih.gov/entrez/jrbrowser.cgi?field=0&regexp=Clinical+Genetics&dispmax=20&dispstart=0

- **Clinical Neurology and Neurosurgery. (Clin Neurol Neurosurg)**
  http://www.ncbi.nlm.nih.gov/entrez/jrbrowser.cgi?field=0&regexp=Clinical+Neurology+and+Neurosurgery&dispmax=20&dispstart=0

- **Clinical Nuclear Medicine. (Clin Nucl Med)**
  http://www.ncbi.nlm.nih.gov/entrez/jrbrowser.cgi?field=0&regexp=Clinical+Nuclear+Medicine&dispmax=20&dispstart=0

- **Clinical Pediatrics. (Clin Pediatr (Phila))**
  http://www.ncbi.nlm.nih.gov/entrez/jrbrowser.cgi?field=0&regexp=Clinical+Pediatrics&dispmax=20&dispstart=0

- **Clinical Rehabilitation. (Clin Rehabil)**
  http://www.ncbi.nlm.nih.gov/entrez/jrbrowser.cgi?field=0&regexp=Clinical+Rehabilitation&dispmax=20&dispstart=0

- **Clinical Rheumatology. (Clin Rheumatol)**
  http://www.ncbi.nlm.nih.gov/entrez/jrbrowser.cgi?field=0&regexp=Clinical+Rheumatology&dispmax=20&dispstart=0

- **Current Opinion in Neurology. (Curr Opin Neurol)**
  http://www.ncbi.nlm.nih.gov/entrez/jrbrowser.cgi?field=0&regexp=Current+Opinion+in+Neurology&dispmax=20&dispstart=0

- **Cytogenetic and Genome Research. (Cytogenet Genome Res)**
  http://www.ncbi.nlm.nih.gov/entrez/jrbrowser.cgi?field=0&regexp=Cytogenetic+and+Genome+Research&dispmax=20&dispstart=0

- **Development (Cambridge, England). (Development)**
  http://www.ncbi.nlm.nih.gov/entrez/jrbrowser.cgi?field=0&regexp=Development+(Cambridge,+England)&dispmax=20&dispstart=0

- **Developmental Medicine and Child Neurology. (Dev Med Child Neurol)**
  http://www.ncbi.nlm.nih.gov/entrez/jrbrowser.cgi?field=0&regexp=Developmental+Medicine+and+Child+Neurology&dispmax=20&dispstart=0

- **Documenta Ophthalmologica. Advances in Ophthalmology. (Doc Ophthalmol)**
  http://www.ncbi.nlm.nih.gov/entrez/jrbrowser.cgi?field=0&regexp=Documenta+Ophthalmologica.+Advances+in+Ophthalmology&dispmax=20&dispstart=0

- **European Heart Journal. (Eur Heart J)**
  http://www.ncbi.nlm.nih.gov/entrez/jrbrowser.cgi?field=0&regexp=European+Heart+Journal&dispmax=20&dispstart=0

- **European Journal of Biochemistry / Febs. (Eur J Biochem)**
  http://www.ncbi.nlm.nih.gov/entrez/jrbrowser.cgi?field=0&regexp=European+Journal+of+Biochemistry+/+Febs&dispmax=20&dispstart=0

- **European Journal of Clinical Investigation. (Eur J Clin Invest)**
  http://www.ncbi.nlm.nih.gov/entrez/jrbrowser.cgi?field=0&regexp=European+Journal+of+Clinical+Investigation&dispmax=20&dispstart=0

- **European Journal of Clinical Nutrition. (Eur J Clin Nutr)**
  http://www.ncbi.nlm.nih.gov/entrez/jrbrowser.cgi?field=0&regexp=European+Journal+of+Clinical+Nutrition&dispmax=20&dispstart=0

- **European Journal of Human Genetics: Ejhg. (Eur J Hum Genet)**
  http://www.ncbi.nlm.nih.gov/entrez/jrbrowser.cgi?field=0&regexp=European+Journal+of+Human+Genetics+:+Ejhg&dispmax=20&dispstart=0

- **European Journal of Paediatric Neurology: Ejpn: Official Journal of the European Paediatric Neurology Society. (Eur J Paediatr Neurol)**
  http://www.ncbi.nlm.nih.gov/entrez/jrbrowser.cgi?field=0&regexp=European+Journal+of+Paediatric+Neurology+:+Ejpn+:+Official+Journal+of+the+European+Paediatric+Neurology+Society&dispmax=20&dispstart=0

- **European Journal of Pediatrics. (Eur J Pediatr)**
  http://www.ncbi.nlm.nih.gov/entrez/jrbrowser.cgi?field=0&regexp=European+Journal+of+Pediatrics&dispmax=20&dispstart=0

- **European Neurology. (Eur Neurol)**
  http://www.ncbi.nlm.nih.gov/entrez/jrbrowser.cgi?field=0&regexp=European+Neurology&dispmax=20&dispstart=0

- **European Radiology. (Eur Radiol)**
  http://www.ncbi.nlm.nih.gov/entrez/jrbrowser.cgi?field=0&regexp=European+Radiology&dispmax=20&dispstart=0

- **Experimental & Molecular Medicine. (Exp Mol Med)**
  http://www.ncbi.nlm.nih.gov/entrez/jrbrowser.cgi?field=0&regexp=Experimental+&+Molecular+Medicine&dispmax=20&dispstart=0

- **Experimental Animals / Japanese Association for Laboratory Animal Science. (Exp Anim)**
  http://www.ncbi.nlm.nih.gov/entrez/jrbrowser.cgi?field=0&regexp=Experimental+Animals+/+Japanese+Association+for+Laboratory+Animal+Science&dispmax=20&dispstart=0

- **Experimental Cell Research. (Exp Cell Res)**
  http://www.ncbi.nlm.nih.gov/entrez/jrbrowser.cgi?field=0&regexp=Experimental+Cell+Research&dispmax=20&dispstart=0

- **Expert Opinion on Biological Therapy. (Expert Opin Biol Ther)**
  http://www.ncbi.nlm.nih.gov/entrez/jrbrowser.cgi?field=0&regexp=Expert+Opinion+on+Biological+Therapy&dispmax=20&dispstart=0

- **Expert Reviews in Molecular Medicine [electronic Resource]. (Expert Rev Mol Med)**
  http://www.ncbi.nlm.nih.gov/entrez/jrbrowser.cgi?field=0&regexp=Expert+Reviews+in+Molecular+Medicine+[electronic+Resource]&dispmax=20&dispstart=0

- **Febs Letters. (FEBS Lett)**
  http://www.ncbi.nlm.nih.gov/entrez/jrbrowser.cgi?field=0&regexp=Febs+Letters&dispmax=20&dispstart=0

- **Gene Therapy. (Gene Ther)**
  http://www.ncbi.nlm.nih.gov/entrez/jrbrowser.cgi?field=0&regexp=Gene+Therapy&dispmax=20&dispstart=0

- **Health & Social Care in the Community. (Health Soc Care Community)**
  http://www.ncbi.nlm.nih.gov/entrez/jrbrowser.cgi?field=0&regexp=Health+&+Social+Care+in+the+Community&dispmax=20&dispstart=0

- **Human Genetics. (Hum Genet)**
  http://www.ncbi.nlm.nih.gov/entrez/jrbrowser.cgi?field=0&regexp=Human+Genetics&dispmax=20&dispstart=0

- **Human Heredity. (Hum Hered)**
  http://www.ncbi.nlm.nih.gov/entrez/jrbrowser.cgi?field=0&regexp=Human+Heredity&dispmax=20&dispstart=0

- **Human Molecular Genetics. (Hum Mol Genet)**
  http://www.ncbi.nlm.nih.gov/entrez/jrbrowser.cgi?field=0&regexp=Human+Molecular+Genetics&dispmax=20&dispstart=0

- **Human Mutation. (Hum Mutat)**
  http://www.ncbi.nlm.nih.gov/entrez/jrbrowser.cgi?field=0&regexp=Human+Mutation&dispmax=20&dispstart=0

- **Indian Journal of Medical Sciences. (Indian J Med Sci)**
  http://www.ncbi.nlm.nih.gov/entrez/jrbrowser.cgi?field=0&regexp=Indian+Journal+of+Medical+Sciences&dispmax=20&dispstart=0

- **Indian Pediatrics. (Indian Pediatr)**
  http://www.ncbi.nlm.nih.gov/entrez/jrbrowser.cgi?field=0&regexp=Indian+Pediatrics&dispmax=20&dispstart=0

- **International Journal of Experimental Pathology. (Int J Exp Pathol)**
  http://www.ncbi.nlm.nih.gov/entrez/jrbrowser.cgi?field=0&regexp=Int
  ernational+Journal+of+Experimental+Pathology&dispmax=20&dispstart
  =0

- **International Journal of Molecular Medicine. (Int J Mol Med)**
  http://www.ncbi.nlm.nih.gov/entrez/jrbrowser.cgi?field=0&regexp=Int
  ernational+Journal+of+Molecular+Medicine&dispmax=20&dispstart=0

- **Journal of Cardiovascular Electrophysiology. (J Cardiovasc Electrophysiol)**
  http://www.ncbi.nlm.nih.gov/entrez/jrbrowser.cgi?field=0&regexp=Jo
  urnal+of+Cardiovascular+Electrophysiology&dispmax=20&dispstart=0

- **Journal of Cellular Physiology. (J Cell Physiol)**
  http://www.ncbi.nlm.nih.gov/entrez/jrbrowser.cgi?field=0&regexp=Jo
  urnal+of+Cellular+Physiology&dispmax=20&dispstart=0

- **Journal of Child Neurology. (J Child Neurol)**
  http://www.ncbi.nlm.nih.gov/entrez/jrbrowser.cgi?field=0&regexp=Jo
  urnal+of+Child+Neurology&dispmax=20&dispstart=0

- **Journal of Clinical Neuroscience: Official Journal of the Neurosurgical Society of Australasia. (J Clin Neurosci)**
  http://www.ncbi.nlm.nih.gov/entrez/jrbrowser.cgi?field=0&regexp=Jo
  urnal+of+Clinical+Neuroscience+:+Official+Journal+of+the+Neurosurgi
  cal+Society+of+Australasia&dispmax=20&dispstart=0

- **Journal of Human Genetics. (J Hum Genet)**
  http://www.ncbi.nlm.nih.gov/entrez/jrbrowser.cgi?field=0&regexp=Jo
  urnal+of+Human+Genetics&dispmax=20&dispstart=0

- **Journal of Immunological Methods. (J Immunol Methods)**
  http://www.ncbi.nlm.nih.gov/entrez/jrbrowser.cgi?field=0&regexp=Jo
  urnal+of+Immunological+Methods&dispmax=20&dispstart=0

- **Journal of Medical Genetics. (J Med Genet)**
  http://www.ncbi.nlm.nih.gov/entrez/jrbrowser.cgi?field=0&regexp=Jo
  urnal+of+Medical+Genetics&dispmax=20&dispstart=0

- **Journal of Neurology. (J Neurol)**
  http://www.ncbi.nlm.nih.gov/entrez/jrbrowser.cgi?field=0&regexp=Journal+of+Neurology&dispmax=20&dispstart=0

- **Journal of Neuro-Ophthalmology: the Official Journal of the North American Neuro-Ophthalmology Society. (J Neuroophthalmol)**
  http://www.ncbi.nlm.nih.gov/entrez/jrbrowser.cgi?field=0&regexp=Journal+of+Neuro-Ophthalmology+:+the+Official+Journal+of+the+North+American+Neuro-Ophthalmology+Society&dispmax=20&dispstart=0

- **Journal of Pediatric Hematology/Oncology: Official Journal of the American Society of Pediatric Hematology/Oncology. (J Pediatr Hematol Oncol)**
  http://www.ncbi.nlm.nih.gov/entrez/jrbrowser.cgi?field=0&regexp=Journal+of+Pediatric+Hematology/Oncology+:+Official+Journal+of+the+American+Society+of+Pediatric+Hematology/Oncology&dispmax=20&dispstart=0

- **Journal of Pediatric Ophthalmology and Strabismus. (J Pediatr Ophthalmol Strabismus)**
  http://www.ncbi.nlm.nih.gov/entrez/jrbrowser.cgi?field=0&regexp=Journal+of+Pediatric+Ophthalmology+and+Strabismus&dispmax=20&dispstart=0

- **Journal of Pediatric Orthopaedics. Part B / European Paediatric Orthopaedic Society, Pediatric Orthopaedic Society of North America. (J Pediatr Orthop B)**
  http://www.ncbi.nlm.nih.gov/entrez/jrbrowser.cgi?field=0&regexp=Journal+of+Pediatric+Orthopaedics.+Part+B+/+European+Paediatric+Orthopaedic+Society,+Pediatric+Orthopaedic+Society+of+North+America&dispmax=20&dispstart=0

- **Journal of Pediatric Orthopedics. (J Pediatr Orthop)**
  http://www.ncbi.nlm.nih.gov/entrez/jrbrowser.cgi?field=0&regexp=Journal+of+Pediatric+Orthopedics&dispmax=20&dispstart=0

- **Journal of Structural Biology. (J Struct Biol)**
  http://www.ncbi.nlm.nih.gov/entrez/jrbrowser.cgi?field=0&regexp=Journal+of+Structural+Biology&dispmax=20&dispstart=0

- **Journal of the American College of Cardiology. (J Am Coll Cardiol)**
  http://www.ncbi.nlm.nih.gov/entrez/jrbrowser.cgi?field=0&regexp=Journal+of+the+American+College+of+Cardiology&dispmax=20&dispstart=0

- **Journal of the Neurological Sciences. (J Neurol Sci)**
  http://www.ncbi.nlm.nih.gov/entrez/jrbrowser.cgi?field=0&regexp=Journal+of+the+Neurological+Sciences&dispmax=20&dispstart=0

- **Journal of the Royal College of Physicians of London. (J R Coll Physicians Lond)**
  http://www.ncbi.nlm.nih.gov/entrez/jrbrowser.cgi?field=0&regexp=Journal+of+the+Royal+College+of+Physicians+of+London&dispmax=20&dispstart=0

- **Methods in Molecular Medicine. (Methods Mol Med)**
  http://www.ncbi.nlm.nih.gov/entrez/jrbrowser.cgi?field=0&regexp=Methods+in+Molecular+Medicine&dispmax=20&dispstart=0

- **Molecular Therapy: the Journal of the American Society of Gene Therapy. (Mol Ther)**
  http://www.ncbi.nlm.nih.gov/entrez/jrbrowser.cgi?field=0&regexp=Molecular+Therapy+:+the+Journal+of+the+American+Society+of+Gene+Therapy&dispmax=20&dispstart=0

- **Muscle & Nerve. (Muscle Nerve)**
  http://www.ncbi.nlm.nih.gov/entrez/jrbrowser.cgi?field=0&regexp=Muscle+&+Nerve&dispmax=20&dispstart=0

- **Nature Genetics. (Nat Genet)**
  http://www.ncbi.nlm.nih.gov/entrez/jrbrowser.cgi?field=0&regexp=Nature+Genetics&dispmax=20&dispstart=0

- **Nature Medicine. (Nat Med)**
  http://www.ncbi.nlm.nih.gov/entrez/jrbrowser.cgi?field=0&regexp=Nature+Medicine&dispmax=20&dispstart=0

- **Neurobiology of Disease. (Neurobiol Dis)**
  http://www.ncbi.nlm.nih.gov/entrez/jrbrowser.cgi?field=0&regexp=Neurobiology+of+Disease&dispmax=20&dispstart=0

- **Neurologic Clinics. (Neurol Clin)**
  http://www.ncbi.nlm.nih.gov/entrez/jrbrowser.cgi?field=0&regexp=Ne
  urologic+Clinics&dispmax=20&dispstart=0

- **Neurological Research. (Neurol Res)**
  http://www.ncbi.nlm.nih.gov/entrez/jrbrowser.cgi?field=0&regexp=Ne
  urological+Research&dispmax=20&dispstart=0

- **Neurology India. (Neurol India)**
  http://www.ncbi.nlm.nih.gov/entrez/jrbrowser.cgi?field=0&regexp=Ne
  urology+India&dispmax=20&dispstart=0

- **Neuromuscular Disorders: Nmd. (Neuromuscul Disord)**
  http://www.ncbi.nlm.nih.gov/entrez/jrbrowser.cgi?field=0&regexp=Ne
  uromuscular+Disorders+:+Nmd&dispmax=20&dispstart=0

- **Neuropathology: Official Journal of the Japanese Society of Neuropathology. (Neuropathology)**
  http://www.ncbi.nlm.nih.gov/entrez/jrbrowser.cgi?field=0&regexp=Ne
  uropathology+:+Official+Journal+of+the+Japanese+Society+of+Neuropa
  thology&dispmax=20&dispstart=0

- **Neuropathology and Applied Neurobiology. (Neuropathol Appl Neurobiol)**
  http://www.ncbi.nlm.nih.gov/entrez/jrbrowser.cgi?field=0&regexp=Ne
  uropathology+and+Applied+Neurobiology&dispmax=20&dispstart=0

- **Neuroscience Letters. (Neurosci Lett)**
  http://www.ncbi.nlm.nih.gov/entrez/jrbrowser.cgi?field=0&regexp=Ne
  uroscience+Letters&dispmax=20&dispstart=0

- **NMR in Biomedicine. (NMR Biomed)**
  http://www.ncbi.nlm.nih.gov/entrez/jrbrowser.cgi?field=0&regexp=N
  mr+in+Biomedicine&dispmax=20&dispstart=0

- **Ophthalmic Surgery and Lasers. (Ophthalmic Surg Lasers)**
  http://www.ncbi.nlm.nih.gov/entrez/jrbrowser.cgi?field=0&regexp=Op
  hthalmic+Surgery+and+Lasers&dispmax=20&dispstart=0

- **Orthodontics & Craniofacial Research. (Orthod Craniofac Res)**
  http://www.ncbi.nlm.nih.gov/entrez/jrbrowser.cgi?field=0&regexp=Or

thodontics+&+Craniofacial+Research&dispmax=20&dispstart=0

- **Osteoporosis International: a Journal Established As Result of Cooperation between the European Foundation for Osteoporosis and the National Osteoporosis Foundation of the Usa. (Osteoporos Int)**
  http://www.ncbi.nlm.nih.gov/entrez/jrbrowser.cgi?field=0&regexp=Os
  teoporosis+International+:+a+Journal+Established+As+Result+of+Coope
  ration+between+the+European+Foundation+for+Osteoporosis+and+the
  +National+Osteoporosis+Foundation+of+the+Usa&dispmax=20&dis

  <Title>Pediatric Cardiology. (Pediatr Cardiol)
  http://www.ncbi.nlm.nih.gov/entrez/jrbrowser.cgi?field=0&regexp=Pe
  diatric+Cardiology&dispmax=20&dispstart=0

- **Pediatric Neurology. (Pediatr Neurol)**
  http://www.ncbi.nlm.nih.gov/entrez/jrbrowser.cgi?field=0&regexp=Pe
  diatric+Neurology&dispmax=20&dispstart=0

- **Pediatric Pulmonology. (Pediatr Pulmonol)**
  http://www.ncbi.nlm.nih.gov/entrez/jrbrowser.cgi?field=0&regexp=Pe
  diatric+Pulmonology&dispmax=20&dispstart=0

- **Physiotherapy Research International: the Journal for Researchers and Clinicians in Physical Therapy. (Physiother Res Int)**
  http://www.ncbi.nlm.nih.gov/entrez/jrbrowser.cgi?field=0&regexp=Ph
  ysiotherapy+Research+International+:+the+Journal+for+Researchers+an
  d+Clinicians+in+Physical+Therapy&dispmax=20&dispstart=0

- **Prenatal Diagnosis. (Prenat Diagn)**
  http://www.ncbi.nlm.nih.gov/entrez/jrbrowser.cgi?field=0&regexp=Pr
  enatal+Diagnosis&dispmax=20&dispstart=0

- **Proceedings of the National Academy of Sciences of the United States of America. (Proc Natl Acad Sci U S A)**
  http://www.ncbi.nlm.nih.gov/entrez/jrbrowser.cgi?field=0&regexp=Pr
  oceedings+of+the+National+Academy+of+Sciences+of+the+United+Stat
  es+of+America&dispmax=20&dispstart=0

- **Respiratory Care. (Respir Care)**
  http://www.ncbi.nlm.nih.gov/entrez/jrbrowser.cgi?field=0&regexp=Re
  spiratory+Care&dispmax=20&dispstart=0

- **Rheumatology (Oxford, England). (Rheumatology (Oxford))**
  http://www.ncbi.nlm.nih.gov/entrez/jrbrowser.cgi?field=0&regexp=Rh
  eumatology+(Oxford,+England)&dispmax=20&dispstart=0

- **Social History of Medicine: the Journal of the Society for the Social History of Medicine / Sshm. (Soc Hist Med)**
  http://www.ncbi.nlm.nih.gov/entrez/jrbrowser.cgi?field=0&regexp=So
  cial+History+of+Medicine+:+the+Journal+of+the+Society+for+the+Socia
  l+History+of+Medicine+/+Sshm&dispmax=20&dispstart=0

- **The American Journal of Cardiology. (Am J Cardiol)**
  http://www.ncbi.nlm.nih.gov/entrez/jrbrowser.cgi?field=0&regexp=Th
  e+American+Journal+of+Cardiology&dispmax=20&dispstart=0

- **The Canadian Journal of Neurological Sciences. Le Journal Canadien Des Sciences Neurologiques. (Can J Neurol Sci)**
  http://www.ncbi.nlm.nih.gov/entrez/jrbrowser.cgi?field=0&regexp=Th
  e+Canadian+Journal+of+Neurological+Sciences.+Le+Journal+Canadien+
  Des+Sciences+Neurologiques&dispmax=20&dispstart=0

- **The Indian Journal of Medical Research. (Indian J Med Res)**
  http://www.ncbi.nlm.nih.gov/entrez/jrbrowser.cgi?field=0&regexp=Th
  e+Indian+Journal+of+Medical+Research&dispmax=20&dispstart=0

- **The Journal of Biological Chemistry. (J Biol Chem)**
  http://www.ncbi.nlm.nih.gov/entrez/jrbrowser.cgi?field=0&regexp=Th
  e+Journal+of+Biological+Chemistry&dispmax=20&dispstart=0

- **The Journal of Bone and Joint Surgery. American Volume. (J Bone Joint Surg Am)**
  http://www.ncbi.nlm.nih.gov/entrez/jrbrowser.cgi?field=0&regexp=Th
  e+Journal+of+Bone+and+Joint+Surgery.+American+Volume&dispmax=
  20&dispstart=0

- **The Journal of Bone and Joint Surgery. British Volume. (J Bone Joint Surg Br)**
  http://www.ncbi.nlm.nih.gov/entrez/jrbrowser.cgi?field=0&regexp=Th
  e+Journal+of+Bone+and+Joint+Surgery.+British+Volume&dispmax=20&
  dispstart=0

- **The Journal of Cell Biology. (J Cell Biol)**
  http://www.ncbi.nlm.nih.gov/entrez/jrbrowser.cgi?field=0&regexp=The+Journal+of+Cell+Biology&dispmax=20&dispstart=0

- **The Journal of Clinical Endocrinology and Metabolism. (J Clin Endocrinol Metab)**
  http://www.ncbi.nlm.nih.gov/entrez/jrbrowser.cgi?field=0&regexp=The+Journal+of+Clinical+Endocrinology+and+Metabolism&dispmax=20&dispstart=0

- **The Journal of Heart and Lung Transplantation: The Official Publication of the International Society for Heart Transplantation. (J Heart Lung Transplant)**
  http://www.ncbi.nlm.nih.gov/entrez/jrbrowser.cgi?field=0&regexp=The+Journal+of+Heart+and+Lung+Transplantation+:+the+Official+Publication+of+the+International+Society+for+Heart+Transplantation&dispmax=20&dispstart=0

- **The Journal of Investigative Dermatology. (J Invest Dermatol)**
  http://www.ncbi.nlm.nih.gov/entrez/jrbrowser.cgi?field=0&regexp=The+Journal+of+Investigative+Dermatology&dispmax=20&dispstart=0

- **The Journal of Pediatrics. (J Pediatr)**
  http://www.ncbi.nlm.nih.gov/entrez/jrbrowser.cgi?field=0&regexp=The+Journal+of+Pediatrics&dispmax=20&dispstart=0

- **The Medical Journal of Australia. (Med J Aust)**
  http://www.ncbi.nlm.nih.gov/entrez/jrbrowser.cgi?field=0&regexp=The+Medical+Journal+of+Australia&dispmax=20&dispstart=0

- **Yonsei Medical Journal. (Yonsei Med J)**
  http://www.ncbi.nlm.nih.gov/entrez/jrbrowser.cgi?field=0&regexp=Yonsei+Medical+Journal&dispmax=20&dispstart=0

Vocabulary Builder

Applicability: A list of the commodities to which the candidate method can be applied as presented or with minor modifications. [NIH]

CHAPTER 7. PHYSICIAN GUIDELINES AND DATABASES

Overview

Doctors and medical researchers rely on a number of information sources to help patients with their conditions. Many will subscribe to journals or newsletters published by their professional associations or refer to specialized textbooks or clinical guides published for the medical profession. In this chapter, we focus on databases and Internet-based guidelines created or written for this professional audience.

NIH Guidelines

For the more common diseases, The National Institutes of Health publish guidelines that are frequently consulted by physicians. Publications are typically written by one or more of the various NIH Institutes. For physician guidelines, commonly referred to as "clinical" or "professional" guidelines, you can visit the following Institutes:

- Office of the Director (OD); guidelines consolidated across agencies available at **http://www.nih.gov/health/consumer/conkey.htm**

- National Institute of General Medical Sciences (NIGMS); fact sheets available at **http://www.nigms.nih.gov/news/facts/**

- National Library of Medicine (NLM); extensive encyclopedia (A.D.A.M., Inc.) with guidelines:
  http://www.nlm.nih.gov/medlineplus/healthtopics.html

- National Institute of Arthritis and Musculoskeletal and Skin Diseases (NIAMS); fact sheets and guidelines available at
  http://www.niams.nih.gov/hi/index.htm

NIH Databases

In addition to the various Institutes of Health that publish professional guidelines, the NIH has designed a number of databases for professionals.[22] Physician-oriented resources provide a wide variety of information related to the biomedical and health sciences, both past and present. The format of these resources varies. Searchable databases, bibliographic citations, full text articles (when available), archival collections, and images are all available. The following are referenced by the National Library of Medicine:[23]

- **Bioethics:** Access to published literature on the ethical, legal and public policy issues surrounding healthcare and biomedical research. This information is provided in conjunction with the Kennedy Institute of Ethics located at Georgetown University, Washington, D.C.: **http://www.nlm.nih.gov/databases/databases_bioethics.html**

- **HIV/AIDS Resources:** Describes various links and databases dedicated to HIV/AIDS research: **http://www.nlm.nih.gov/pubs/factsheets/aidsinfs.html**

- **NLM Online Exhibitions:** Describes "Exhibitions in the History of Medicine": **http://www.nlm.nih.gov/exhibition/exhibition.html**. Additional resources for historical scholarship in medicine: **http://www.nlm.nih.gov/hmd/hmd.html**

- **Biotechnology Information:** Access to public databases. The National Center for Biotechnology Information conducts research in computational biology, develops software tools for analyzing genome data, and disseminates biomedical information for the better understanding of molecular processes affecting human health and disease: **http://www.ncbi.nlm.nih.gov/**

- **Population Information:** The National Library of Medicine provides access to worldwide coverage of population, family planning, and related health issues, including family planning technology and programs, fertility, and population law and policy: **http://www.nlm.nih.gov/databases/databases_population.html**

- **Cancer Information:** Access to caner-oriented databases: **http://www.nlm.nih.gov/databases/databases_cancer.html**

---

[22] Remember, for the general public, the National Library of Medicine recommends the databases referenced in MEDLINE*plus* (**http://medlineplus.gov/** or **http://www.nlm.nih.gov/medlineplus/databases.html**).
[23] See **http://www.nlm.nih.gov/databases/databases.html**.

- **Profiles in Science:** Offering the archival collections of prominent twentieth-century biomedical scientists to the public through modern digital technology: **http://www.profiles.nlm.nih.gov/**

- **Chemical Information:** Provides links to various chemical databases and references: **http://sis.nlm.nih.gov/Chem/ChemMain.html**

- **Clinical Alerts:** Reports the release of findings from the NIH-funded clinical trials where such release could significantly affect morbidity and mortality: **http://www.nlm.nih.gov/databases/alerts/clinical_alerts.html**

- **Space Life Sciences:** Provides links and information to space-based research (including NASA): **http://www.nlm.nih.gov/databases/databases_space.html**

- **MEDLINE:** Bibliographic database covering the fields of medicine, nursing, dentistry, veterinary medicine, the healthcare system, and the pre-clinical sciences: **http://www.nlm.nih.gov/databases/databases_medline.html**

- **Toxicology and Environmental Health Information (TOXNET):** Databases covering toxicology and environmental health: **http://sis.nlm.nih.gov/Tox/ToxMain.html**

- **Visible Human Interface:** Anatomically detailed, three-dimensional representations of normal male and female human bodies: **http://www.nlm.nih.gov/research/visible/visible_human.html**

While all of the above references may be of interest to physicians who study and treat muscular dystrophy, the following are particularly noteworthy.

The NLM Gateway[24]

The NLM (National Library of Medicine) Gateway is a Web-based system that lets users search simultaneously in multiple retrieval systems at the U.S. National Library of Medicine (NLM). It allows users of NLM services to initiate searches from one Web interface, providing "one-stop searching" for many of NLM's information resources or databases.[25] One target audience for the Gateway is the Internet user who is new to NLM's online resources and does not know what information is available or how best to search for it. This audience may include physicians and other healthcare providers,

---

[24] Adapted from NLM: **http://gateway.nlm.nih.gov/gw/Cmd?Overview.x**.

[25] The NLM Gateway is currently being developed by the Lister Hill National Center for Biomedical Communications (LHNCBC) at the National Library of Medicine (NLM) of the National Institutes of Health (NIH).

researchers, librarians, students, and, increasingly, patients, their families, and the public.[26] To use the NLM Gateway, simply go to the search site at **http://gateway.nlm.nih.gov/gw/Cmd**. Type "muscular dystrophy" (or synonyms) into the search box and click "Search." The results will be presented in a tabular form, indicating the number of references in each database category.

Results Summary

Category	Items Found
Journal Articles	18735
Books / Periodicals / Audio Visual	227
Consumer Health	192
Meeting Abstracts	6
Other Collections	262
Total	19422

HSTAT[27]

HSTAT is a free, Web-based resource that provides access to full-text documents used in healthcare decision-making.[28] HSTAT's audience includes healthcare providers, health service researchers, policy makers, insurance companies, consumers, and the information professionals who serve these groups. HSTAT provides access to a wide variety of publications, including clinical practice guidelines, quick-reference guides for clinicians, consumer health brochures, evidence reports and technology assessments from the Agency for Healthcare Research and Quality (AHRQ), as well as AHRQ's Put Prevention Into Practice.[29] Simply search by "muscular dystrophy" (or synonyms) at the following Web site: **http://text.nlm.nih.gov**.

---

[26] Other users may find the Gateway useful for an overall search of NLM's information resources. Some searchers may locate what they need immediately, while others will utilize the Gateway as an adjunct tool to other NLM search services such as PubMed® and MEDLINEplus®. The Gateway connects users with multiple NLM retrieval systems while also providing a search interface for its own collections. These collections include various types of information that do not logically belong in PubMed, LOCATORplus, or other established NLM retrieval systems (e.g., meeting announcements and pre-1966 journal citations). The Gateway will provide access to the information found in an increasing number of NLM retrieval systems in several phases.

[27] Adapted from HSTAT: **http://www.nlm.nih.gov/pubs/factsheets/hstat.html**.

[28] The HSTAT URL is **http://hstat.nlm.nih.gov/**.

[29] Other important documents in HSTAT include: the National Institutes of Health (NIH) Consensus Conference Reports and Technology Assessment Reports; the HIV/AIDS Treatment Information Service (ATIS) resource documents; the Substance Abuse and Mental Health Services Administration's Center for Substance Abuse Treatment (SAMHSA/CSAT)

Coffee Break: Tutorials for Biologists[30]

Some patients may wish to have access to a general healthcare site that takes a scientific view of the news and covers recent breakthroughs in biology that may one day assist physicians in developing treatments. To this end, we recommend "Coffee Break," a collection of short reports on recent biological discoveries. Each report incorporates interactive tutorials that demonstrate how bioinformatics tools are used as a part of the research process. Currently, all Coffee Breaks are written by NCBI staff.[31] Each report is about 400 words and is usually based on a discovery reported in one or more articles from recently published, peer-reviewed literature.[32] This site has new articles every few weeks, so it can be considered an online magazine of sorts, and intended for general background information. You can access Coffee Break at **http://www.ncbi.nlm.nih.gov/Coffeebreak/**.

Other Commercial Databases

In addition to resources maintained by official agencies, other databases exist that are commercial ventures addressing medical professionals. Here are some examples that may interest you:

- **CliniWeb International:** Index and table of contents to selected clinical information on the Internet; see **http://www.ohsu.edu/cliniweb/**.

- **Medical World Search:** Searches full text from thousands of selected medical sites on the Internet; see **http://www.mwsearch.com/**.

Treatment Improvement Protocols (TIP) and Center for Substance Abuse Prevention (SAMHSA/CSAP) Prevention Enhancement Protocols System (PEPS); the Public Health Service (PHS) Preventive Services Task Force's *Guide to Clinical Preventive Services*; the independent, nonfederal Task Force on Community Services *Guide to Community Preventive Services*; and the Health Technology Advisory Committee (HTAC) of the Minnesota Health Care Commission (MHCC) health technology evaluations.

[30] Adapted from **http://www.ncbi.nlm.nih.gov/Coffeebreak/Archive/FAQ**.html.

[31] The figure that accompanies each article is frequently supplied by an expert external to NCBI, in which case the source of the figure is cited. The result is an interactive tutorial that tells a biological story.

[32] After a brief introduction that sets the work described into a broader context, the report focuses on how a molecular understanding can provide explanations of observed biology and lead to therapies for diseases. Each vignette is accompanied by a figure and hypertext links that lead to a series of pages that interactively show how NCBI tools and resources are used in the research process.

The Genome Project and Muscular Dystrophy

With all the discussion in the press about the Human Genome Project, it is only natural that physicians, researchers, and patients want to know about how human genes relate to muscular dystrophy. In the following section, we will discuss databases and references used by physicians and scientists who work in this area.

Online Mendelian Inheritance in Man (OMIM)

The Online Mendelian Inheritance in Man (OMIM) database is a catalog of human genes and genetic disorders authored and edited by Dr. Victor A. McKusick and his colleagues at Johns Hopkins and elsewhere. OMIM was developed for the World Wide Web by the National Center for Biotechnology Information (NCBI).[33] The database contains textual information, pictures, and reference information. It also contains copious links to NCBI's Entrez database of MEDLINE articles and sequence information.

Go to **http://www.ncbi.nlm.nih.gov/Omim/searchomim.html** to search the database. If too many results appear, you can narrow the search by adding the word "clinical." Each report will have additional links to related research and databases. By following these links, especially the link titled "Database Links," you will be exposed to numerous specialized databases that are largely used by the scientific community. These databases are overly technical and seldom used by the general public, but offer an abundance of information. The following is an example of the results you can obtain from the OMIM for muscular dystrophy:

- **Facioscapulohumeral Muscular Dystrophy 1a**
  Web site:
  http://www.ncbi.nlm.nih.gov/entrez/dispomim.cgi?id=158900

- **Facioscapulohumeral Muscular Dystrophy 1b**
  Web site:
  http://www.ncbi.nlm.nih.gov/entrez/dispomim.cgi?id=158901

---

[33] Adapted from **http://www.ncbi.nlm.nih.gov/**. Established in 1988 as a national resource for molecular biology information, NCBI creates public databases, conducts research in computational biology, develops software tools for analyzing genome data, and disseminates biomedical information--all for the better understanding of molecular processes affecting human health and disease.

- **Rigid Spine Muscular Dystrophy 1**
  Web site:
  http://www.ncbi.nlm.nih.gov/entrez/dispomim.cgi?id=602771

Genes and Disease (NCBI - Map)

The Genes and Disease database is produced by the National Center for Biotechnology Information of the National Library of Medicine at the National Institutes of Health. This Web site categorizes each disorder by the system of the body. Go to **http://www.ncbi.nlm.nih.gov/disease/**, and browse the system pages to have a full view of important conditions linked to human genes. Since this site is regularly updated, you may wish to re-visit it from time to time. The following systems and associated disorders are addressed:

- **Muscle and Bone:** Movement and growth.
  Examples: Duchenne muscular dystrophy, Ellis-van Creveld syndrome, Marfan syndrome, myotonic dystrophy, spinal muscular atrophy.
  Web site: **http://www.ncbi.nlm.nih.gov/disease/Muscle.html**

- **Nervous System:** Mind and body.
  Examples: Alzheimer disease, Amyotrophic lateral sclerosis, Angelman syndrome, Charcot-Marie-Tooth disease, epilepsy, essential tremor, Fragile X syndrome, Friedreich's ataxia, Huntington disease, Niemann-Pick disease, Parkinson disease, Prader-Willi syndrome, Rett syndrome, Spinocerebellar atrophy, Williams syndrome.
  Web site: **http://www.ncbi.nlm.nih.gov/disease/Brain.html**

- **Signals:** Cellular messages.
  Examples: Ataxia telangiectasia, Baldness, Cockayne syndrome, Glaucoma, SRY: sex determination, Tuberous sclerosis, Waardenburg syndrome, Werner syndrome.
  Web site: **http://www.ncbi.nlm.nih.gov/disease/Signals.html**

- **Transporters:** Pumps and channels.
  Examples: Cystic Fibrosis, deafness, diastrophic dysplasia, Hemophilia A, long-QT syndrome, Menkes syndrome, Pendred syndrome, polycystic kidney disease, sickle cell anemia, Wilson's disease, Zellweger syndrome.
  Web site: **http://www.ncbi.nlm.nih.gov/disease/Transporters.html**

Entrez

Entrez is a search and retrieval system that integrates several linked databases at the National Center for Biotechnology Information (NCBI). These databases include nucleotide sequences, protein sequences, macromolecular structures, whole genomes, and MEDLINE through PubMed. Entrez provides access to the following databases:

- **3D Domains:** Domains from Entrez Structure,
  Web site: **http://www.ncbi.nlm.nih.gov/entrez/query.fcgi?db=geo**

- **Books:** Online books,
  Web site: **http://www.ncbi.nlm.nih.gov/entrez/query.fcgi?db=books**

- **Genome:** Complete genome assemblies,
  Web site: **http://www.ncbi.nlm.nih.gov/entrez/query.fcgi?db=Genome**

- **NCBI's Protein Sequence Information Survey Results:**
  Web site: **http://www.ncbi.nlm.nih.gov/About/proteinsurvey/**

- **Nucleotide Sequence Database (Genbank):**
  Web site:
  http://www.ncbi.nlm.nih.gov/entrez/query.fcgi?db=Nucleotide

- **OMIM:** Online Mendelian Inheritance in Man,
  Web site: **http://www.ncbi.nlm.nih.gov/entrez/query.fcgi?db=OMIM**

- **PopSet:** Population study data sets,
  Web site: **http://www.ncbi.nlm.nih.gov/entrez/query.fcgi?db=Popset**

- **ProbeSet:** Gene Expression Omnibus (GEO),
  Web site: **http://www.ncbi.nlm.nih.gov/entrez/query.fcgi?db=geo**

- **Protein Sequence Database:**
  Web site: **http://www.ncbi.nlm.nih.gov/entrez/query.fcgi?db=Protein**

- **PubMed:** Biomedical literature (PubMed),
  Web site: **http://www.ncbi.nlm.nih.gov/entrez/query.fcgi?db=PubMed**

- **Structure:** Three-dimensional macromolecular structures,
  Web site: **http://www.ncbi.nlm.nih.gov/entrez/query.fcgi?db=Structure**

- **Taxonomy:** Organisms in GenBank,
  Web site:
  http://www.ncbi.nlm.nih.gov/entrez/query.fcgi?db=Taxonomy

Access the Entrez system of the NCBI at the following hyperlink: **http://www.ncbi.nlm.nih.gov/entrez/query.fcgi?CMD=search&DB=genome**, and then select the database that you would like to search. The databases available are listed in the drop box next to "Search." In the box next to "for," enter "muscular dystrophy" (or synonyms) and click "Go."

Jablonski's Multiple Congenital Anomaly/Mental Retardation (MCA/MR) Syndromes Database[34]

This online resource can be quite useful. It has been developed to facilitate the identification and differentiation of syndromic entities. Special attention is given to the type of information that is usually limited or completely omitted in existing reference sources due to space limitations of the printed form.

You can search across syndromes using an alphabetical index at **http://www.nlm.nih.gov/mesh/jablonski/syndrome_toc/toc_a.html.** At **http://www.nlm.nih.gov/mesh/jablonski/syndrome_db.html**, search by keyword.

The Genome Database[35]

Established at Johns Hopkins University in Baltimore, Maryland in 1990, the Genome Database (GDB) is the official central repository for genomic mapping data resulting from the Human Genome Initiative. In the spring of 1999, the Bioinformatics Supercomputing Centre (BiSC) at the Hospital for Sick Children in Toronto, Ontario assumed the management of GDB. The Human Genome Initiative is a worldwide research effort focusing on structural analysis of human DNA to determine the location and sequence of the estimated 100,000 human genes. In support of this project, GDB stores and curates data generated by researchers worldwide who are engaged in the mapping effort of the Human Genome Project (HGP). GDB's mission is to provide scientists with an encyclopedia of the human genome which is continually revised and updated to reflect the current state of scientific knowledge. Although GDB has historically focused on gene mapping, its focus will broaden as the Genome Project moves from mapping to sequence, and finally, to functional analysis.

To access the GDB, simply go to the following hyperlink: **http://www.gdb.org/**. Search "All Biological Data" by "Keyword." Type

---

[34] Adapted from the National Library of Medicine: **http://www.nlm.nih.gov/mesh/jablonski/about_syndrome.html**.
[35] Adapted from the Genome Database: **http://gdbwww.gdb.org/gdb/aboutGDB.html#mission**.

"muscular dystrophy" (or synonyms) into the search box, and review the results. If more than one word is used in the search box, then separate each one with the word "and" or "or" (using "or" might be useful when using synonyms). This database is extremely technical as it was created for specialists. The articles are the results which are the most accessible to non-professionals and often listed under the heading "Citations." The contact names are also accessible to non-professionals.

Specialized References

The following books are specialized references written for professionals interested in muscular dystrophy (sorted alphabetically by title, hyperlinks provide rankings, information, and reviews at Amazon.com):

- **Approach to the Patient with a Musculoskeletal Disorder** by Warren D. Blackburn; Paperback, 2nd edition (August 15, 2002), Professional Communications; ISBN: 188473572X; http://www.amazon.com/exec/obidos/ASIN/188473572X/icongroupinterna

- **Connective Tissue and Its Heritable Disorders: Molecular, Genetic, and Medical Aspects** by Peter M. Royce (Editor), Beat Steinmann (Editor); Hardcover, 2nd edition (December 15, 2001), John Wiley & Sons; ISBN: 0471251852; http://www.amazon.com/exec/obidos/ASIN/0471251852/icongroupinterna

- **Current Diagnosis & Treatment in Orthopedics** by Harry B. Skinner; Paperback - 720 pages, 2nd edition (May 26, 2000), McGraw-Hill Professional Publishing; ISBN: 0838503632; http://www.amazon.com/exec/obidos/ASIN/0838503632/icongroupinterna

- **Current Topics in Musculoskeletal Medicine: A Case Study Approach (Athletic Training Library)** by Mark Decarlo (Editor), Kathy Oneacre, M.A. ATC (Editor); Paperback (March 15, 2001), Slack, Inc.; ISBN: 1556424345; http://www.amazon.com/exec/obidos/ASIN/1556424345/icongroupinterna

- **Diagnosis and Treatment of Movement Impairment Syndromes** by Shirley Sahrmann; Hardcover - 384 pages, 1st edition (August 20, 2001), Mosby, Inc.; ISBN: 0801672058; http://www.amazon.com/exec/obidos/ASIN/0801672058/icongroupinterna

- **Diagnosis of Bone and Joint Disorders (5-Volume Set)** by Donald Resnick; Hardcover - 5472 pages, 4th edition (March 8, 2002); W B Saunders Co; ISBN: 0721689213; http://www.amazon.com/exec/obidos/ASIN/0721689213/icongroupinterna

- **Essentials of Musculoskeletal Care** by Walter B. Greene, MD (Editor), Robert K. Snider; Hardcover, 2nd edition (January 15, 2001), American Academy of Orthopaedic; ISBN: 0892032170; http://www.amazon.com/exec/obidos/ASIN/0892032170/icongroupinterna

- **Examination & Diagnosis of Musculoskeletal Disorders** by Miranda Castrp; Hardcover, 1st edition (February 15, 2001), Thieme Medical Pub; ISBN: 0865777411; http://www.amazon.com/exec/obidos/ASIN/0865777411/icongroupinterna

- **Examination and Diagnosis of Musculoskeletal Disorders: Clinical Examination - Imaging Modalities** by William H. M. Castro, et al; Hardcover - 464 pages, 1st edition (January 15, 2001), Thieme Medical Pub; ISBN: 1588900320; http://www.amazon.com/exec/obidos/ASIN/1588900320/icongroupinterna

- **Mechanical Loading of Bones and Joints** by Hideaki Takahashi (Editor); Hardcover - 324 pages, 1st edition (July 15, 1999), Springer Verlag; ISBN: 4431702423; http://www.amazon.com/exec/obidos/ASIN/4431702423/icongroupinterna

- **Musculoskeletal Assessment: Joint Range of Motion and Manual Muscle Strength** by Hazel M. Clarkson; Spiral-bound - 432 pages, 2nd edition (January 15, 2000), Lippincott Williams & Wilkins Publishers; ISBN: 0683303848; http://www.amazon.com/exec/obidos/ASIN/0683303848/icongroupinterna

- **Musculoskeletal Disorders: A Practical Guide for Diagnosis and Rehabilitation** by Ralph M. Buschbacher (Editor); Hardcover, 2nd edition (March 15, 2002), Butterworth-Heinemann; ISBN: 0750673575; http://www.amazon.com/exec/obidos/ASIN/0750673575/icongroupinterna

- **Musculoskeletal Examination** by Jeffrey Gross, et al; Paperback, 2nd edition (March 2002), Blackwell Science Inc; ISBN: 0632045582;

http://www.amazon.com/exec/obidos/ASIN/0632045582/icongroupinter
na

- **Orthopedic Biomechanics** by Paul Brinckmann, et al; Hardcover (March 2002), Thieme Medical Pub; ISBN: 1588900800;
http://www.amazon.com/exec/obidos/ASIN/1588900800/icongroupinter
na

- **Orthopaedic Pathology** by Vincent J. Vigorita, Bernard Ghelman; Hardcover - 718 pages (February 15, 1999), Lippincott Williams & Wilkins Publishers; ISBN: 078170040X;
http://www.amazon.com/exec/obidos/ASIN/078170040X/icongroupinter
na

- **Pathology of Skeletal Muscle** by Stirling Carpenter, George Karpati; Hardcover, 2nd edition (January 15, 2001), Oxford University Press; ISBN: 0195063643;
http://www.amazon.com/exec/obidos/ASIN/0195063643/icongroupinter
na

- **Skeletal Trauma: Basic Science, Management, and Reconstruction** by Bruce D. Browner (Editor); Hardcover, 3rd edition (August 2002), W B Saunders Co; ISBN: 0721694810;
http://www.amazon.com/exec/obidos/ASIN/0721694810/icongroupinter
na

Vocabulary Builder

The following vocabulary builder provides definitions of words used in this chapter that have not been defined in previous chapters:

Essential Tremor: A rhythmic, involuntary, purposeless, oscillating movement resulting from the alternate contraction and relaxation of opposing groups of muscles. [NIH]

Rett Syndrome: A neurological disorder seen almost exclusively in females, and found in a variety of racial and ethnic groups worldwide. [NIH]

CHAPTER 8. DISSERTATIONS ON MUSCULAR DYSTROPHY

Overview

University researchers are active in studying almost all known diseases. The result of research is often published in the form of Doctoral or Master's dissertations. You should understand, therefore, that applied diagnostic procedures and/or therapies can take many years to develop after the thesis that proposed the new technique or approach was written.

In this chapter, we will give you a bibliography on recent dissertations relating to muscular dystrophy. You can read about these in more detail using the Internet or your local medical library. We will also provide you with information on how to use the Internet to stay current on dissertations.

Dissertations on Muscular Dystrophy

ProQuest Digital Dissertations is the largest archive of academic dissertations available. From this archive, we have compiled the following list covering dissertations devoted to muscular dystrophy. You will see that the information provided includes the dissertation's title, its author, and the author's institution. To read more about the following, simply use the Internet address indicated. The following covers recent dissertations dealing with muscular dystrophy:

- **A study of selected variables in relation to accidents of muscular dystrophy children in special schools.** by NEMARICH, SAMUEL PETER, PHD from New York University, 1975, 168 pages
  http://wwwlib.umi.com/dissertations/fullcit/7601746

- **Energy metabolism in progressive muscular dystrophy studies on oxidative phosphorylation of genetically determined muscular dystrophy in mice and hamsters** by Wrogemann, Klaus, ADVDEG from The University of Manitoba (Canada), 1969
  http://wwwlib.umi.com/dissertations/fullcit/NK04482

- **Maximal isometric strength on the kinetic communicator system for Duchenne muscular dystrophy patients** by Xie, Xiaoqing (Steven), DA from Middle Tennessee State University, 2001, 123 pages
  http://wwwlib.umi.com/dissertations/fullcit/3030580

- **Parents' perspectives on Duchenne/Becker muscular dystrophy and specific learning disabilities: A grounded theory study** by Webb, Carol Lee, PhD from Ohio University, 2002, 170 pages
  http://wwwlib.umi.com/dissertations/fullcit/3062177

- **The effect of physostigmine on language processes in boys with Duchenne muscular dystrophy (memory)** by Cameron, Thomas Hartley, PhD from The University of North Carolina at Chapel Hill, 1985, 108 pages
  http://wwwlib.umi.com/dissertations/fullcit/8527184

Keeping Current

As previously mentioned, an effective way to stay current on dissertations dedicated to muscular dystrophy is to use the database called *ProQuest Digital Dissertations* via the Internet, located at the following Web address: **http://wwwlib.umi.com/dissertations**. The site allows you to freely access the last two years of citations and abstracts. Ask your medical librarian if the library has full and unlimited access to this database. From the library, you should be able to do more complete searches than with the limited 2-year access available to the general public.

PART III. APPENDICES

ABOUT PART III

Part III is a collection of appendices on general medical topics which may be of interest to patients with muscular dystrophy and related conditions.

APPENDIX A. RESEARCHING YOUR MEDICATIONS

Overview

There are a number of sources available on new or existing medications which could be prescribed to patients with muscular dystrophy. While a number of hard copy or CD-Rom resources are available to patients and physicians for research purposes, a more flexible method is to use Internet-based databases. In this chapter, we will begin with a general overview of medications. We will then proceed to outline official recommendations on how you should view your medications. You may also want to research medications that you are currently taking for other conditions as they may interact with medications for muscular dystrophy. Research can give you information on the side effects, interactions, and limitations of prescription drugs used in the treatment of muscular dystrophy. Broadly speaking, there are two sources of information on approved medications: public sources and private sources. We will emphasize free-to-use public sources.

Your Medications: The Basics[36]

The Agency for Health Care Research and Quality has published extremely useful guidelines on how you can best participate in the medication aspects of muscular dystrophy. Taking medicines is not always as simple as swallowing a pill. It can involve many steps and decisions each day. The AHCRQ recommends that patients with muscular dystrophy take part in treatment decisions. Do not be afraid to ask questions and talk about your concerns. By taking a moment to ask questions early, you may avoid

---

[36] This section is adapted from AHCRQ: **http://www.ahcpr.gov/consumer/ncpiebro.htm.**

problems later. Here are some points to cover each time a new medicine is prescribed:

- Ask about all parts of your treatment, including diet changes, exercise, and medicines.

- Ask about the risks and benefits of each medicine or other treatment you might receive.

- Ask how often you or your doctor will check for side effects from a given medication.

Do not hesitate to ask what is important to you about your medicines. You may want a medicine with the fewest side effects, or the fewest doses to take each day. You may care most about cost, or how the medicine might affect how you live or work. Or, you may want the medicine your doctor believes will work the best. Telling your doctor will help him or her select the best treatment for you.

Do not be afraid to "bother" your doctor with your concerns and questions about medications for muscular dystrophy. You can also talk to a nurse or a pharmacist. They can help you better understand your treatment plan. Feel free to bring a friend or family member with you when you visit your doctor. Talking over your options with someone you trust can help you make better choices, especially if you are not feeling well. Specifically, ask your doctor the following:

- The name of the medicine and what it is supposed to do.

- How and when to take the medicine, how much to take, and for how long.

- What food, drinks, other medicines, or activities you should avoid while taking the medicine.

- What side effects the medicine may have, and what to do if they occur.

- If you can get a refill, and how often.

- About any terms or directions you do not understand.

- What to do if you miss a dose.

- If there is written information you can take home (most pharmacies have information sheets on your prescription medicines; some even offer large-print or Spanish versions).

Do not forget to tell your doctor about all the medicines you are currently taking (not just those for muscular dystrophy). This includes prescription medicines and the medicines that you buy over the counter. Then your doctor can avoid giving you a new medicine that may not work well with the medications you take now. When talking to your doctor, you may wish to prepare a list of medicines you currently take, the reason you take them, and how you take them. Be sure to include the following information for each:

- Name of medicine

- Reason taken

- Dosage

- Time(s) of day

Also include any over-the-counter medicines, such as:

- Laxatives

- Diet pills

- Vitamins

- Cold medicine

- Aspirin or other pain, headache, or fever medicine

- Cough medicine

- Allergy relief medicine

- Antacids

- Sleeping pills

- Others (include names)

Learning More about Your Medications

Because of historical investments by various organizations and the emergence of the Internet, it has become rather simple to learn about the medications your doctor has recommended for muscular dystrophy. One such source is the United States Pharmacopeia. In 1820, eleven physicians met in Washington, D.C. to establish the first compendium of standard drugs for the United States. They called this compendium the "U.S. Pharmacopeia (USP)." Today, the USP is a non-profit organization consisting of 800 volunteer scientists, eleven elected officials, and 400 representatives of state associations and colleges of medicine and pharmacy. The USP is located in Rockville, Maryland, and its home page is located at **www.usp.org**. The USP currently provides standards for over 3,700 medications. The resulting USP DI® Advice for the Patient® can be accessed through the National Library of

Medicine of the National Institutes of Health. The database is partially derived from lists of federally approved medications in the Food and Drug Administration's (FDA) Drug Approvals database.[37]

While the FDA database is rather large and difficult to navigate, the Phamacopeia is both user-friendly and free to use. It covers more than 9,000 prescription and over-the-counter medications. To access this database, simply type the following hyperlink into your Web browser: **http://www.nlm.nih.gov/medlineplus/druginformation.html**. To view examples of a given medication (brand names, category, description, preparation, proper use, precautions, side effects, etc.), simply follow the hyperlinks indicated within the United States Pharmacopeia (USP).

Of course, we as editors cannot be certain as to what medications you are taking. Therefore, we have compiled a list of medications associated with the treatment of muscular dystrophy. Once again, due to space limitations, we only list a sample of medications and provide hyperlinks to ample documentation (e.g. typical dosage, side effects, drug-interaction risks, etc.). The following drugs have been mentioned in the Pharmacopeia and other sources as being potentially applicable to muscular dystrophy:

Anticonvulsants, Hydantoin

- **Systemic - U.S. Brands:** Cerebyx; Dilantin; Dilantin Infatabs; Dilantin Kapseals; Dilantin-125; Mesantoin; Peganone; Phenytek http://www.nlm.nih.gov/medlineplus/druginfo/uspdi/202052.html

Clofibrate

- **Systemic - U.S. Brands:** Abitrate; Atromid-S http://www.nlm.nih.gov/medlineplus/druginfo/uspdi/202150.html

Dantrolene

- **Systemic - U.S. Brands:** Dantrium; Dantrium Intravenous http://www.nlm.nih.gov/medlineplus/druginfo/uspdi/202181.html

Lithium

- **Systemic - U.S. Brands:** Cibalith-S; Eskalith; Eskalith CR; Lithane; Lithobid; Lithonate; Lithotabs

---

[37] Though cumbersome, the FDA database can be freely browsed at the following site: **www.fda.gov/cder/da/da.htm.**

http://www.nlm.nih.gov/medlineplus/druginfo/uspdi/202330.html

Vitamin E

- **Systemic - U.S. Brands:** Amino-Opti-E; Aquasol E; E-1000 I.U. Softgels; E-200 I.U. Softgels; E-400 I.U. in a Water Soluble Base; E-Complex-600; E-Vitamin Succinate; Liqui-E; Pheryl-E; Vita Plus E http://www.nlm.nih.gov/medlineplus/druginfo/uspdi/202598.html

Commercial Databases

In addition to the medications listed in the USP above, a number of commercial sites are available by subscription to physicians and their institutions. You may be able to access these sources from your local medical library or your doctor's office.

Reuters Health Drug Database

The Reuters Health Drug Database can be searched by keyword at the hyperlink: **http://www.reutershealth.com/frame2/drug.html**.

Mosby's GenRx

Mosby's GenRx database (also available on CD-Rom and book format) covers 45,000 drug products including generics and international brands. It provides prescribing information, drug interactions, and patient information. Information can be obtained at the following hyperlink: **http://www.genrx.com/Mosby/PhyGenRx/group.html**.

PDR*health*

The PDR*health* database is a free-to-use, drug information search engine that has been written for the public in layman's terms. It contains FDA-approved drug information adapted from the Physicians' Desk Reference (PDR) database. PDR*health* can be searched by brand name, generic name, or indication. It features multiple drug interactions reports. Search PDR*health* at **http://www.pdrhealth.com/drug_info/index.html**.

Other Web Sites

A number of additional Web sites discuss drug information. As an example, you may like to look at **www.drugs.com** which reproduces the information in the Pharmacopeia as well as commercial information. You may also want to consider the Web site of the Medical Letter, Inc. which allows users to download articles on various drugs and therapeutics for a nominal fee: **http://www.medletter.com/**.

Researching Orphan Drugs

Orphan drugs are a special class of pharmaceuticals used by patients who are unaffected by existing treatments or with illnesses for which no known drug is effective. Orphan drugs are most commonly prescribed or developed for "rare" diseases or conditions.[38] According to the FDA, an orphan drug (or biological) may already be approved, or it may still be experimental. A drug becomes an "orphan" when it receives orphan designation from the Office of Orphan Products Development at the FDA.[39] Orphan designation qualifies the sponsor to receive certain benefits from the U.S. Government in exchange for developing the drug. The drug must then undergo the new drug approval process as any other drug would. To date, over 1000 orphan products have been designated, and over 200 have been approved for marketing. Historically, the approval time for orphan products as a group has been considerably shorter than the approval time for other drugs. This is due to the fact that many orphan products receive expedited review because they are developed for serious or life-threatening diseases.

The cost of orphan products is determined by the sponsor of the drug and can vary greatly. Reimbursement rates for drug expenses are set by each insurance company and outlined in your policy. Insurance companies will generally reimburse for orphan products that have been approved for marketing, but may not reimburse for products that are considered experimental. Consult your insurance company about specific reimbursement policies. If an orphan product has been approved for

---

[38] The U.S. Food and Drug Administration defines a rare disease or condition as "any disease or condition which affects less than 200,000 persons in the United States, or affects more than 200,000 in the United States and for which there is no reasonable expectation that the cost of developing and making available in the United States a drug for such disease or condition will be recovered from sales in the United States of such drug." Adapted from the U.S. Food and Drug Administration: **http://www.fda.gov/opacom/laws/orphandg.htm**.
[39] The following is adapted from the U.S. Food and Drug Administration: **http://www.fda.gov/orphan/faq/index.htm**.

marketing, it will be available through the normal pharmaceutical supply channels. If the product has not been approved, the sponsor may make the product available on a compassionate-use basis.[40]

Although the list of orphan drugs is revised on a daily basis, you can quickly research orphan drugs that might be applicable to muscular dystrophy using the database managed by the National Organization for Rare Disorders, Inc. (NORD), located at **www.raredisease.org**. Simply go to their general search page and select "Orphan Drug Designation Database." On this page (**http://www.rarediseases.org/search/noddsearch.html**), type "muscular dystrophy" or a synonym into the search box and click "Submit Query." When you see a list of drugs, understand that not all of the drugs may be relevant. Some may have been withdrawn from orphan status. Write down or print out the name of each drug and the relevant contact information. Visit the Pharmacopeia Web site and type the name of each orphan drug into the search box on **http://www.nlm.nih.gov/medlineplus/druginformation.html**. Read about each drug in detail and consult your doctor to find out if you might benefit from these medications. You or your physician may need to contact the sponsor or NORD.

NORD conducts "early access programs for investigational new drugs (IND) under the Food and Drug Administration's (FDA's) approval 'Treatment INDs' programs which allow for a limited number of individuals to receive investigational drugs before FDA marketing approval." If the orphan product about which you are seeking information is approved for marketing, information on side effects can be found on the product's label. If the product is not approved, you or your physician should consult the sponsor.

The following is a list of orphan drugs currently listed in the NORD Orphan Drug Designation Database for muscular dystrophy or related conditions:

- **Mazindol (trade name: Sanorex)**
  http://www.rarediseases.org/nord/search/nodd_full?code=148

- **Oxandrolone (trade name: Oxandrin)**
  http://www.rarediseases.org/nord/search/nodd_full?code=890

---

[40] For contact information on sponsors of orphan products, contact the Office of Orphan Products Development (**http://www.fda.gov/orphan/**). General inquiries may be routed to the main office: Office of Orphan Products Development (HF-35); Food and Drug Administration, 5600 Fishers Lane, Rockville, MD 20857; Voice: (301) 827-3666 or (800) 300-7469; FAX: (301) 443-4915.

Contraindications and Interactions (Hidden Dangers)

Some of the medications mentioned in the previous discussions can be problematic for patients with muscular dystrophy--not because they are used in the treatment process, but because of contraindications, or side effects. Medications with contraindications are those that could react with drugs used to treat muscular dystrophy or potentially create deleterious side effects in patients with muscular dystrophy. You should ask your physician about any contraindications, especially as these might apply to other medications that you may be taking for common ailments.

Drug-drug interactions occur when two or more drugs react with each other. This drug-drug interaction may cause you to experience an unexpected side effect. Drug interactions may make your medications less effective, cause unexpected side effects, or increase the action of a particular drug. Some drug interactions can even be harmful to you.

Be sure to read the label every time you use a nonprescription or prescription drug, and take the time to learn about drug interactions. These precautions may be critical to your health. You can reduce the risk of potentially harmful drug interactions and side effects with a little bit of knowledge and common sense.

Drug labels contain important information about ingredients, uses, warnings, and directions which you should take the time to read and understand. Labels also include warnings about possible drug interactions. Further, drug labels may change as new information becomes available. This is why it's especially important to read the label every time you use a medication. When your doctor prescribes a new drug, discuss all over-the-counter and prescription medications, dietary supplements, vitamins, botanicals, minerals and herbals you take as well as the foods you eat. Ask your pharmacist for the package insert for each prescription drug you take. The package insert provides more information about potential drug interactions.

A Final Warning

At some point, you may hear of alternative medications from friends, relatives, or in the news media. Advertisements may suggest that certain alternative drugs can produce positive results for patients with muscular dystrophy. Exercise caution--some of these drugs may have fraudulent claims, and others may actually hurt you. The Food and Drug Administration (FDA) is the official U.S. agency charged with discovering which medications are likely to improve the health of patients with muscular dystrophy. The FDA warns patients to watch out for[41]:

- Secret formulas (real scientists share what they know)

- Amazing breakthroughs or miracle cures (real breakthroughs don't happen very often; when they do, real scientists do not call them amazing or miracles)

- Quick, painless, or guaranteed cures

- If it sounds too good to be true, it probably isn't true.

If you have any questions about any kind of medical treatment, the FDA may have an office near you. Look for their number in the blue pages of the phone book. You can also contact the FDA through its toll-free number, 1-888-INFO-FDA (1-888-463-6332), or on the World Wide Web at **www.fda.gov**.

General References

In addition to the resources provided earlier in this chapter, the following general references describe medications (sorted alphabetically by title; hyperlinks provide rankings, information and reviews at Amazon.com):

- **Complete Guide to Prescription and Nonprescription Drugs 2001 (Complete Guide to Prescription and Nonprescription Drugs, 2001)** by H. Winter Griffith, Paperback 16th edition (2001), Medical Surveillance; ISBN: 0942447417;
http://www.amazon.com/exec/obidos/ASIN/039952634X/icongroupinterna

- **The Essential Guide to Prescription Drugs, 2001** by James J. Rybacki, James W. Long; Paperback - 1274 pages (2001), Harper Resource; ISBN: 0060958162;
http://www.amazon.com/exec/obidos/ASIN/0060958162/icongroupinterna

- **Handbook of Commonly Prescribed Drugs** by G. John Digregorio, Edward J. Barbieri; Paperback 16th edition (2001), Medical Surveillance; ISBN: 0942447417;
http://www.amazon.com/exec/obidos/ASIN/0942447417/icongroupinterna

---

[41] This section has been adapted from **http://www.fda.gov/opacom/lowlit/medfraud.html**.

- **Johns Hopkins Complete Home Encyclopedia of Drugs 2nd ed.** by Simeon Margolis (Ed.), Johns Hopkins; Hardcover - 835 pages (2000), Rebus; ISBN: 0929661583;
http://www.amazon.com/exec/obidos/ASIN/0929661583/icongroupinterna

- **Medical Pocket Reference: Drugs 2002** by Springhouse Paperback 1st edition (2001), Lippincott Williams & Wilkins Publishers; ISBN: 1582550964;
http://www.amazon.com/exec/obidos/ASIN/1582550964/icongroupinterna

- **PDR** by Medical Economics Staff, Medical Economics Staff Hardcover - 3506 pages 55th edition (2000), Medical Economics Company; ISBN: 1563633752;
http://www.amazon.com/exec/obidos/ASIN/1563633752/icongroupinterna

- **Pharmacy Simplified: A Glossary of Terms** by James Grogan; Paperback - 432 pages, 1st edition (2001), Delmar Publishers; ISBN: 0766828581;
http://www.amazon.com/exec/obidos/ASIN/0766828581/icongroupinterna

- **Physician Federal Desk Reference** by Christine B. Fraizer; Paperback 2nd edition (2001), Medicode Inc; ISBN: 1563373971;
http://www.amazon.com/exec/obidos/ASIN/1563373971/icongroupinterna

- **Physician's Desk Reference Supplements** Paperback - 300 pages, 53 edition (1999), ISBN: 1563632950;
http://www.amazon.com/exec/obidos/ASIN/1563632950/icongroupinterna

Vocabulary Builder

Compassionate: A process for providing experimental drugs to very sick patients who have no treatment options. [NIH]

Contraindications: Any factor or sign that it is unwise to pursue a certain kind of action or treatment, e. g. giving a general anesthetic to a person with pneumonia. [NIH]

Dilantin: A drug that is often used to control seizures. [NIH]

Appendix B. Researching Alternative Medicine

Overview

Complementary and alternative medicine (CAM) is one of the most contentious aspects of modern medical practice. You may have heard of these treatments on the radio or on television. Maybe you have seen articles written about these treatments in magazines, newspapers, or books. Perhaps your friends or doctor have mentioned alternatives.

In this chapter, we will begin by giving you a broad perspective on complementary and alternative therapies. Next, we will introduce you to official information sources on CAM relating to muscular dystrophy. Finally, at the conclusion of this chapter, we will provide a list of readings on muscular dystrophy from various authors. We will begin, however, with the National Center for Complementary and Alternative Medicine's (NCCAM) overview of complementary and alternative medicine.

What Is CAM?[42]

Complementary and alternative medicine (CAM) covers a broad range of healing philosophies, approaches, and therapies. Generally, it is defined as those treatments and healthcare practices which are not taught in medical schools, used in hospitals, or reimbursed by medical insurance companies. Many CAM therapies are termed "holistic," which generally means that the healthcare practitioner considers the whole person, including physical, mental, emotional, and spiritual health. Some of these therapies are also known as "preventive," which means that the practitioner educates and

---

[42] Adapted from the NCCAM: **http://nccam.nih.gov/health/whatiscam/#4**.

treats the person to prevent health problems from arising, rather than treating symptoms after problems have occurred.

People use CAM treatments and therapies in a variety of ways. Therapies are used alone (often referred to as alternative), in combination with other alternative therapies, or in addition to conventional treatment (sometimes referred to as complementary). Complementary and alternative medicine, or "integrative medicine," includes a broad range of healing philosophies, approaches, and therapies. Some approaches are consistent with physiological principles of Western medicine, while others constitute healing systems with non-Western origins. While some therapies are far outside the realm of accepted Western medical theory and practice, others are becoming established in mainstream medicine.

Complementary and alternative therapies are used in an effort to prevent illness, reduce stress, prevent or reduce side effects and symptoms, or control or cure disease. Some commonly used methods of complementary or alternative therapy include mind/body control interventions such as visualization and relaxation, manual healing including acupressure and massage, homeopathy, vitamins or herbal products, and acupuncture.

What Are the Domains of Alternative Medicine?[43]

The list of CAM practices changes continually. The reason being is that these new practices and therapies are often proved to be safe and effective, and therefore become generally accepted as "mainstream" healthcare practices. Today, CAM practices may be grouped within five major domains: (1) alternative medical systems, (2) mind-body interventions, (3) biologically-based treatments, (4) manipulative and body-based methods, and (5) energy therapies. The individual systems and treatments comprising these categories are too numerous to list in this sourcebook. Thus, only limited examples are provided within each.

Alternative Medical Systems

Alternative medical systems involve complete systems of theory and practice that have evolved independent of, and often prior to, conventional biomedical approaches. Many are traditional systems of medicine that are

---

[43] Adapted from the NCCAM: **http://nccam.nih.gov/health/whatiscam/#4**.

practiced by individual cultures throughout the world, including a number of venerable Asian approaches.

Traditional oriental medicine emphasizes the balance or disturbances of qi (pronounced chi) or vital energy in health and disease, respectively. Traditional oriental medicine consists of a group of techniques and methods including acupuncture, herbal medicine, oriental massage, and qi gong (a form of energy therapy). Acupuncture involves stimulating specific anatomic points in the body for therapeutic purposes, usually by puncturing the skin with a thin needle.

Ayurveda is India's traditional system of medicine. Ayurvedic medicine (meaning "science of life") is a comprehensive system of medicine that places equal emphasis on body, mind, and spirit. Ayurveda strives to restore the innate harmony of the individual. Some of the primary Ayurvedic treatments include diet, exercise, meditation, herbs, massage, exposure to sunlight, and controlled breathing.

Other traditional healing systems have been developed by the world's indigenous populations. These populations include Native American, Aboriginal, African, Middle Eastern, Tibetan, and Central and South American cultures. Homeopathy and naturopathy are also examples of complete alternative medicine systems.

Homeopathic medicine is an unconventional Western system that is based on the principle that "like cures like," i.e., that the same substance that in large doses produces the symptoms of an illness, in very minute doses cures it. Homeopathic health practitioners believe that the more dilute the remedy, the greater its potency. Therefore, they use small doses of specially prepared plant extracts and minerals to stimulate the body's defense mechanisms and healing processes in order to treat illness.

Naturopathic medicine is based on the theory that disease is a manifestation of alterations in the processes by which the body naturally heals itself and emphasizes health restoration rather than disease treatment. Naturopathic physicians employ an array of healing practices, including the following: diet and clinical nutrition, homeopathy, acupuncture, herbal medicine, hydrotherapy (the use of water in a range of temperatures and methods of applications), spinal and soft-tissue manipulation, physical therapies (such as those involving electrical currents, ultrasound, and light), therapeutic counseling, and pharmacology.

Mind-Body Interventions

Mind-body interventions employ a variety of techniques designed to facilitate the mind's capacity to affect bodily function and symptoms. Only a select group of mind-body interventions having well-documented theoretical foundations are considered CAM. For example, patient education and cognitive-behavioral approaches are now considered "mainstream." On the other hand, complementary and alternative medicine includes meditation, certain uses of hypnosis, dance, music, and art therapy, as well as prayer and mental healing.

Biological-Based Therapies

This category of CAM includes natural and biological-based practices, interventions, and products, many of which overlap with conventional medicine's use of dietary supplements. This category includes herbal, special dietary, orthomolecular, and individual biological therapies.

Herbal therapy employs an individual herb or a mixture of herbs for healing purposes. An herb is a plant or plant part that produces and contains chemical substances that act upon the body. Special diet therapies, such as those proposed by Drs. Atkins, Ornish, Pritikin, and Weil, are believed to prevent and/or control illness as well as promote health. Orthomolecular therapies aim to treat disease with varying concentrations of chemicals such as magnesium, melatonin, and mega-doses of vitamins. Biological therapies include, for example, the use of laetrile and shark cartilage to treat cancer and the use of bee pollen to treat autoimmune and inflammatory diseases.

Manipulative and Body-Based Methods

This category includes methods that are based on manipulation and/or movement of the body. For example, chiropractors focus on the relationship between structure and function, primarily pertaining to the spine, and how that relationship affects the preservation and restoration of health. Chiropractors use manipulative therapy as an integral treatment tool.

In contrast, osteopaths place particular emphasis on the musculoskeletal system and practice osteopathic manipulation. Osteopaths believe that all of the body's systems work together and that disturbances in one system may have an impact upon function elsewhere in the body. Massage therapists manipulate the soft tissues of the body to normalize those tissues.

Energy Therapies

Energy therapies focus on energy fields originating within the body (biofields) or those from other sources (electromagnetic fields). Biofield therapies are intended to affect energy fields (the existence of which is not yet experimentally proven) that surround and penetrate the human body. Some forms of energy therapy manipulate biofields by applying pressure and/or manipulating the body by placing the hands in or through these fields. Examples include Qi gong, Reiki and Therapeutic Touch.

Qi gong is a component of traditional oriental medicine that combines movement, meditation, and regulation of breathing to enhance the flow of vital energy (qi) in the body, improve blood circulation, and enhance immune function. Reiki, the Japanese word representing Universal Life Energy, is based on the belief that, by channeling spiritual energy through the practitioner, the spirit is healed and, in turn, heals the physical body. Therapeutic Touch is derived from the ancient technique of "laying-on of hands." It is based on the premises that the therapist's healing force affects the patient's recovery and that healing is promoted when the body's energies are in balance. By passing their hands over the patient, these healers identify energy imbalances.

Bioelectromagnetic-based therapies involve the unconventional use of electromagnetic fields to treat illnesses or manage pain. These therapies are often used to treat asthma, cancer, and migraine headaches. Types of electromagnetic fields which are manipulated in these therapies include pulsed fields, magnetic fields, and alternating current or direct current fields.

Can Alternatives Affect My Treatment?

A critical issue in pursuing complementary alternatives mentioned thus far is the risk that these might have undesirable interactions with your medical treatment. It becomes all the more important to speak with your doctor who can offer advice on the use of alternatives. Official sources confirm this view. Though written for women, we find that the National Women's Health Information Center's advice on pursuing alternative medicine is appropriate for patients of both genders and all ages.[44]

---

[44] Adapted from **http://www.4woman.gov/faq/alternative.htm**.

Is It Okay to Want Both Traditional and Alternative or Complementary Medicine?

Should you wish to explore non-traditional types of treatment, be sure to discuss all issues concerning treatments and therapies with your healthcare provider, whether a physician or practitioner of complementary and alternative medicine. Competent healthcare management requires knowledge of both conventional and alternative therapies you are taking for the practitioner to have a complete picture of your treatment plan.

The decision to use complementary and alternative treatments is an important one. Consider before selecting an alternative therapy, the safety and effectiveness of the therapy or treatment, the expertise and qualifications of the healthcare practitioner, and the quality of delivery. These topics should be considered when selecting any practitioner or therapy.

National Center for Complementary and Alternative Medicine

The National Center for Complementary and Alternative Medicine (NCCAM) of the National Institutes of Health (**http://nccam.nih.gov**) has created a link to the National Library of Medicine's databases to allow patients to search for articles that specifically relate to muscular dystrophy and complementary medicine. To search the database, go to **www.nlm.nih.gov/nccam/camonpubmed.html**. Select "CAM on PubMed." Enter "muscular dystrophy" (or synonyms) into the search box. Click "Go." The following references provide information on particular aspects of complementary and alternative medicine (CAM) that are related to muscular dystrophy:

- **A case of ventricular fibrillation in the prone position during back stabilisation surgery in a boy with Duchenne's muscular dystrophy.**
  Author(s): Reid JM, Appleton PJ.
  Source: Anaesthesia. 1999 April; 54(4): 364-7.
  http://www.ncbi.nlm.nih.gov/entrez/query.fcgi?cmd=Retrieve&db=pubmed&dopt=Abstract&list_uids=10455837

- **Activity of creatine kinase in sera from healthy women, carriers of Duchenne muscular dystrophy and cord blood, determined by the "European" recommended method with NAC-EDTA activation.**
  Author(s): Moss DW, Whitaker KB, Parmar C, Heckmatt J, Wikowski J, Sewry C, Dubowitz V.

Source: Clinica Chimica Acta; International Journal of Clinical Chemistry. 1981 October 26; 116(2): 209-16.
http://www.ncbi.nlm.nih.gov/entrez/query.fcgi?cmd=Retrieve&db=pubmed&dopt=Abstract&list_uids=6794955

- **Actomyosin alterations in Duchenne muscular dystrophy.**
  Author(s): Samaha FJ.
  Source: Archives of Neurology. 1973 June; 28(6): 405-7.
  http://www.ncbi.nlm.nih.gov/entrez/query.fcgi?cmd=Retrieve&db=pubmed&dopt=Abstract&list_uids=4267103

- **Breathing exercises for children with pseudohypertrophic muscular dystrophy.**
  Author(s): Houser CR, Johnson DM.
  Source: Physical Therapy. 1971 July; 51(7): 751-9.
  http://www.ncbi.nlm.nih.gov/entrez/query.fcgi?cmd=Retrieve&db=pubmed&dopt=Abstract&list_uids=4933570

- **Ca2+ transport in erythrocytes from patients with Duchenne muscular dystrophy.**
  Author(s): Pijst HL, Scholte HR.
  Source: Journal of the Neurological Sciences. 1983 August-September; 60(3): 411-7.
  http://www.ncbi.nlm.nih.gov/entrez/query.fcgi?cmd=Retrieve&db=pubmed&dopt=Abstract&list_uids=6138395

- **Canadian pilot study in music therapy with muscular dystrophy children.**
  Author(s): KORSON F.
  Source: Can J Occup Ther. 1959 June; 26(2): 45-9. No Abstract Available.
  http://www.ncbi.nlm.nih.gov/entrez/query.fcgi?cmd=Retrieve&db=pubmed&dopt=Abstract&list_uids=13662904

- **Cell transplantation as an experimental treatment for Duchenne muscular dystrophy.**
  Author(s): Law PK, Goodwin TG, Fang Q, Deering MB, Duggirala V, Larkin C, Florendo JA, Kirby DS, Li HJ, Chen M, et al.
  Source: Cell Transplantation. 1993 November-December; 2(6): 485-505.
  http://www.ncbi.nlm.nih.gov/entrez/query.fcgi?cmd=Retrieve&db=pubmed&dopt=Abstract&list_uids=8167934

- **Clinical trial of high dosage vitamin E in human muscular dystrophy.**
  Author(s): BERNESKE GM, BUTSON AR, GAULD EN, LEVY D.
  Source: Can Med Assoc J. 1960 February 20; 82: 418-21. No Abstract Available.
  http://www.ncbi.nlm.nih.gov/entrez/query.fcgi?cmd=Retrieve&db=pubmed&dopt=Abstract&list_uids=13799736

- **Comparative effects of sodium selenite and selenomethionine upon nutritional muscular dystrophy, selenium-dependent glutathione peroxidase, and tissue selenium concentrations of turkey poults.**
  Author(s): Cantor AH, Moorhead PD, Musser MA.
  Source: Poultry Science. 1982 March; 61(3): 478-84.
  http://www.ncbi.nlm.nih.gov/entrez/query.fcgi?cmd=Retrieve&db=pubmed&dopt=Abstract&list_uids=7088800

- **Corticosteroids in Duchenne muscular dystrophy: a reappraisal.**
  Author(s): Wong BL, Christopher C.
  Source: Journal of Child Neurology. 2002 March; 17(3): 183-90. Review.
  http://www.ncbi.nlm.nih.gov/entrez/query.fcgi?cmd=Retrieve&db=pubmed&dopt=Abstract&list_uids=12026233

- **Cultural differences in family communication about Duchenne muscular dystrophy.**
  Author(s): Fitzpatrick C, Barry C.
  Source: Developmental Medicine and Child Neurology. 1990 November; 32(11): 967-73.
  http://www.ncbi.nlm.nih.gov/entrez/query.fcgi?cmd=Retrieve&db=pubmed&dopt=Abstract&list_uids=2269406

- **Deficiency of a 180-kDa extracellular matrix protein in Fukuyama type congenital muscular dystrophy skeletal muscle.**
  Author(s): Sunada Y, Saito F, Higuchi I, Matsumura K, Shimizu T.
  Source: Neuromuscular Disorders: Nmd. 2002 February; 12(2): 117-20.
  http://www.ncbi.nlm.nih.gov/entrez/query.fcgi?cmd=Retrieve&db=pubmed&dopt=Abstract&list_uids=11738352

- **Detection of glucocorticoid-like activity in traditional Chinese medicine used for the treatment of Duchenne muscular dystrophy.**
  Author(s): Courdier-Fruh I, Barman L, Wettstein P, Meier T.

Source: Neuromuscular Disorders: Nmd. 2003 November; 13(9): 699-704.
http://www.ncbi.nlm.nih.gov/entrez/query.fcgi?cmd=Retrieve&db=pu
bmed&dopt=Abstract&list_uids=14561491

- **Dose-dependent effect of individualized respiratory muscle training in children with Duchenne muscular dystrophy.**
  Author(s): Topin N, Matecki S, Le Bris S, Rivier F, Echenne B, Prefaut C, Ramonatxo M.
  Source: Neuromuscular Disorders: Nmd. 2002 August; 12(6): 576-83.
  http://www.ncbi.nlm.nih.gov/entrez/query.fcgi?cmd=Retrieve&db=pu
  bmed&dopt=Abstract&list_uids=12117483

- **Duchenne muscular dystrophy and concomitant metastatic alveolar rhabdomyosarcoma.**
  Author(s): Rossbach HC, Lacson A, Grana NH, Barbosa JL.
  Source: Journal of Pediatric Hematology/Oncology: Official Journal of the American Society of Pediatric Hematology/Oncology. 1999 November-December; 21(6): 528-30.
  http://www.ncbi.nlm.nih.gov/entrez/query.fcgi?cmd=Retrieve&db=pu
  bmed&dopt=Abstract&list_uids=10598666

- **Duchenne muscular dystrophy--parental perceptions.**
  Author(s): Bothwell JE, Dooley JM, Gordon KE, MacAuley A, Camfield PR, MacSween J.
  Source: Clinical Pediatrics. 2002 March; 41(2): 105-9.
  http://www.ncbi.nlm.nih.gov/entrez/query.fcgi?cmd=Retrieve&db=pu
  bmed&dopt=Abstract&list_uids=11931326

- **Effects of electrical stimulation on muscles of children with Duchenne and Becker muscular dystrophy.**
  Author(s): Zupan A, Gregoric M, Valencic V, Vandot S.
  Source: Neuropediatrics. 1993 August; 24(4): 189-92.
  http://www.ncbi.nlm.nih.gov/entrez/query.fcgi?cmd=Retrieve&db=pu
  bmed&dopt=Abstract&list_uids=8232775

- **Effects of iron deprivation on the pathology and stress protein expression in murine X-linked muscular dystrophy.**
  Author(s): Bornman L, Rossouw H, Gericke GS, Polla BS.
  Source: Biochemical Pharmacology. 1998 September 15; 56(6): 751-7.
  http://www.ncbi.nlm.nih.gov/entrez/query.fcgi?cmd=Retrieve&db=pu
  bmed&dopt=Abstract&list_uids=9751080

- **Effects of physical therapy program on vital capacity of patients with muscular dystrophy.**
Author(s): Adams MA, Chandler LS.
Source: Physical Therapy. 1974 May; 54(5): 494-6.
http://www.ncbi.nlm.nih.gov/entrez/query.fcgi?cmd=Retrieve&db=pubmed&dopt=Abstract&list_uids=4607793

- **Efficacy of drug regimen exceeds electrostimulation in treatment of avian muscular dystrophy.**
Author(s): Hudecki MS, Povoski SP, Gregorio CC, Granchelli JA, Pollina CM.
Source: Journal of Applied Physiology (Bethesda, Md.: 1985). 1995 June; 78(6): 2014-9.
http://www.ncbi.nlm.nih.gov/entrez/query.fcgi?cmd=Retrieve&db=pubmed&dopt=Abstract&list_uids=7665393

- **Erythrocyte membrane autophosphorylation in Duchenne muscular dystrophy: effect of two methods of erythrocyte ghost preparation on results.**
Author(s): Roses AD.
Source: Clinica Chimica Acta; International Journal of Clinical Chemistry. 1979 July 2; 95(1): 69-73.
http://www.ncbi.nlm.nih.gov/entrez/query.fcgi?cmd=Retrieve&db=pubmed&dopt=Abstract&list_uids=509731

- **Feasibility, safety, and efficacy of myoblast transfer therapy on Duchenne muscular dystrophy boys.**
Author(s): Law PK, Goodwin TG, Fang Q, Duggirala V, Larkin C, Florendo JA, Kirby DS, Deering MB, Li HJ, Chen M, et al.
Source: Cell Transplantation. 1992; 1(2-3): 235-44.
http://www.ncbi.nlm.nih.gov/entrez/query.fcgi?cmd=Retrieve&db=pubmed&dopt=Abstract&list_uids=1344295

- **Hearing acuity in patients with muscular dystrophy.**
Author(s): Allen NR.
Source: Developmental Medicine and Child Neurology. 1973 August; 15(4): 500-5.
http://www.ncbi.nlm.nih.gov/entrez/query.fcgi?cmd=Retrieve&db=pubmed&dopt=Abstract&list_uids=4732900

- **Hyperbaric oxygen therapy for muscular dystrophy.**
Author(s): Hirotani H, Kuyama T.

Source: Nippon Geka Hokan. 1974 March; 43(2): 161-7. No Abstract Available.
http://www.ncbi.nlm.nih.gov/entrez/query.fcgi?cmd=Retrieve&db=pubmed&dopt=Abstract&list_uids=4473049

- **Inspiratory muscle training in patients with Duchenne muscular dystrophy.**
Author(s): Wanke T, Toifl K, Merkle M, Formanek D, Lahrmann H, Zwick H.
Source: Chest. 1994 February; 105(2): 475-82.
http://www.ncbi.nlm.nih.gov/entrez/query.fcgi?cmd=Retrieve&db=pubmed&dopt=Abstract&list_uids=8306750

- **Looking under every rock: Duchenne muscular dystrophy and traditional Chinese medicine.**
Author(s): Urtizberea JA, Fan QS, Vroom E, Recan D, Kaplan JC.
Source: Neuromuscular Disorders: Nmd. 2003 November; 13(9): 705-7.
http://www.ncbi.nlm.nih.gov/entrez/query.fcgi?cmd=Retrieve&db=pubmed&dopt=Abstract&list_uids=14561492

- **Muscle blood flow in Duchenne type muscular dystrophy, limb-girdle dystrophy, polymyositis, and in normal controls.**
Author(s): Paulson OB, Engel AG, Gomez MR.
Source: Journal of Neurology, Neurosurgery, and Psychiatry. 1974 June; 37(6): 685-90.
http://www.ncbi.nlm.nih.gov/entrez/query.fcgi?cmd=Retrieve&db=pubmed&dopt=Abstract&list_uids=4210685

- **Muscular dystrophy: multidisciplinary approach to management.**
Author(s): Siegel IM.
Source: Postgraduate Medicine. 1981 February; 69(2): 124-8, 131-3.
http://www.ncbi.nlm.nih.gov/entrez/query.fcgi?cmd=Retrieve&db=pubmed&dopt=Abstract&list_uids=7454643

- **Myotilin, the limb-girdle muscular dystrophy 1A (LGMD1A) protein, cross-links actin filaments and controls sarcomere assembly.**
Author(s): Salmikangas P, van der Ven PF, Lalowski M, Taivainen A, Zhao F, Suila H, Schroder R, Lappalainen P, Furst DO, Carpen O.
Source: Human Molecular Genetics. 2003 January 15; 12(2): 189-203.
http://www.ncbi.nlm.nih.gov/entrez/query.fcgi?cmd=Retrieve&db=pubmed&dopt=Abstract&list_uids=12499399

- **Na+ + K+ ATPase of erythrocyte membranes in Duchenne muscular dystrophy.**
  Author(s): Mawatari S, Igisu H, Kuroiwa Y, Miyoshino S.
  Source: Neurology. 1981 March; 31(3): 293-7.
  http://www.ncbi.nlm.nih.gov/entrez/query.fcgi?cmd=Retrieve&db=pubmed&dopt=Abstract&list_uids=6259557

- **Novel therapies for Duchenne muscular dystrophy.**
  Author(s): Kapsa R, Kornberg AJ, Byrne E.
  Source: Lancet. Neurology. 2003 May; 2(5): 299-310. Review.
  http://www.ncbi.nlm.nih.gov/entrez/query.fcgi?cmd=Retrieve&db=pubmed&dopt=Abstract&list_uids=12849184

- **Ocular muscular dystrophy. A cause of curare sensitivity.**
  Author(s): Robertson JA.
  Source: Anaesthesia. 1984 March; 39(3): 251-3.
  http://www.ncbi.nlm.nih.gov/entrez/query.fcgi?cmd=Retrieve&db=pubmed&dopt=Abstract&list_uids=6703294

- **On the mechanism of a calcium-associated defect of oxidative phosphorylation in progessive muscular dystrophy.**
  Author(s): Wrogemann K, Jacobson BE, Blanchaer MC.
  Source: Archives of Biochemistry and Biophysics. 1973 November; 159(1): 267-78.
  http://www.ncbi.nlm.nih.gov/entrez/query.fcgi?cmd=Retrieve&db=pubmed&dopt=Abstract&list_uids=4361547

- **Oral creatine supplementation in Duchenne muscular dystrophy: a clinical and 31P magnetic resonance spectroscopy study.**
  Author(s): Felber S, Skladal D, Wyss M, Kremser C, Koller A, Sperl W.
  Source: Neurological Research. 2000 March; 22(2): 145-50.
  http://www.ncbi.nlm.nih.gov/entrez/query.fcgi?cmd=Retrieve&db=pubmed&dopt=Abstract&list_uids=10763500

- **Paraffin wax embedded muscle is suitable for the diagnosis of muscular dystrophy.**
  Author(s): Sheriffs IN, Rampling D, Smith VV.
  Source: Journal of Clinical Pathology. 2001 July; 54(7): 517-20.
  http://www.ncbi.nlm.nih.gov/entrez/query.fcgi?cmd=Retrieve&db=pubmed&dopt=Abstract&list_uids=11429422

- **Progressive muscular dystrophy--Duchenne type. Controversies of the kinesitherapy treatment.**
  Author(s): de Araujo Leitao AV, Duro LA, de Andrade Penque GM.
  Source: Sao Paulo Medical Journal = Revista Paulista De Medicina. 1995 September-October; 113(5): 995-9.
  http://www.ncbi.nlm.nih.gov/entrez/query.fcgi?cmd=Retrieve&db=pubmed&dopt=Abstract&list_uids=8729744

- **Pulmonary problems in Duchenne muscular dystrophy. Diagnosis, prophylaxis, and treatment.**
  Author(s): Siegel IM.
  Source: Physical Therapy. 1975 February; 55(2): 160-2.
  http://www.ncbi.nlm.nih.gov/entrez/query.fcgi?cmd=Retrieve&db=pubmed&dopt=Abstract&list_uids=1096180

- **Pursed lips breathing improves ventilation in myotonic muscular dystrophy.**
  Author(s): Ugalde V, Breslin EH, Walsh SA, Bonekat HW, Abresch RT, Carter GT.
  Source: Archives of Physical Medicine and Rehabilitation. 2000 April; 81(4): 472-8.
  http://www.ncbi.nlm.nih.gov/entrez/query.fcgi?cmd=Retrieve&db=pubmed&dopt=Abstract&list_uids=10768538

- **Pyruvic and lactic acid metabolism in muscular dystrophy, neuropathies and other neuromuscular disorders.**
  Author(s): Goto I, Peters HA, Reese HH.
  Source: The American Journal of the Medical Sciences. 1967 April; 253(4): 431-48.
  http://www.ncbi.nlm.nih.gov/entrez/query.fcgi?cmd=Retrieve&db=pubmed&dopt=Abstract&list_uids=4290040

- **Relating familial stress to the psychosocial adjustment of adolescents with Duchenne muscular dystrophy.**
  Author(s): Reid DT, Renwick RM.
  Source: International Journal of Rehabilitation Research. Internationale Zeitschrift Fur Rehabilitationsforschung. Revue Internationale De Recherches De Readaptation. 2001 June; 24(2): 83-93.
  http://www.ncbi.nlm.nih.gov/entrez/query.fcgi?cmd=Retrieve&db=pubmed&dopt=Abstract&list_uids=11421396

- **Report on the muscular dystrophy campaign workshop: exercise in neuromuscular diseases Newcastle, January 2002.**
  Author(s): Eagle M.
  Source: Neuromuscular Disorders: Nmd. 2002 December; 12(10): 975-83.
  http://www.ncbi.nlm.nih.gov/entrez/query.fcgi?cmd=Retrieve&db=pubmed&dopt=Abstract&list_uids=12467755

- **Respiratory muscle training in Duchenne muscular dystrophy.**
  Author(s): Rodillo E, Noble-Jamieson CM, Aber V, Heckmatt JZ, Muntoni F, Dubowitz V.
  Source: Archives of Disease in Childhood. 1989 May; 64(5): 736-8.
  http://www.ncbi.nlm.nih.gov/entrez/query.fcgi?cmd=Retrieve&db=pubmed&dopt=Abstract&list_uids=2658856

- **Respiratory muscle training in Duchenne muscular dystrophy.**
  Author(s): Smith PE, Coakley JH, Edwards RH.
  Source: Muscle & Nerve. 1988 July; 11(7): 784-5.
  http://www.ncbi.nlm.nih.gov/entrez/query.fcgi?cmd=Retrieve&db=pubmed&dopt=Abstract&list_uids=3405245

- **Reversal of impaired oxidative phosphorylation and calcium overloading in the in vitro cardiac mitochondria of CHF-146 dystrophic hamsters with hereditary muscular dystrophy.**
  Author(s): Bhattacharya SK, Johnson PL, Thakar JH.
  Source: Journal of the Neurological Sciences. 1993 December 15; 120(2): 180-6.
  http://www.ncbi.nlm.nih.gov/entrez/query.fcgi?cmd=Retrieve&db=pubmed&dopt=Abstract&list_uids=8138808

- **Selenium metabolism and supplementation in patients with muscular dystrophy.**
  Author(s): Jackson MJ, Coakley J, Stokes M, Edwards RH, Oster O.
  Source: Neurology. 1989 May; 39(5): 655-9.
  http://www.ncbi.nlm.nih.gov/entrez/query.fcgi?cmd=Retrieve&db=pubmed&dopt=Abstract&list_uids=2540451

- **Selenium supplementation in X-linked muscular dystrophy. Effects on erythrocyte and serum selenium and on erythrocyte glutathione peroxidase activity.**
  Author(s): Gebre-Medhin M, Gustavson KH, Gamstorp I, Plantin LO.

Source: Acta Paediatr Scand. 1985 November; 74(6): 886-90.
http://www.ncbi.nlm.nih.gov/entrez/query.fcgi?cmd=Retrieve&db=pubmed&dopt=Abstract&list_uids=4090964

- **Serum enzyme changes, muscular dystrophy and erythrocyte abnormalities in lambs fed on diets containing cod-liver oil and maize oil, and the therapeutic effect of vitamin E.**
  Author(s): Boyd JW.
  Source: The British Journal of Nutrition. 1968 September; 22(3): 411-22.
  http://www.ncbi.nlm.nih.gov/entrez/query.fcgi?cmd=Retrieve&db=pubmed&dopt=Abstract&list_uids=5677207

- **Spectrin extractability from erythrocytes in Duchenne muscular dystrophy patients and carriers and in other myopathies.**
  Author(s): Gargioni G, Chiaffoni G, Bonadonna G, Corradini P, Lechi C, de Grandis D, Zatti M.
  Source: Clinica Chimica Acta; International Journal of Clinical Chemistry. 1985 February 15; 145(3): 259-65.
  http://www.ncbi.nlm.nih.gov/entrez/query.fcgi?cmd=Retrieve&db=pubmed&dopt=Abstract&list_uids=3987029

- **Stem cell therapy for muscular dystrophy.**
  Author(s): Sohn RL, Gussoni E.
  Source: Expert Opinion on Biological Therapy. 2004 January; 4(1): 1-9. Review.
  http://www.ncbi.nlm.nih.gov/entrez/query.fcgi?cmd=Retrieve&db=pubmed&dopt=Abstract&list_uids=14680464

- **Therapies in muscular dystrophy: current concepts and future prospects.**
  Author(s): Urtizberea JA.
  Source: European Neurology. 2000; 43(3): 127-32. Review.
  http://www.ncbi.nlm.nih.gov/entrez/query.fcgi?cmd=Retrieve&db=pubmed&dopt=Abstract&list_uids=10765050

- **Update on Duchenne muscular dystrophy.**
  Author(s): Siegel IM.
  Source: Compr Ther. 1989 March; 15(3): 45-52. Review.
  http://www.ncbi.nlm.nih.gov/entrez/query.fcgi?cmd=Retrieve&db=pubmed&dopt=Abstract&list_uids=2650976

- **Use of child's kapok life preserver in reversed position in rehabilitation of children with pseudohypertrophic muscular dystrophy.**
  Author(s): PIERCE DS.
  Source: Archives of Physical Medicine and Rehabilitation. 1962 November; 43: 574-5.
  http://www.ncbi.nlm.nih.gov/entrez/query.fcgi?cmd=Retrieve&db=pubmed&dopt=Abstract&list_uids=13943395

- **Using a novel exercise programme for patients with muscular dystrophy. Part I: a qualitative study.**
  Author(s): Wenneberg S, Gunnarsson LG, Ahlstrom G.
  Source: Disability and Rehabilitation. 2004 May 20; 26(10): 586-94.
  http://www.ncbi.nlm.nih.gov/entrez/query.fcgi?cmd=Retrieve&db=pubmed&dopt=Abstract&list_uids=15204512

- **Using a novel exercise programme for patients with muscular dystrophy. Part II: a quantitative study.**
  Author(s): Wenneberg S, Gunnarsson LG, Ahlstrom G.
  Source: Disability and Rehabilitation. 2004 May 20; 26(10): 595-602.
  http://www.ncbi.nlm.nih.gov/entrez/query.fcgi?cmd=Retrieve&db=pubmed&dopt=Abstract&list_uids=15204513

- **Weaning from mechanical ventilation: successful use of modified inspiratory resistive training in muscular dystrophy.**
  Author(s): Aldrich TK, Uhrlass RM.
  Source: Critical Care Medicine. 1987 March; 15(3): 247-9.

Additional Web Resources

A number of additional Web sites offer encyclopedic information covering CAM and related topics. The following is a representative sample:

- Alternative Medicine Foundation, Inc.: **http://www.herbmed.org/**

- AOL: **http://search.aol.com/cat.adp?id=169&layer=&from=subcats**

- Chinese Medicine: **http://www.newcenturynutrition.com/**

- Family Village: **http://www.familyvillage.wisc.edu/med_altn.htm**

- Google: **http://directory.google.com/Top/Health/Alternative/**

- Open Directory Project: **http://dmoz.org/Health/Alternative/**

- TPN.com: **http://www.tnp.com/**

- Yahoo.com: **http://dir.yahoo.com/Health/Alternative_Medicine/**

- WebMD®Health: **http://my.webmd.com/drugs_and_herbs**

- WholeHealthMD.com:
  http://www.wholehealthmd.com/reflib/0,1529,,00.html

The following is a specific Web list relating to muscular dystrophy; please note that any particular subject below may indicate either a therapeutic use, or a contraindication (potential danger), and does not reflect an official recommendation:

- **General Overview**

    Dysphagia
    Source: Integrative Medicine Communications; www.drkoop.com

    Muscular Dystrophy
    Source: Integrative Medicine Communications; www.drkoop.com

- **Alternative Therapy**

    Trager Approach
    Source: WholeHealthMD.com, LLC.; www.wholehealthmd.com
    Hyperlink:
    http://www.wholehealthmd.com/refshelf/substances_view/0,1525,
    741,00.html

- **Herbs and Supplements**

    Allopurinol
    Source: Healthnotes, Inc.; www.healthnotes.com

    BCAAs
    Source: Prima Communications, Inc.www.personalhealthzone.com

    Coenzyme Q10
    Source: Healthnotes, Inc.; www.healthnotes.com

    Coenzyme Q10
    Source: Integrative Medicine Communications; www.drkoop.com

Coenzyme Q10 (CoQ10)
Source: Prima Communications, Inc.www.personalhealthzone.com

Coq10
Source: Integrative Medicine Communications; www.drkoop.com

Glycyrrhiza
Alternative names: Licorice; Glycyrrhiza glabra L.
Source: Alternative Medicine Foundation, Inc.;
www.amfoundation.org

General References

A good place to find general background information on CAM is the National Library of Medicine. It has prepared within the MEDLINEplus system an information topic page dedicated to complementary and alternative medicine. To access this page, go to the MEDLINEplus site at: **www.nlm.nih.gov/medlineplus/alternativemedicine.html.** This Web site provides a general overview of various topics and can lead to a number of general sources. The following additional references describe, in broad terms, alternative and complementary medicine (sorted alphabetically by title; hyperlinks provide rankings, information, and reviews at Amazon.com):

- **Acupunture Treatment for Musculoskeletal Pain: A Textbook for Orthopedics and Anesthesia** by Harris Gellman (Editor); Hardcover (May 2001), Harwood Academic Pub; ISBN: 9057025167; http://www.amazon.com/exec/obidos/ASIN/9057025167/icongroupinterna

- **Homeopathy for Musculoskeletal Healing** by Asa Hershoff; Paperback - 300 pages (January 1997), North Atlantic Books; ISBN: 1556432372; http://www.amazon.com/exec/obidos/ASIN/1556432372/icongroupinterna

- **Joint Pains: A Guide to Successful Herbal Remedies** by Penelope Ody; Paperback - 172 pages (April 2002), Souvenir Press Ltd; ISBN: 0285636227; http://www.amazon.com/exec/obidos/ASIN/0285636227/icongroupinterna

- **Kinesiology of the Musculoskeletal System** by Neumann, et al; Hardcover - 624 pages, 1st edition (March 22, 2002), Mosby, Inc.; ISBN:

0815163495;
http://www.amazon.com/exec/obidos/ASIN/0815163495/icongroupinterna

- **Applied Kinesiology: A Training Manual and Reference Book of Basic Principles and Practices** by Robert Frost, George J. Goodheart; Paperback - 300 pages, 1st edition (March 21, 2002), Publishers Group West; ISBN: 1556433743;
http://www.amazon.com/exec/obidos/ASIN/1556433743/icongroupinterna

- **Musculoskeletal Disorders: Healing Methods from Chinese Medicine, Orthopaedic Medicine and Osteopathy** by Alon Marcus; Hardcover - 650 pages (January 1999), North Atlantic Books; ISBN: 1556432828;
http://www.amazon.com/exec/obidos/ASIN/1556432828/icongroupinterna

- **The Posture Prescription: A Doctor's Rx for Eliminating Back, Muscle, and Joint Pain, Achieving Optimum Strength and Mobility, Living a Life of Fitne b**y Arthur White, MD, et al; Paperback - 256 pages, 1st edition (January 8, 2002), Three Rivers Pr; ISBN: 0609806319;
http://www.amazon.com/exec/obidos/ASIN/0609806319/icongroupinterna

For additional information on complementary and alternative medicine, ask your doctor or write to:

National Center for Complementary and Alternative Medicine Clearinghouse
National Institutes of Health
P. O. Box 8218
Silver Spring, MD 20907-8218

APPENDIX C. RESEARCHING NUTRITION

Overview

Since the time of Hippocrates, doctors have understood the importance of diet and nutrition to patients' health and well-being. Since then, they have accumulated an impressive archive of studies and knowledge dedicated to this subject. Based on their experience, doctors and healthcare providers may recommend particular dietary supplements to patients with muscular dystrophy. Any dietary recommendation is based on a patient's age, body mass, gender, lifestyle, eating habits, food preferences, and health condition. It is therefore likely that different patients with muscular dystrophy may be given different recommendations. Some recommendations may be directly related to muscular dystrophy, while others may be more related to the patient's general health. These recommendations, themselves, may differ from what official sources recommend for the average person.

In this chapter we will begin by briefly reviewing the essentials of diet and nutrition that will broadly frame more detailed discussions of muscular dystrophy. We will then show you how to find studies dedicated specifically to nutrition and muscular dystrophy.

Food and Nutrition: General Principles

What Are Essential Foods?

Food is generally viewed by official sources as consisting of six basic elements: (1) fluids, (2) carbohydrates, (3) protein, (4) fats, (5) vitamins, and (6) minerals. Consuming a combination of these elements is considered to be a healthy diet:

- **Fluids** are essential to human life as 80-percent of the body is composed of water. Water is lost via urination, sweating, diarrhea, vomiting, diuretics (drugs that increase urination), caffeine, and physical exertion.

- **Carbohydrates** are the main source for human energy (thermoregulation) and the bulk of typical diets. They are mostly classified as being either simple or complex. Simple carbohydrates include sugars which are often consumed in the form of cookies, candies, or cakes. Complex carbohydrates consist of starches and dietary fibers. Starches are consumed in the form of pastas, breads, potatoes, rice, and other foods. Soluble fibers can be eaten in the form of certain vegetables, fruits, oats, and legumes. Insoluble fibers include brown rice, whole grains, certain fruits, wheat bran and legumes.

- **Proteins** are eaten to build and repair human tissues. Some foods that are high in protein are also high in fat and calories. Food sources for protein include nuts, meat, fish, cheese, and other dairy products.

- **Fats** are consumed for both energy and the absorption of certain vitamins. There are many types of fats, with many general publications recommending the intake of unsaturated fats or those low in cholesterol.

Vitamins and minerals are fundamental to human health, growth, and, in some cases, disease prevention. Most are consumed in your diet (exceptions being vitamins K and D which are produced by intestinal bacteria and sunlight on the skin, respectively). Each vitamin and mineral plays a different role in health. The following outlines essential vitamins:

- **Vitamin A** is important to the health of your eyes, hair, bones, and skin; sources of vitamin A include foods such as eggs, carrots, and cantaloupe.

- **Vitamin B^1**, also known as thiamine, is important for your nervous system and energy production; food sources for thiamine include meat, peas, fortified cereals, bread, and whole grains.

- **Vitamin B^2**, also known as riboflavin, is important for your nervous system and muscles, but is also involved in the release of proteins from nutrients; food sources for riboflavin include dairy products, leafy vegetables, meat, and eggs.

- **Vitamin B^3**, also known as niacin, is important for healthy skin and helps the body use energy; food sources for niacin include peas, peanuts, fish, and whole grains

- **Vitamin B^6**, also known as pyridoxine, is important for the regulation of cells in the nervous system and is vital for blood formation; food sources for pyridoxine include bananas, whole grains, meat, and fish.

- **Vitamin B¹²** is vital for a healthy nervous system and for the growth of red blood cells in bone marrow; food sources for vitamin B¹² include yeast, milk, fish, eggs, and meat.

- **Vitamin C** allows the body's immune system to fight various diseases, strengthens body tissue, and improves the body's use of iron; food sources for vitamin C include a wide variety of fruits and vegetables.

- **Vitamin D** helps the body absorb calcium which strengthens bones and teeth; food sources for vitamin D include oily fish and dairy products.

- **Vitamin E** can help protect certain organs and tissues from various degenerative diseases; food sources for vitamin E include margarine, vegetables, eggs, and fish.

- **Vitamin K** is essential for bone formation and blood clotting; common food sources for vitamin K include leafy green vegetables.

- **Folic Acid** maintains healthy cells and blood and, when taken by a pregnant woman, can prevent her fetus from developing neural tube defects; food sources for folic acid include nuts, fortified breads, leafy green vegetables, and whole grains.

It should be noted that it is possible to overdose on certain vitamins which become toxic if consumed in excess (e.g. vitamin A, D, E and K).

Like vitamins, minerals are chemicals that are required by the body to remain in good health. Because the human body does not manufacture these chemicals internally, we obtain them from food and other dietary sources. The more important minerals include:

- **Calcium** is needed for healthy bones, teeth, and muscles, but also helps the nervous system function; food sources for calcium include dry beans, peas, eggs, and dairy products.

- **Chromium** is helpful in regulating sugar levels in blood; food sources for chromium include egg yolks, raw sugar, cheese, nuts, beets, whole grains, and meat.

- **Fluoride** is used by the body to help prevent tooth decay and to reinforce bone strength; sources of fluoride include drinking water and certain brands of toothpaste.

- **Iodine** helps regulate the body's use of energy by synthesizing into the hormone thyroxine; food sources include leafy green vegetables, nuts, egg yolks, and red meat.

- **Iron** helps maintain muscles and the formation of red blood cells and certain proteins; food sources for iron include meat, dairy products, eggs, and leafy green vegetables.

- **Magnesium** is important for the production of DNA, as well as for healthy teeth, bones, muscles, and nerves; food sources for magnesium include dried fruit, dark green vegetables, nuts, and seafood.

- **Phosphorous** is used by the body to work with calcium to form bones and teeth; food sources for phosphorous include eggs, meat, cereals, and dairy products.

- **Selenium** primarily helps maintain normal heart and liver functions; food sources for selenium include wholegrain cereals, fish, meat, and dairy products.

- **Zinc** helps wounds heal, the formation of sperm, and encourage rapid growth and energy; food sources include dried beans, shellfish, eggs, and nuts.

The United States government periodically publishes recommended diets and consumption levels of the various elements of food. Again, your doctor may encourage deviations from the average official recommendation based on your specific condition. To learn more about basic dietary guidelines, visit the Web site: **http://www.health.gov/dietaryguidelines/**. Based on these guidelines, many foods are required to list the nutrition levels on the food's packaging. Labeling Requirements are listed at the following site maintained by the Food and Drug Administration: **http://www.cfsan.fda.gov/~dms/lab-cons.html**. When interpreting these requirements, the government recommends that consumers become familiar with the following abbreviations before reading FDA literature:[45]

- **DVs (Daily Values):** A new dietary reference term that will appear on the food label. It is made up of two sets of references, DRVs and RDIs.

- **DRVs (Daily Reference Values):** A set of dietary references that applies to fat, saturated fat, cholesterol, carbohydrate, protein, fiber, sodium, and potassium.

- **RDIs (Reference Daily Intakes):** A set of dietary references based on the Recommended Dietary Allowances for essential vitamins and minerals and, in selected groups, protein. The name "RDI" replaces the term "U.S. RDA."

---

[45] Adapted from the FDA: **http://www.fda.gov/fdac/special/foodlabel/dvs.html**.

- **RDAs (Recommended Dietary Allowances):** A set of estimated nutrient allowances established by the National Academy of Sciences. It is updated periodically to reflect current scientific knowledge.

What Are Dietary Supplements?[46]

Dietary supplements are widely available through many commercial sources, including health food stores, grocery stores, pharmacies, and by mail. Dietary supplements are provided in many forms including tablets, capsules, powders, gel-tabs, extracts, and liquids. Historically in the United States, the most prevalent type of dietary supplement was a multivitamin/mineral tablet or capsule that was available in pharmacies, either by prescription or "over the counter." Supplements containing strictly herbal preparations were less widely available. Currently in the United States, a wide array of supplement products are available, including vitamin, mineral, other nutrients, and botanical supplements as well as ingredients and extracts of animal and plant origin.

The Office of Dietary Supplements (ODS) of the National Institutes of Health is the official agency of the United States which has the expressed goal of acquiring "new knowledge to help prevent, detect, diagnose, and treat disease and disability, from the rarest genetic disorder to the common cold."[47] According to the ODS, dietary supplements can have an important impact on the prevention and management of disease and on the maintenance of health.[48] The ODS notes that considerable research on the effects of dietary supplements has been conducted in Asia and Europe where the use of plant products, in particular, has a long tradition. However, the overwhelming majority of supplements have not been studied scientifically. To explore the role of dietary supplements in the improvement of health care, the ODS plans, organizes, and supports conferences, workshops, and

---

[46] This discussion has been adapted from the NIH: **http://ods.od.nih.gov/showpage.aspx?pageid=46.**

[47] Contact: The Office of Dietary Supplements, National Institutes of Health, Building 31, Room 1B29, 31 Center Drive, MSC 2086, Bethesda, Maryland 20892-2086, Tel: (301) 435-2920, Fax: (301) 480-1845, E-mail: ods@nih.gov.

[48] Adapted from **http://ods.od.nih.gov/showpage.aspx?pageid=2.** The Dietary Supplement Health and Education Act defines dietary supplements as "a product (other than tobacco) intended to supplement the diet that bears or contains one or more of the following dietary ingredients: a vitamin, mineral, amino acid, herb or other botanical; or a dietary substance for use to supplement the diet by increasing the total dietary intake; or a concentrate, metabolite, constituent, extract, or combination of any ingredient described above; and intended for ingestion in the form of a capsule, powder, softgel, or gelcap, and not represented as a conventional food or as a sole item of a meal or the diet."

symposia on scientific topics related to dietary supplements. The ODS often works in conjunction with other NIH Institutes and Centers, other government agencies, professional organizations, and public advocacy groups.

To learn more about official information on dietary supplements, visit the ODS site at **http://dietary-supplements.info.nih.gov/**. Or contact:

> **The Office of Dietary Supplements**
> National Institutes of Health
> Building 31, Room 1B29
> 31 Center Drive, MSC 2086
> Bethesda, Maryland 20892-2086
> Tel: (301) 435-2920
> Fax: (301) 480-1845
> E-mail: ods@nih.gov

Finding Studies on Muscular Dystrophy

The NIH maintains an office dedicated to patient nutrition and diet. The National Institutes of Health's Office of Dietary Supplements (ODS) offers a searchable bibliographic database called the IBIDS (International Bibliographic Information on Dietary Supplements). The IBIDS contains over 460,000 scientific citations and summaries about dietary supplements and nutrition as well as references to published international, scientific literature on dietary supplements such as vitamins, minerals, and botanicals.[49] IBIDS is available to the public free of charge through the ODS Internet page: **http://ods.od.nih.gov/databases/ibids.html**.

After entering the search area, you have three choices: (1) IBIDS Consumer Database, (2) Full IBIDS Database, or (3) Peer Reviewed Citations Only. We recommend that you start with the Consumer Database. While you may not find references for the topics that are of most interest to you, check back periodically as this database is frequently updated. More studies can be found by searching the Full IBIDS Database. Healthcare professionals and researchers generally use the third option, which lists peer-reviewed citations. In all cases, we suggest that you take advantage of the "Advanced

---

[49] Adapted from **http://ods.od.nih.gov**. IBIDS is produced by the Office of Dietary Supplements (ODS) at the National Institutes of Health to assist the public, healthcare providers, educators, and researchers in locating credible, scientific information on dietary supplements. IBIDS was developed and will be maintained through an interagency partnership with the Food and Nutrition Information Center of the National Agricultural Library, U.S. Department of Agriculture.

Search" option that allows you to retrieve up to 100 fully explained references in a comprehensive format. Type "muscular dystrophy" (or synonyms) into the search box. To narrow the search, you can also select the "Title" field.

The following information is typical of that found when using the "Full IBIDS Database" when searching using "muscular dystrophy" (or a synonym):

- **Abnormal calcium homeostasis in Duchenne muscular dystrophy myotubes contracting in vitro.**
  Author(s): Laboratoire de Physiologie Generale, URA CNRS 1869, Universite de Poitiers, France.
  Source: Imbert, N Cognard, C Duport, G Guillou, C Raymond, G Cell-Calcium. 1995 September; 18(3): 177-86 0143-4160

- **Becker and limb-girdle muscular dystrophy associated with pituitary dwarfism.**
  Author(s): Department of Neurology, University of Florence, Italy.
  Source: Marconi, G Taiuti, R Sbrilli, C Pizzi, A J-Neurol. 1987 August; 234(6): 430-2 0340-5354

- **Biochemical effect of naturally and experimental induced nutritional muscular dystrophy on copper and iron levels in plasmas of suckling Egyptian buffalo calves.**
  Source: El Neweehy, T.K. Amer, H.A. Abd el Salam, S.A. Arch-Exp-Veterinarmed. Leipzig, E. Ger.: S. Hirzel. 1985. volume 39 (6) page 859-863. 0003-9055

- **Calcium homeostasis and ultrastructural studies in a patient with limb girdle muscular dystrophy type 2C.**
  Author(s): Muscular Dystrophy Research Laboratories, Newcastle General Hospital, Newcastle upon Tyne, UK.
  Source: Hassoni, A A Cullen, M J Neuropathol-Appl-Neurobiol. 1999 June; 25(3): 244-53 0305-1846

- **Changes in cytosolic resting ionized calcium level and in calcium transients during in vitro development of normal and Duchenne muscular dystrophy cultured skeletal muscle measured by laser cytofluorimetry using indo-1.**
  Author(s): Laboratoire de Physiologie Generale, URA CNRS n 290, Universite de Poitiers, France.
  Source: Rivet Bastide, M Imbert, N Cognard, C Duport, G Rideau, Y Raymond, G Cell-Calcium. 1993 July; 14(7): 563-71 0143-4160

- **Duchenne muscular dystrophy and concomitant metastatic alveolar rhabdomyosarcoma.**
  Author(s): Division of Pediatric Hematology/Oncology, All Children's Hospital, University of South Florida College of Medicine, St. Petersburg, USA.
  Source: Rossbach, H C Lacson, A Grana, N H Barbosa, J L J-Pediatr-Hematol-Oncol. 1999 Nov-December; 21(6): 528-30 1077-4114

- **Intraruminal selenium pellet for control of nutritional muscular dystrophy in cattle.**
  Source: Hidiroglou, M. Proulx, J. Jolette, J. J-Dairy-Sci. Champaign, Ill.: American Dairy Science Association. January 1985. volume 68 (1) page 57-66. 0022-0302

- **Nutritional muscular dystrophy in calves. Effect of administreing intraruminally Selenium pellets to pregnant cattle.**
  Source: Hidiroglou, M. Proulx, J. Jolette, J. Trace elements in man and animals: TEMA 5: proceedings of the fifth International Symposium on Trace Elements in Man and Animals / editors C.F. Mills, I. Bremner, & J.K. Chesters. Farnham Royal, Slough: Commonwealth Agricultural Bureaux, c1985. page 744-748. ISBN: 085198553X

- **Some studies on nutritional muscular dystrophy in Qassim region in Saudi Arabia. Effect of administration of vitamin E-selenium preparation to pregnant ewes on serum muscle-specific enzymes in their lambs.**
  Source: El Neweehy, T.K. Abdel Rahman, H.A. Al Qarawi, A.A. Small-rumin-res. Amsterdam; New York: Elsevier,. July 2001. volume 41 (1) page 87-89. 0921-4488

- **The stabilizing effect of bestatin on the resting membrane potentials of X-linked muscular dystrophy mice.**
  Author(s): Fourth Department of Medicine, Toho University School of Medicine, Tokyo, Japan.
  Source: Kishi, M Kurihara, T Hidaka, T Kinoshita, M Jpn-J-Psychiatry-Neurol. 1990 September; 44(3): 595-600 0912-2036

- **Urinary excretion of selenium and other minerals in patients with Duchenne muscular dystrophy (M.D.) and Werdnig-Hoffman (W-H) spinal atrophy.**
  Source: Ahlrot Westerlund, B. Carlmark, B. Nutr-Res. Elmsford, N.Y.: Pergamon Press. 1985. (suppl. 1) page 406-409. ill. 0271-5317

Federal Resources on Nutrition

In addition to the IBIDS, the United States Department of Health and Human Services (HHS) and the United States Department of Agriculture (USDA) provide many sources of information on general nutrition and health. Recommended resources include:

- healthfinder®, HHS's gateway to health information, including diet and nutrition:
  http://www.healthfinder.gov/scripts/SearchContext.asp?topic=238&page=0

- The United States Department of Agriculture's Web site dedicated to nutrition information: **www.nutrition.gov**

- The Food and Drug Administration's Web site for federal food safety information: **www.foodsafety.gov**

- The National Action Plan on Overweight and Obesity sponsored by the United States Surgeon General:
  http://www.surgeongeneral.gov/topics/obesity/

- The Center for Food Safety and Applied Nutrition has an Internet site sponsored by the Food and Drug Administration and the Department of Health and Human Services: **http://vm.cfsan.fda.gov/**

- Center for Nutrition Policy and Promotion sponsored by the United States Department of Agriculture: **http://www.usda.gov/cnpp/**

- Food and Nutrition Information Center, National Agricultural Library sponsored by the United States Department of Agriculture:
  http://www.nal.usda.gov/fnic/

- Food and Nutrition Service sponsored by the United States Department of Agriculture: **http://www.fns.usda.gov/fns/**

Additional Web Resources

A number of additional Web sites offer encyclopedic information covering food and nutrition. The following is a representative sample:

- AOL: **http://search.aol.com/cat.adp?id=174&layer=&from=subcats**

- Family Village: **http://www.familyvillage.wisc.edu/med_nutrition.html**

- Google: **http://directory.google.com/Top/Health/Nutrition/**

- Open Directory Project: **http://dmoz.org/Health/Nutrition/**

- Yahoo.com: **http://dir.yahoo.com/Health/Nutrition/**

- WebMD®Health: **http://my.webmd.com/nutrition**

- WholeHealthMD.com:
  http://www.wholehealthmd.com/reflib/0,1529,,00.html

The following is a specific Web list relating to muscular dystrophy; please note that any particular subject below may indicate either a therapeutic use, or a contraindication (potential danger), and does not reflect an official recommendation:

- **Minerals**

  Biotin
  Source: Integrative Medicine Communications; www.drkoop.com

  Carnitine
  Source: Prima Communications, Inc.www.personalhealthzone.com

  Creatine
  Source: WholeHealthMD.com, LLC.; www.wholehealthmd.com
  Hyperlink:
  http://www.wholehealthmd.com/refshelf/substances_view/0,1525, 10020,00.html

  Creatine Monohydrate
  Source: Healthnotes, Inc.; www.healthnotes.com

  Vitamin H (Biotin)
  Source: Integrative Medicine Communications; www.drkoop.com

APPENDIX D. FINDING MEDICAL LIBRARIES

Overview

At a medical library you can find medical texts and reference books, consumer health publications, specialty newspapers and magazines, as well as medical journals. In this Appendix, we show you how to quickly find a medical library in your area.

Preparation

Before going to the library, highlight the references mentioned in this sourcebook that you find interesting. Focus on those items that are not available via the Internet, and ask the reference librarian for help with your search. He or she may know of additional resources that could be helpful to you. Most importantly, your local public library and medical libraries have Interlibrary Loan programs with the National Library of Medicine (NLM), one of the largest medical collections in the world. According to the NLM, most of the literature in the general and historical collections of the National Library of Medicine is available on interlibrary loan to any library. NLM's interlibrary loan services are only available to libraries. If you would like to access NLM medical literature, then visit a library in your area that can request the publications for you.[50]

---

[50] Adapted from the NLM: **http://www.nlm.nih.gov/psd/cas/interlibrary.html**.

Finding a Local Medical Library

The quickest method to locate medical libraries is to use the Internet-based directory published by the National Network of Libraries of Medicine (NN/LM). This network includes 4626 members and affiliates that provide many services to librarians, health professionals, and the public. To find a library in your area, simply visit **http://nnlm.gov/members/adv.html** or call 1-800-338-7657.

Medical Libraries in the U.S. and Canada

In addition to the NN/LM, the National Library of Medicine (NLM) lists a number of libraries with reference facilities that are open to the public. The following is the NLM's list and includes hyperlinks to each library's Web site. These Web pages can provide information on hours of operation and other restrictions. The list below is a small sample of libraries recommended by the National Library of Medicine (sorted alphabetically by name of the U.S. state or Canadian province where the library is located)[51]:

- **Alabama:** Health InfoNet of Jefferson County (Jefferson County Library Cooperative, Lister Hill Library of the Health Sciences), **http://www.uab.edu/infonet/**

- **Alabama:** Richard M. Scrushy Library (American Sports Medicine Institute)

- **Arizona:** Samaritan Regional Medical Center: The Learning Center (Samaritan Health System, Phoenix, Arizona), **http://www.samaritan.edu/library/bannerlibs.htm**

- **California:** Kris Kelly Health Information Center (St. Joseph Health System, Humboldt), **http://www.humboldt1.com/~kkhic/index.html**

- **California:** Community Health Library of Los Gatos, **http://www.healthlib.org/orgresources.html**

- **California:** Consumer Health Program and Services (CHIPS) (County of Los Angeles Public Library, Los Angeles County Harbor-UCLA Medical Center Library) - Carson, CA, **http://www.colapublib.org/services/chips.html**

- **California:** Gateway Health Library (Sutter Gould Medical Foundation)

- **California:** Health Library (Stanford University Medical Center), **http://www-med.stanford.edu/healthlibrary/**

---

[51] Abstracted from **http://www.nlm.nih.gov/medlineplus/libraries.html**.

- **California:** Patient Education Resource Center - Health Information and Resources (University of California, San Francisco), **http://sfghdean.ucsf.edu/barnett/PERC/default.asp**

- **California:** Redwood Health Library (Petaluma Health Care District), **http://www.phcd.org/rdwdlib.html**

- **California:** Los Gatos PlaneTree Health Library, **http://planetreesanjose.org/**

- **California:** Sutter Resource Library (Sutter Hospitals Foundation, Sacramento), **http://suttermedicalcenter.org/library/**

- **California:** Health Sciences Libraries (University of California, Davis), **http://www.lib.ucdavis.edu/healthsci/**

- **California:** ValleyCare Health Library & Ryan Comer Cancer Resource Center (ValleyCare Health System, Pleasanton), **http://gaelnet.stmarys-ca.edu/other.libs/gbal/east/vchl.html**

- **California:** Washington Community Health Resource Library (Fremont), **http://www.healthlibrary.org/**

- **Colorado:** William V. Gervasini Memorial Library (Exempla Healthcare), **http://www.saintjosephdenver.org/yourhealth/libraries/**

- **Connecticut:** Hartford Hospital Health Science Libraries (Hartford Hospital), **http://www.harthosp.org/library/**

- **Connecticut:** Healthnet: Connecticut Consumer Health Information Center (University of Connecticut Health Center, Lyman Maynard Stowe Library), **http://library.uchc.edu/departm/hnet/**

- **Connecticut:** Waterbury Hospital Health Center Library (Waterbury Hospital, Waterbury), **http://www.waterburyhospital.com/library/consumer.shtml**

- **Delaware:** Consumer Health Library (Christiana Care Health System, Eugene du Pont Preventive Medicine & Rehabilitation Institute, Wilmington), **http://www.christianacare.org/health_guide/health_guide_pmri_health_info.cfm**

- **Delaware:** Lewis B. Flinn Library (Delaware Academy of Medicine, Wilmington), **http://www.delamed.org/chls.html**

- **Georgia:** Family Resource Library (Medical College of Georgia, Augusta), **http://cmc.mcg.edu/kids_families/fam_resources/fam_res_lib/frl.htm**

- **Georgia:** Health Resource Center (Medical Center of Central Georgia, Macon), **http://www.mccg.org/hrc/hrchome.asp**

- **Hawaii:** Hawaii Medical Library: Consumer Health Information Service (Hawaii Medical Library, Honolulu), **http://hml.org/CHIS/**

- **Idaho:** DeArmond Consumer Health Library (Kootenai Medical Center, Coeur d'Alene), **http://www.nicon.org/DeArmond/index.htm**

- **Illinois:** Health Learning Center of Northwestern Memorial Hospital (Chicago), **http://www.nmh.org/health_info/hlc.html**

- **Illinois:** Medical Library (OSF Saint Francis Medical Center, Peoria), **http://www.osfsaintfrancis.org/general/library/**

- **Kentucky:** Medical Library - Services for Patients, Families, Students & the Public (Central Baptist Hospital, Lexington), **http://www.centralbap.com/education/community/library.cfm**

- **Kentucky:** University of Kentucky - Health Information Library (Chandler Medical Center, Lexington), **http://www.mc.uky.edu/PatientEd/**

- **Louisiana:** Alton Ochsner Medical Foundation Library (Alton Ochsner Medical Foundation, New Orleans), **http://www.ochsner.org/library/**

- **Louisiana:** Louisiana State University Health Sciences Center Medical Library-Shreveport, **http://lib-sh.lsuhsc.edu/**

- **Maine:** Franklin Memorial Hospital Medical Library (Franklin Memorial Hospital, Farmington), **http://www.fchn.org/fmh/lib.htm**

- **Maine:** Gerrish-True Health Sciences Library (Central Maine Medical Center, Lewiston), **http://www.cmmc.org/library/library.html**

- **Maine:** Hadley Parrot Health Science Library (Eastern Maine Healthcare, Bangor), **http://www.emh.org/hll/hpl/guide.htm**

- **Maine:** Maine Medical Center Library (Maine Medical Center, Portland), **http://www.mmc.org/library/**

- **Maine:** Parkview Hospital (Brunswick), **http://www.parkviewhospital.org/**

- **Maine:** Southern Maine Medical Center Health Sciences Library (Southern Maine Medical Center, Biddeford), **http://www.smmc.org/services/service.php3?choice=10**

- **Maine:** Stephens Memorial Hospital's Health Information Library (Western Maine Health, Norway), **http://www.wmhcc.org/Library/**

- **Manitoba, Canada:** Consumer & Patient Health Information Service (University of Manitoba Libraries), **http://www.umanitoba.ca/libraries/units/health/reference/chis.html**

- **Manitoba, Canada:** J.W. Crane Memorial Library (Deer Lodge Centre, Winnipeg), http://www.deerlodge.mb.ca/crane_library/about.asp

- **Maryland:** Health Information Center at the Wheaton Regional Library (Montgomery County, Dept. of Public Libraries, Wheaton Regional Library), http://www.mont.lib.md.us/healthinfo/hic.asp

- **Massachusetts:** Baystate Medical Center Library (Baystate Health System), http://www.baystatehealth.com/1024/

- **Massachusetts:** Boston University Medical Center Alumni Medical Library (Boston University Medical Center), http://med-libwww.bu.edu/library/lib.html

- **Massachusetts:** Lowell General Hospital Health Sciences Library (Lowell General Hospital, Lowell), http://www.lowellgeneral.org/library/HomePageLinks/WWW.htm

- **Massachusetts:** Paul E. Woodard Health Sciences Library (New England Baptist Hospital, Boston), http://www.nebh.org/health_lib.asp

- **Massachusetts:** St. Luke's Hospital Health Sciences Library (St. Luke's Hospital, Southcoast Health System, New Bedford), http://www.southcoast.org/library/

- **Massachusetts:** Treadwell Library Consumer Health Reference Center (Massachusetts General Hospital), http://www.mgh.harvard.edu/library/chrcindex.html

- **Massachusetts:** UMass HealthNet (University of Massachusetts Medical School, Worchester), http://healthnet.umassmed.edu/

- **Michigan:** Botsford General Hospital Library - Consumer Health (Botsford General Hospital, Library & Internet Services), http://www.botsfordlibrary.org/consumer.htm

- **Michigan:** Helen DeRoy Medical Library (Providence Hospital and Medical Centers), http://www.providence-hospital.org/library/

- **Michigan:** Marquette General Hospital - Consumer Health Library (Marquette General Hospital, Health Information Center), http://www.mgh.org/center.html

- **Michigan:** Patient Education Resouce Center - University of Michigan Cancer Center (University of Michigan Comprehensive Cancer Center, Ann Arbor), http://www.cancer.med.umich.edu/learn/leares.htm

- **Michigan:** Sladen Library & Center for Health Information Resources - Consumer Health Information (Detroit), http://www.henryford.com/body.cfm?id=39330

- **Montana:** Center for Health Information (St. Patrick Hospital and Health Sciences Center, Missoula)

- **National:** Consumer Health Library Directory (Medical Library Association, Consumer and Patient Health Information Section), **http://caphis.mlanet.org/directory/index.html**

- **National:** National Network of Libraries of Medicine (National Library of Medicine) - provides library services for health professionals in the United States who do not have access to a medical library, **http://nnlm.gov/**

- **National:** NN/LM List of Libraries Serving the Public (National Network of Libraries of Medicine), **http://nnlm.gov/members/**

- **Nevada:** Health Science Library, West Charleston Library (Las Vegas-Clark County Library District, Las Vegas), **http://www.lvccld.org/special_collections/medical/index.htm**

- **New Hampshire:** Dartmouth Biomedical Libraries (Dartmouth College Library, Hanover), **http://www.dartmouth.edu/~biomed/resources.htmld/conshealth.htmld**

- **New Jersey:** Consumer Health Library (Rahway Hospital, Rahway), **http://www.rahwayhospital.com/library.htm**

- **New Jersey:** Dr. Walter Phillips Health Sciences Library (Englewood Hospital and Medical Center, Englewood), **http://www.englewoodhospital.com/links/index.htm**

- **New Jersey:** Meland Foundation (Englewood Hospital and Medical Center, Englewood), **http://www.geocities.com/ResearchTriangle/9360/**

- **New York:** Choices in Health Information (New York Public Library) - NLM Consumer Pilot Project participant, **http://www.nypl.org/branch/health/links.html**

- **New York:** Health Information Center (Upstate Medical University, State University of New York, Syracuse), **http://www.upstate.edu/library/hic/**

- **New York:** Health Sciences Library (Long Island Jewish Medical Center, New Hyde Park), **http://www.lij.edu/library/library.html**

- **New York:** ViaHealth Medical Library (Rochester General Hospital), **http://www.nyam.org/library/**

- **Ohio:** Consumer Health Library (Akron General Medical Center, Medical & Consumer Health Library), **http://www.akrongeneral.org/hwlibrary.htm**

- **Oklahoma:** The Health Information Center at Saint Francis Hospital (Saint Francis Health System, Tulsa), **http://www.sfh-tulsa.com/services/healthinfo.asp**

- **Oregon:** Planetree Health Resource Center (Mid-Columbia Medical Center, The Dalles), **http://www.mcmc.net/phrc/**

- **Pennsylvania:** Community Health Information Library (Milton S. Hershey Medical Center, Hershey), **http://www.hmc.psu.edu/commhealth/**

- **Pennsylvania:** Community Health Resource Library (Geisinger Medical Center, Danville), **http://www.geisinger.edu/education/commlib.shtml**

- **Pennsylvania:** HealthInfo Library (Moses Taylor Hospital, Scranton), **http://www.mth.org/healthwellness.html**

- **Pennsylvania:** Hopwood Library (University of Pittsburgh, Health Sciences Library System, Pittsburgh), **http://www.hsls.pitt.edu/guides/chi/hopwood/index_html**

- **Pennsylvania:** Koop Community Health Information Center (College of Physicians of Philadelphia), **http://www.collphyphil.org/kooppg1.shtml**

- **Pennsylvania:** Learning Resources Center - Medical Library (Susquehanna Health System, Williamsport), **http://www.shscares.org/services/lrc/index.asp**

- **Pennsylvania:** Medical Library (UPMC Health System, Pittsburgh), **http://www.upmc.edu/passavant/library.htm**

- **Quebec, Canada:** Medical Library (Montreal General Hospital), **http://www.mghlib.mcgill.ca/**

- **South Dakota:** Rapid City Regional Hospital Medical Library (Rapid City Regional Hospital), **http://www.rcrh.org/Services/Library/Default.asp**

- **Texas:** Houston HealthWays (Houston Academy of Medicine-Texas Medical Center Library), **http://hhw.library.tmc.edu/**

- **Washington:** Community Health Library (Kittitas Valley Community Hospital), **http://www.kvch.com/**

- **Washington:** Southwest Washington Medical Center Library (Southwest Washington Medical Center, Vancouver), **http://www.swmedicalcenter.com/body.cfm?id=72**

APPENDIX E. YOUR RIGHTS AND INSURANCE

Overview

Any patient with muscular dystrophy faces a series of issues related more to the healthcare industry than to the medical condition itself. This appendix covers two important topics in this regard: your rights and responsibilities as a patient, and how to get the most out of your medical insurance plan.

Your Rights as a Patient

The President's Advisory Commission on Consumer Protection and Quality in the Healthcare Industry has created the following summary of your rights as a patient.[52]

Information Disclosure

Consumers have the right to receive accurate, easily understood information. Some consumers require assistance in making informed decisions about health plans, health professionals, and healthcare facilities. Such information includes:

- *Health plans.* Covered benefits, cost-sharing, and procedures for resolving complaints, licensure, certification, and accreditation status, comparable measures of quality and consumer satisfaction, provider network composition, the procedures that govern access to specialists and emergency services, and care management information.

---

[52]Adapted from Consumer Bill of Rights and Responsibilities:
http://www.hcqualitycommission.gov/press/cbor.html#head1.

- *Health professionals.* Education, board certification, and recertification, years of practice, experience performing certain procedures, and comparable measures of quality and consumer satisfaction.

- *Healthcare facilities.* Experience in performing certain procedures and services, accreditation status, comparable measures of quality, worker, and consumer satisfaction, and procedures for resolving complaints.

- *Consumer assistance programs.* Programs must be carefully structured to promote consumer confidence and to work cooperatively with health plans, providers, payers, and regulators. Desirable characteristics of such programs are sponsorship that ensures accountability to the interests of consumers and stable, adequate funding.

Choice of Providers and Plans

Consumers have the right to a choice of healthcare providers that is sufficient to ensure access to appropriate high-quality healthcare. To ensure such choice, the Commission recommends the following:

- *Provider network adequacy.* All health plan networks should provide access to sufficient numbers and types of providers to assure that all covered services will be accessible without unreasonable delay -- including access to emergency services 24 hours a day and 7 days a week. If a health plan has an insufficient number or type of providers to provide a covered benefit with the appropriate degree of specialization, the plan should ensure that the consumer obtains the benefit outside the network at no greater cost than if the benefit were obtained from participating providers.

- *Women's health services.* Women should be able to choose a qualified provider offered by a plan -- such as gynecologists, certified nurse midwives, and other qualified healthcare providers -- for the provision of covered care necessary to provide routine and preventative women's healthcare services.

- *Access to specialists.* Consumers with complex or serious medical conditions who require frequent specialty care should have direct access to a qualified specialist of their choice within a plan's network of providers. Authorizations, when required, should be for an adequate number of direct access visits under an approved treatment plan.

- *Transitional care.* Consumers who are undergoing a course of treatment for a chronic or disabling condition (or who are in the second or third trimester of a pregnancy) at the time they involuntarily change health plans or at a time when a provider is terminated by a plan for other than cause should be able to continue seeing their current specialty providers for up to 90 days (or through completion of postpartum care) to allow for transition of care.

- *Choice of health plans.* Public and private group purchasers should, wherever feasible, offer consumers a choice of high-quality health insurance plans.

Access to Emergency Services

Consumers have the right to access emergency healthcare services when and where the need arises. Health plans should provide payment when a consumer presents to an emergency department with acute symptoms of sufficient severity--including severe pain--such that a "prudent layperson" could reasonably expect the absence of medical attention to result in placing that consumer's health in serious jeopardy, serious impairment to bodily functions, or serious dysfunction of any bodily organ or part.

Participation in Treatment Decisions

Consumers have the right and responsibility to fully participate in all decisions related to their healthcare. Consumers who are unable to fully participate in treatment decisions have the right to be represented by parents, guardians, family members, or other conservators. Physicians and other health professionals should:

- Provide patients with sufficient information and opportunity to decide among treatment options consistent with the informed consent process.

- Discuss all treatment options with a patient in a culturally competent manner, including the option of no treatment at all.

- Ensure that persons with disabilities have effective communications with members of the health system in making such decisions.

- Discuss all current treatments a consumer may be undergoing.

- Discuss all risks, benefits, and consequences to treatment or nontreatment.

- Give patients the opportunity to refuse treatment and to express preferences about future treatment decisions.

- Discuss the use of advance directives -- both living wills and durable powers of attorney for healthcare -- with patients and their designated family members.

- Abide by the decisions made by their patients and/or their designated representatives consistent with the informed consent process.

Health plans, health providers, and healthcare facilities should:

- Disclose to consumers factors -- such as methods of compensation, ownership of or interest in healthcare facilities, or matters of conscience -- that could influence advice or treatment decisions.

- Assure that provider contracts do not contain any so-called "gag clauses" or other contractual mechanisms that restrict healthcare providers' ability to communicate with and advise patients about medically necessary treatment options.

- Be prohibited from penalizing or seeking retribution against healthcare professionals or other health workers for advocating on behalf of their patients.

Respect and Nondiscrimination

Consumers have the right to considerate, respectful care from all members of the healthcare industry at all times and under all circumstances. An environment of mutual respect is essential to maintain a quality healthcare system. To assure that right, the Commission recommends the following:

- Consumers must not be discriminated against in the delivery of healthcare services consistent with the benefits covered in their policy, or as required by law, based on race, ethnicity, national origin, religion, sex, age, mental or physical disability, sexual orientation, genetic information, or source of payment.

- Consumers eligible for coverage under the terms and conditions of a health plan or program, or as required by law, must not be discriminated against in marketing and enrollment practices based on race, ethnicity, national origin, religion, sex, age, mental or physical disability, sexual orientation, genetic information, or source of payment.

Confidentiality of Health Information

Consumers have the right to communicate with healthcare providers in confidence and to have the confidentiality of their individually identifiable healthcare information protected. Consumers also have the right to review and copy their own medical records and request amendments to their records.

Complaints and Appeals

Consumers have the right to a fair and efficient process for resolving differences with their health plans, healthcare providers, and the institutions that serve them, including a rigorous system of internal review and an independent system of external review. A free copy of the Patient's Bill of Rights is available from the American Hospital Association.[53]

Patient Responsibilities

Treatment is a two-way street between you and your healthcare providers. To underscore the importance of finance in modern healthcare as well as your responsibility for the financial aspects of your care, the President's Advisory Commission on Consumer Protection and Quality in the Healthcare Industry has proposed that patients understand the following "Consumer Responsibilities."[54] In a healthcare system that protects consumers' rights, it is reasonable to expect and encourage consumers to assume certain responsibilities. Greater individual involvement by the consumer in his or her care increases the likelihood of achieving the best outcome and helps support a quality-oriented, cost-conscious environment. Such responsibilities include:

- Take responsibility for maximizing healthy habits such as exercising, not smoking, and eating a healthy diet.

- Work collaboratively with healthcare providers in developing and carrying out agreed-upon treatment plans.

- Disclose relevant information and clearly communicate wants and needs.

- Use your health insurance plan's internal complaint and appeal processes to address your concerns.

- Avoid knowingly spreading disease.

---

[53] To order your free copy of the Patient's Bill of Rights, telephone 312-422-3000 or visit the American Hospital Association's Web site: **http://www.aha.org**. Click on "Resource Center," go to "Search" at bottom of page, and then type in "Patient's Bill of Rights." The Patient's Bill of Rights is also available from Fax on Demand, at 312-422-2020, document number 471124.

[54] Adapted from **http://www.hcqualitycommission.gov/press/cbor.html#head1**.

- Recognize the reality of risks, the limits of the medical science, and the human fallibility of the healthcare professional.

- Be aware of a healthcare provider's obligation to be reasonably efficient and equitable in providing care to other patients and the community.

- Become knowledgeable about your health plan's coverage and options (when available) including all covered benefits, limitations, and exclusions, rules regarding use of network providers, coverage and referral rules, appropriate processes to secure additional information, and the process to appeal coverage decisions.

- Show respect for other patients and health workers.

- Make a good-faith effort to meet financial obligations.

- Abide by administrative and operational procedures of health plans, healthcare providers, and Government health benefit programs.

Choosing an Insurance Plan

There are a number of official government agencies that help consumers understand their healthcare insurance choices.[55] The U.S. Department of Labor, in particular, recommends ten ways to make your health benefits choices work best for you.[56]

1. Your options are important. There are many different types of health benefit plans. Find out which one your employer offers, then check out the plan, or plans, offered. Your employer's human resource office, the health plan administrator, or your union can provide information to help you match your needs and preferences with the available plans. The more information you have, the better your healthcare decisions will be.

2. Reviewing the benefits available. Do the plans offered cover preventive care, well-baby care, vision or dental care? Are there deductibles? Answers to these questions can help determine the out-of-pocket expenses you may face. Matching your needs and those of your family members will result in the best possible benefits. Cheapest may not always be best. Your goal is high quality health benefits.

---

[55] More information about quality across programs is provided at the following AHRQ Web site: http://www.ahrq.gov/consumer/qntascii/qnthplan.htm.
[56] Adapted from the Department of Labor: http://www.dol.gov/dol/pwba/public/pubs/health/top10-text.html.

3. Look for quality. The quality of healthcare services varies, but quality can be measured. You should consider the quality of healthcare in deciding among the healthcare plans or options available to you. Not all health plans, doctors, hospitals and other providers give the highest quality care. Fortunately, there is quality information you can use right now to help you compare your healthcare choices. Find out how you can measure quality. Consult the U.S. Department of Health and Human Services publication "Your Guide to Choosing Quality Health Care" on the Internet at **www.ahcpr.gov/consumer**.

4. Your plan's summary plan description (SPD) provides a wealth of information. Your health plan administrator can provide you with a copy of your plan's SPD. It outlines your benefits and your legal rights under the Employee Retirement Income Security Act (ERISA), the federal law that protects your health benefits. It should contain information about the coverage of dependents, what services will require a co-pay, and the circumstances under which your employer can change or terminate a health benefits plan. Save the SPD and all other health plan brochures and documents, along with memos or correspondence from your employer relating to health benefits.

5. Assess your benefit coverage as your family status changes. Marriage, divorce, childbirth or adoption, and the death of a spouse are all life events that may signal a need to change your health benefits. You, your spouse and dependent children may be eligible for a special enrollment period under provisions of the Health Insurance Portability and Accountability Act (HIPAA). Even without life-changing events, the information provided by your employer should tell you how you can change benefits or switch plans, if more than one plan is offered. If your spouse's employer also offers a health benefits package, consider coordinating both plans for maximum coverage.

6. Changing jobs and other life events can affect your health benefits. Under the Consolidated Omnibus Budget Reconciliation Act (COBRA), you, your covered spouse, and your dependent children may be eligible to purchase extended health coverage under your employer's plan if you lose your job, change employers, get divorced, or upon occurrence of certain other events. Coverage can range from 18 to 36 months depending on your situation. COBRA applies to most employers with 20 or more workers and requires your plan to notify you of your rights. Most plans require eligible individuals to make their COBRA election within 60 days of the plan's notice. Be sure to follow up with your plan sponsor if you don't receive notice, and make sure you respond within the allotted time.

7. HIPAA can also help if you are changing jobs, particularly if you have a medical condition. HIPAA generally limits pre-existing condition exclusions to a maximum of 12 months (18 months for late enrollees). HIPAA also requires this maximum period to be reduced by the length of time you had prior "creditable coverage." You should receive a certificate documenting your prior creditable coverage from your old plan when coverage ends.

8. Plan for retirement. Before you retire, find out what health benefits, if any, extend to you and your spouse during your retirement years. Consult with your employer's human resources office, your union, the plan administrator, and check your SPD. Make sure there is no conflicting information among these sources about the benefits you will receive or the circumstances under which they can change or be eliminated. With this information in hand, you can make other important choices, like finding out if you are eligible for Medicare and Medigap insurance coverage.

9. Know how to file an appeal if your health benefits claim is denied. Understand how your plan handles grievances and where to make appeals of the plan's decisions. Keep records and copies of correspondence. Check your health benefits package and your SPD to determine who is responsible for handling problems with benefit claims. Contact PWBA for customer service assistance if you are unable to obtain a response to your complaint.

10. You can take steps to improve the quality of the healthcare and the health benefits you receive. Look for and use things like Quality Reports and Accreditation Reports whenever you can. Quality reports may contain consumer ratings -- how satisfied consumers are with the doctors in their plan, for instance-- and clinical performance measures -- how well a healthcare organization prevents and treats illness. Accreditation reports provide information on how accredited organizations meet national standards, and often include clinical performance measures. Look for these quality measures whenever possible. Consult "Your Guide to Choosing Quality Health Care" on the Internet at **www.ahcpr.gov/consumer**.

Medicare and Medicaid

Illness strikes both rich and poor families. For low-income families, Medicaid is available to defer the costs of treatment. The Health Care Financing Administration (HCFA) administers Medicare, the nation's largest health insurance program, which covers 39 million Americans. In the following pages, you will learn the basics about Medicare insurance as well as useful contact information on how to find more in-depth information about Medicaid.[57]

Who Is Eligible for Medicare?

Generally, you are eligible for Medicare if you or your spouse worked for at least 10 years in Medicare-covered employment and you are 65 years old and a citizen or permanent resident of the United States. You might also qualify for coverage if you are under age 65 but have a disability or End-Stage Renal disease (permanent kidney failure requiring dialysis or transplant). Here are some simple guidelines:

You can get Part A at age 65 without having to pay premiums if:

- You are already receiving retirement benefits from Social Security or the Railroad Retirement Board.

- You are eligible to receive Social Security or Railroad benefits but have not yet filed for them.

- You or your spouse had Medicare-covered government employment.

If you are under 65, you can get Part A without having to pay premiums if:

- You have received Social Security or Railroad Retirement Board disability benefit for 24 months.

- You are a kidney dialysis or kidney transplant patient.

Medicare has two parts:

- Part A (Hospital Insurance). Most people do not have to pay for Part A.

- Part B (Medical Insurance). Most people pay monthly for Part B.

Part A (Hospital Insurance)

Helps Pay For: Inpatient hospital care, care in critical access hospitals (small facilities that give limited outpatient and inpatient services to people in rural areas) and skilled nursing facilities, hospice care, and some home healthcare.

---

[57] This section has been adapted from the Official U.S. Site for Medicare Information: **http://www.medicare.gov/Basics/Overview.asp**.

Cost: Most people get Part A automatically when they turn age 65. You do not have to pay a monthly payment called a premium for Part A because you or a spouse paid Medicare taxes while you were working.

If you (or your spouse) did not pay Medicare taxes while you were working and you are age 65 or older, you still may be able to buy Part A. If you are not sure you have Part A, look on your red, white, and blue Medicare card. It will show "Hospital Part A" on the lower left corner of the card. You can also call the Social Security Administration toll free at 1-800-772-1213 or call your local Social Security office for more information about buying Part A. If you get benefits from the Railroad Retirement Board, call your local RRB office or 1-800-808-0772. For more information, call your Fiscal Intermediary about Part A bills and services. The phone number for the Fiscal Intermediary office in your area can be obtained from the following Web site: **http://www.medicare.gov/Contacts/home.asp**.

Part B (Medical Insurance)

Helps Pay For: Doctors, services, outpatient hospital care, and some other medical services that Part A does not cover, such as the services of physical and occupational therapists, and some home healthcare. Part B helps pay for covered services and supplies when they are medically necessary.

Cost: As of 2001, you pay the Medicare Part B premium of $50.00 per month. In some cases this amount may be higher if you did not choose Part B when you first became eligible at age 65. The cost of Part B may go up 10% for each 12-month period that you were eligible for Part B but declined coverage, except in special cases. You will have to pay the extra 10% cost for the rest of your life.

Enrolling in Part B is your choice. You can sign up for Part B anytime during a 7-month period that begins 3 months before you turn 65. Visit your local Social Security office, or call the Social Security Administration at 1-800-772-1213 to sign up. If you choose to enroll in Part B, the premium is usually taken out of your monthly Social Security, Railroad Retirement, or Civil Service Retirement payment. If you do not receive any of the above payments, Medicare sends you a bill for your part B premium every 3 months. You should receive your Medicare premium bill in the mail by the 10th of the month. If you do not, call the Social Security Administration at 1-800-772-1213, or your local Social Security office. If you get benefits from the Railroad Retirement Board, call your local RRB office or 1-800-808-0772. For more information, call your Medicare carrier about bills and services. The phone number for the Medicare carrier in your area can be found at the following Web site: **http://www.medicare.gov/Contacts/home.asp**. You may have choices in how you get your healthcare including the Original Medicare Plan, Medicare Managed Care Plans (like HMOs), and Medicare Private Fee-for-Service Plans.

Medicaid

Medicaid is a joint federal and state program that helps pay medical costs for some people with low incomes and limited resources. Medicaid programs vary from state to state. People on Medicaid may also get coverage for nursing home care and outpatient prescription drugs which are not covered by Medicare. You can find more information about Medicaid on the HCFA.gov Web site at **http://www.hcfa.gov/medicaid/medicaid.htm**.

States also have programs that pay some or all of Medicare's premiums and may also pay Medicare deductibles and coinsurance for certain people who have Medicare and a low income. To qualify, you must have:

- Part A (Hospital Insurance),
- Assets, such as bank accounts, stocks, and bonds that are not more than $4,000 for a single person, or $6,000 for a couple, and
- A monthly income that is below certain limits.

For more information, look at the Medicare Savings Programs brochure, **http://www.medicare.gov/Library/PDFNavigation/PDFInterim.asp?Langua ge=English&Type=Pub&PubID=10126**. There are also Prescription Drug Assistance Programs available. Find information on these programs which offer discounts or free medications to individuals in need at **http://www.medicare.gov/Prescription/Home.asp**.

NORD's Medication Assistance Programs

Finally, the National Organization for Rare Disorders, Inc. (NORD) administers medication programs sponsored by humanitarian-minded pharmaceutical and biotechnology companies to help uninsured or under-insured individuals secure life-saving or life-sustaining drugs.[58] NORD programs ensure that certain vital drugs are available "to those individuals whose income is too high to qualify for Medicaid but too low to pay for their

---

[58] Adapted from NORD: **http://www.rarediseases.org/programs/medication**.

prescribed medications." The program has standards for fairness, equity, and unbiased eligibility. It currently covers some 14 programs for nine pharmaceutical companies. NORD also offers early access programs for investigational new drugs (IND) under the approved "Treatment INDs" programs of the Food and Drug Administration (FDA). In these programs, a limited number of individuals can receive investigational drugs that have yet to be approved by the FDA. These programs are generally designed for rare diseases or disorders. For more information, visit **www.rarediseases.org**.

Additional Resources

In addition to the references already listed in this chapter, you may need more information on health insurance, hospitals, or the healthcare system in general. The NIH has set up an excellent guidance Web site that addresses these and other issues. Topics include:[59]

- Health Insurance:
  http://www.nlm.nih.gov/medlineplus/healthinsurance.html

- Health Statistics:
  http://www.nlm.nih.gov/medlineplus/healthstatistics.html

- HMO and Managed Care:
  http://www.nlm.nih.gov/medlineplus/managedcare.html

- Hospice Care: **http://www.nlm.nih.gov/medlineplus/hospicecare.html**

- Medicaid: **http://www.nlm.nih.gov/medlineplus/medicaid.html**

- Medicare: **http://www.nlm.nih.gov/medlineplus/medicare.html**

- Nursing Homes and Long-Term Care:
  http://www.nlm.nih.gov/medlineplus/nursinghomes.html

- Patient's Rights, Confidentiality, Informed Consent, Ombudsman Programs, Privacy and Patient Issues:
  http://www.nlm.nih.gov/medlineplus/patientissues.html

- Veteran's Health, Persian Gulf War, Gulf War Syndrome, Agent Orange:
  http://www.nlm.nih.gov/medlineplus/veteranshealth.html

---

[59] You can access this information at
http://www.nlm.nih.gov/medlineplus/healthsystem.html.

ONLINE GLOSSARIES

The Internet provides access to a number of free-to-use medical dictionaries and glossaries. The National Library of Medicine has compiled the following list of online dictionaries:

- ADAM Medical Encyclopedia (A.D.A.M., Inc.), comprehensive medical reference: **http://www.nlm.nih.gov/medlineplus/encyclopedia.html**

- MedicineNet.com Medical Dictionary (MedicineNet, Inc.): **http://www.medterms.com/Script/Main/hp.asp**

- Merriam-Webster Medical Dictionary (Inteli-Health, Inc.): **http://www.intelihealth.com/IH/**

- Multilingual Glossary of Technical and Popular Medical Terms in Eight European Languages (European Commission) - Danish, Dutch, English, French, German, Italian, Portuguese, and Spanish: **http://allserv.rug.ac.be/~rvdstich/eugloss/welcome.html**

- On-line Medical Dictionary (CancerWEB): **http://www.graylab.ac.uk/omd/**

- Technology Glossary (National Library of Medicine) - Health Care Technology: **http://www.nlm.nih.gov/nichsr/ta101/ta10108.htm**

- Terms and Definitions (Office of Rare Diseases): **http://rarediseases.info.nih.gov/ord/glossary_a-e.html**

Beyond these, MEDLINEplus contains a very user-friendly encyclopedia covering every aspect of medicine (licensed from A.D.A.M., Inc.). The ADAM Medical Encyclopedia can be accessed via the following Web site address: **http://www.nlm.nih.gov/medlineplus/encyclopedia.html**. ADAM is also available on commercial Web sites such as Web MD (**http://my.webmd.com/adam/asset/adam_disease_articles/a_to_z/a**) and drkoop.com (**http://www.drkoop.com/**). Topics of interest can be researched by using keywords before continuing elsewhere, as these basic definitions and concepts will be useful in more advanced areas of research. You may choose to print various pages specifically relating to muscular dystrophy and keep them on file. The NIH, in particular, suggests that patients with muscular dystrophy visit the following Web sites in the ADAM Medical Encyclopedia:

- **Basic Guidelines for Muscular Dystrophy**

  Muscular dystrophy
  Web site:
  http://www.nlm.nih.gov/medlineplus/ency/article/001190.htm

  Muscular dystrophy - resources
  Web site:
  http://www.nlm.nih.gov/medlineplus/ency/article/002154.htm

- **Signs & Symptoms for Muscular Dystrophy**

  Drooling
  Web site:
  http://www.nlm.nih.gov/medlineplus/ency/article/003048.htm

  Eyelid drooping
  Web site:
  http://www.nlm.nih.gov/medlineplus/ency/article/003035.htm

  Hearing loss
  Web site:
  http://www.nlm.nih.gov/medlineplus/ency/article/003044.htm

  Hyperthermia
  Web site:
  http://www.nlm.nih.gov/medlineplus/ency/article/003090.htm

  Hypotonia
  Web site:
  http://www.nlm.nih.gov/medlineplus/ency/article/003298.htm

  Lordosis
  Web site:
  http://www.nlm.nih.gov/medlineplus/ency/article/003278.htm

  Muscle contractures
  Web site:
  http://www.nlm.nih.gov/medlineplus/ency/article/003193.htm

  Muscle weakness
  Web site:
  http://www.nlm.nih.gov/medlineplus/ency/article/003174.htm

Problems walking
Web site:
http://www.nlm.nih.gov/medlineplus/ency/article/003199.htm

Wasting
Web site:
http://www.nlm.nih.gov/medlineplus/ency/article/003188.htm

Weakness
Web site:
http://www.nlm.nih.gov/medlineplus/ency/article/003174.htm

- **Diagnostics and Tests for Muscular Dystrophy**

Aldolase
Web site:
http://www.nlm.nih.gov/medlineplus/ency/article/003566.htm

ALT
Web site:
http://www.nlm.nih.gov/medlineplus/ency/article/003473.htm

ANA
Web site:
http://www.nlm.nih.gov/medlineplus/ency/article/003535.htm

AST
Web site:
http://www.nlm.nih.gov/medlineplus/ency/article/003472.htm

Biopsy
Web site:
http://www.nlm.nih.gov/medlineplus/ency/article/003416.htm

Chorionic villus sampling
Web site:
http://www.nlm.nih.gov/medlineplus/ency/article/003406.htm

CPK
Web site:
http://www.nlm.nih.gov/medlineplus/ency/article/003503.htm

CPK isoenzymes
Web site:
http://www.nlm.nih.gov/medlineplus/ency/article/003504.htm

Creatine kinase
Web site:
http://www.nlm.nih.gov/medlineplus/ency/article/003503.htm

Creatinine
Web site:
http://www.nlm.nih.gov/medlineplus/ency/article/003475.htm

Creatinine - urine
Web site:
http://www.nlm.nih.gov/medlineplus/ency/article/003610.htm

Differential
Web site:
http://www.nlm.nih.gov/medlineplus/ency/article/003657.htm

ECG
Web site:
http://www.nlm.nih.gov/medlineplus/ency/article/003868.htm

Electromyography
Web site:
http://www.nlm.nih.gov/medlineplus/ency/article/003929.htm

EMG
Web site:
http://www.nlm.nih.gov/medlineplus/ency/article/003929.htm

FSH
Web site:
http://www.nlm.nih.gov/medlineplus/ency/article/003710.htm

LDH
Web site:
http://www.nlm.nih.gov/medlineplus/ency/article/003471.htm

LDH isoenzymes
Web site:
http://www.nlm.nih.gov/medlineplus/ency/article/003499.htm

MRI
Web site:
http://www.nlm.nih.gov/medlineplus/ency/article/003335.htm

Muscle biopsy
Web site:
http://www.nlm.nih.gov/medlineplus/ency/article/003924.htm

Myoglobin - serum
Web site:
http://www.nlm.nih.gov/medlineplus/ency/article/003663.htm

Myoglobin - urine
Web site:
http://www.nlm.nih.gov/medlineplus/ency/article/003664.htm

Serum CPK
Web site:
http://www.nlm.nih.gov/medlineplus/ency/article/003503.htm

- **Background Topics for Muscular Dystrophy**

Gene
Web site:
http://www.nlm.nih.gov/medlineplus/ency/article/002371.htm

Genes
Web site:
http://www.nlm.nih.gov/medlineplus/ency/article/002371.htm

Genetic counseling
Web site:
http://www.nlm.nih.gov/medlineplus/ency/article/002053.htm

Inheritance
Web site:
http://www.nlm.nih.gov/medlineplus/ency/article/002048.htm

Muscular dystrophy - support group
Web site:
http://www.nlm.nih.gov/medlineplus/ency/article/002154.htm

Prenatal diagnosis
Web site:
http://www.nlm.nih.gov/medlineplus/ency/article/002053.htm

Proximal
Web site:
http://www.nlm.nih.gov/medlineplus/ency/article/002287.htm

Respiratory
Web site:
http://www.nlm.nih.gov/medlineplus/ency/article/002290.htm

Online Dictionary Directories

The following are additional online directories compiled by the National Library of Medicine, including a number of specialized medical dictionaries and glossaries:

- Medical Dictionaries: Medical & Biological (World Health Organization):
  http://www.who.int/hlt/virtuallibrary/English/diction.htm#Medical

- MEL-Michigan Electronic Library List of Online Health and Medical Dictionaries (Michigan Electronic Library):
  http://mel.lib.mi.us/health/health-dictionaries.html

- Patient Education: Glossaries (DMOZ Open Directory Project):
  http://dmoz.org/Health/Education/Patient_Education/Glossaries/

- Web of Online Dictionaries (Bucknell University):
  http://www.yourdictionary.com/diction5.html#medicine

MUSCULAR DYSTROPHY GLOSSARY

The following is a complete glossary of terms used in this sourcebook. The definitions are derived from official public sources including the National Institutes of Health [NIH] and the European Union [EU]. After this glossary, we list a number of additional hardbound and electronic glossaries and dictionaries that you may wish to consult.

Adjustment: The dynamic process wherein the thoughts, feelings, behavior, and biophysiological mechanisms of the individual continually change to adjust to the environment. [NIH]

Ameliorating: A changeable condition which prevents the consequence of a failure or accident from becoming as bad as it otherwise would. [NIH]

Amplification: The production of additional copies of a chromosomal DNA sequence, found as either intrachromosomal or extrachromosomal DNA. [NIH]

Apnea: Cessation of breathing. [NIH]

Applicability: A list of the commodities to which the candidate method can be applied as presented or with minor modifications. [NIH]

ATP: ATP an abbreviation for adenosine triphosphate, a compound which serves as a carrier of energy for cells. [NIH]

Attenuated: Strain with weakened or reduced virulence. [NIH]

Audiologist: Study of hearing including treatment of persons with hearing defects. [NIH]

Avian: A plasmodial infection in birds. [NIH]

Axonal: Condition associated with metabolic derangement of the entire neuron and is manifest by degeneration of the distal portion of the nerve fiber. [NIH]

Bell's palsy: Paralysis of the upper and lower muscles of the face on one side, due to inflammation of the facial nerve within the stylomastoid foramen. [NIH]

Bernstein: A sensitive means of determining whether acid reflux is the cause of pain, but may be falsely negative in the patient receiving treatment. [NIH]

Bioengineering: The application of engineering principles to the solution of biological problems, for example, remote-handling devices, life-support systems, controls, and displays. [NIH]

Biophysics: The science of physical phenomena and processes in living organisms. [NIH]

Blot: To transfer DNA, RNA, or proteins to an immobilizing matrix such as nitrocellulose. [NIH]

Bowen: Intraepithelial epithelioma affecting the skin and sometimes the mucous membranes. [NIH]

Brace: Any form of splint or appliance used to support the limbs or trunk. [NIH]

Caspase: Enzyme released by the cell at a crucial stage in apoptosis in order to shred all cellular proteins. [NIH]

Cataracts: In medicine, an opacity of the crystalline lens of the eye obstructing partially or totally its transmission of light. [NIH]

CDNA: Synthetic DNA reverse transcribed from a specific RNA through the action of the enzyme reverse transcriptase. DNA synthesized by reverse transcriptase using RNA as a template. [NIH]

Chaos: Complex behavior that seems random but actually has some hidden order. [NIH]

Cloning: The production of a number of genetically identical individuals; in genetic engineering, a process for the efficient replication of a great number of identical DNA molecules. [NIH]

CMV: A virus that belongs to the herpes virus group. [NIH]

Codons: Any triplet of nucleotides (coding unit) in DNA or RNA (if RNA is the carrier of primary genetic information as in some viruses) that codes for particular amino acid or signals the beginning or end of the message. [NIH]

Compassionate: A process for providing experimental drugs to very sick patients who have no treatment options. [NIH]

Complementation: The production of a wild-type phenotype when two different mutations are combined in a diploid or a heterokaryon and tested in trans-configuration. [NIH]

Consultation: A deliberation between two or more physicians concerning the diagnosis and the proper method of treatment in a case. [NIH]

Continuum: An area over which the vegetation or animal population is of constantly changing composition so that homogeneous, separate communities cannot be distinguished. [NIH]

Contraindications: Any factor or sign that it is unwise to pursue a certain kind of action or treatment, e. g. giving a general anesthetic to a person with pneumonia. [NIH]

Crawford: Variation of the luminosity of a light stimulus with position of entry of the light pencil through the pupil. [NIH]

Cytotoxicity: Quality of being capable of producing a specific toxic action upon cells of special organs. [NIH]

Deletion: A genetic rearrangement through loss of segments of DNA (chromosomes), bringing sequences, which are normally separated, into close proximity. [NIH]

Density: The logarithm to the base 10 of the opacity of an exposed and processed film. [NIH]

Diaphragm: Contraceptive intra-uterine device. [NIH]

Dilantin: A drug that is often used to control seizures. [NIH]

Diploid: Having two sets of chromosomes. [NIH]

Dissection: Cutting up of an organism for study. [NIH]

Dystrophic: Pertaining to toxic habitats low in nutrients. [NIH]

EEG: A graphic recording of the changes in electrical potential associated with the activity of the cerebral cortex made with the electroencephalogram. [NIH]

Effector: It is often an enzyme that converts an inactive precursor molecule into an active second messenger. [NIH]

Egger: Line formed by the attachment of the hyaloideo-capsular ligament to the posterior capsule of the crystalline lens, in a ring of about 9 mm in diameter. [NIH]

ELISA: A sensitive analytical technique in which an enzyme is complexed to an antigen or antibody. A substrate is then added which generates a color proportional to the amount of binding. This method can be adapted to a solid-phase technique. [NIH]

Enhancer: Transcriptional element in the virus genome. [NIH]

Enzymatic: Phase where enzyme cuts the precursor protein. [NIH]

Eosinophil: A polymorphonuclear leucocyte with large eosinophilic granules in its cytoplasm, which plays a role in hypersensitivity reactions. [NIH]

Epitope: A molecule or portion of a molecule capable of binding to the combining site of an antibody. For every given antigenic determinant, the body can construct a variety of antibody-combining sites, some of which fit almost perfectly, and others which barely fit. [NIH]

Escalation: Progressive use of more harmful drugs. [NIH]

Essential Tremor: A rhythmic, involuntary, purposeless, oscillating movement resulting from the alternate contraction and relaxation of opposing groups of muscles. [NIH]

Eukaryote: An organism (or a cell) that carries its genetic material physically constrained within a nuclear membrane, separate from the cytoplasm. [NIH]

Excitability: Property of a cardiac cell whereby, when the cell is depolarized to a critical level (called threshold), the membrane becomes permeable and a regenerative inward current causes an action potential. [NIH]

Excitotoxicity: Excessive exposure to glutamate or related compounds can kill brain neurons, presumably by overstimulating them. [NIH]

Exon: The part of the DNA that encodes the information for the actual amino acid sequence of the protein. In many eucaryotic genes, the coding sequences consist of a series of exons alternating with intron sequences. [NIH]

Extensor: A muscle whose contraction tends to straighten a limb; the antagonist of a flexor. [NIH]

Extraocular: External to or outside of the eye. [NIH]

Fibronectin: An adhesive glycoprotein. One form circulates in plasma, acting as an opsonin; another is a cell-surface protein which mediates cellular adhesive interactions. [NIH]

Frameshift: A type of mutation which causes out-of-phase transcription of the base sequence; such mutations arise from the addition or delection of nucleotide(s) in numbers other than 3 or multiples of 3. [NIH]

Fuchs: A spur of indented, iridic, posterior pigment epithelium into the posterior surface of the sphincter pupillae muscle, about midway along its length, associated with the junction of a few fibers of the dilator pupillae muscle. [NIH]

Genetics: The biological science that deals with the phenomena and mechanisms of heredity. [NIH]

Grafting: The operation of transfer of tissue from one site to another. [NIH]

GTPase: Enzyme that hydrolyzes guanosine triphosphate (GTP). [NIH]

Hammer: The largest of the three ossicles of the ear. [NIH]

Handicap: A handicap occurs as a result of disability, but disability does not always constitute a handicap. A handicap may be said to exist when a disability causes a substantial and continuing reduction in a person's capacity to function socially and vocationally. [NIH]

Hereditary: Of, relating to, or denoting factors that can be transmitted genetically from one generation to another. [NIH]

Heterogeneity: The property of one or more samples or populations which implies that they are not identical in respect of some or all of their parameters, e. g. heterogeneity of variance. [NIH]

Heterozygotes: Having unlike alleles at one or more corresponding loci on homologous chromosomes. [NIH]

Holt: An empirical method for computing compensation for loss of vision, based on the assumption that the total loss of vision of one eye is an 18% loss of the total function of the body. [NIH]

Homodimer: Protein-binding "activation domains" always combine with identical proteins. [NIH]

Hospice: Institution dedicated to caring for the terminally ill. [NIH]

Hybrid: Cross fertilization between two varieties or, more usually, two species of vines, see also crossing. [NIH]

Immunofluorescence: A technique for identifying molecules present on the surfaces of cells or in tissues using a highly fluorescent substance coupled to a specific antibody. [NIH]

Impairment: In the context of health experience, an impairment is any loss or abnormality of psychological, physiological, or anatomical structure or function. [NIH]

Infancy: The period of complete dependency prior to the acquisition of competence in walking, talking, and self-feeding. [NIH]

Infections: The illnesses caused by an organism that usually does not cause disease in a person with a normal immune system. [NIH]

Initiation: Mutation induced by a chemical reactive substance causing cell changes; being a step in a carcinogenic process. [NIH]

Insight: The capacity to understand one's own motives, to be aware of one's own psychodynamics, to appreciate the meaning of symbolic behavior. [NIH]

Involuntary: Reaction occurring without intention or volition. [NIH]

Koch: It was an early form of tuberculin of low specificity, devised by Robert Koch and made by heat concentration of a broth culture of Mycobacterium tuberculosis. [NIH]

Ligands: A RNA simulation method developed by the MIT. [NIH]

Linkage: The tendency of two or more genes in the same chromosome to remain together from one generation to the next more frequently than expected according to the law of independent assortment. [NIH]

Migration: The systematic movement of genes between populations of the same species, geographic race, or variety. [NIH]

Mitotic: Cell resulting from mitosis. [NIH]

Modeling: A treatment procedure whereby the therapist presents the target behavior which the learner is to imitate and make part of his repertoire. [NIH]

Modification: A change in an organism, or in a process in an organism, that is acquired from its own activity or environment. [NIH]

Monitor: An apparatus which automatically records such physiological signs as respiration, pulse, and blood pressure in an anesthetized patient or one undergoing surgical or other procedures. [NIH]

Monoclonal: An antibody produced by culturing a single type of cell. It therefore consists of a single species of immunoglobulin molecules. [NIH]

Morphological: Relating to the configuration or the structure of live organs. [NIH]

MRNA: The RNA molecule that conveys from the DNA the information that is to be translated into the structure of a particular polypeptide molecule. [NIH]

Nerve: A cordlike structure of nervous tissue that connects parts of the nervous system with other tissues of the body and conveys nervous impulses to, or away from, these tissues. [NIH]

Networks: Pertaining to a nerve or to the nerves, a meshlike structure of interlocking fibers or strands. [NIH]

Noguchi: A medium composed of fresh rabbit kidney tissue in sterile ascitic fluid under vaseline in narrow tubes. [NIH]

Nucleus: A body of specialized protoplasm found in nearly all cells and containing the chromosomes. [NIH]

Orbicularis: A thin layer of fibers that originates at the posterior lacrimal crest and passes outward and forward, dividing into two slips which surround the canaliculi. [NIH]

Orderly: A male hospital attendant. [NIH]

Outpatient: A patient who is not an inmate of a hospital but receives diagnosis or treatment in a clinic or dispensary connected with the hospital. [NIH]

Patch: A piece of material used to cover or protect a wound, an injured part, etc.: a patch over the eye. [NIH]

Pathologies: The study of abnormality, especially the study of diseases. [NIH]

Pediatrics: The branch of medical science concerned with children and their diseases. [NIH]

Pharmacodynamic: Is concerned with the response of living tissues to chemical stimuli, that is, the action of drugs on the living organism in the absence of disease. [NIH]

Pharmacokinetic: The mathematical analysis of the time courses of absorption, distribution, and elimination of drugs. [NIH]

Phenotypes: An organism as observed, i. e. as judged by its visually perceptible characters resulting from the interaction of its genotype with the environment. [NIH]

Phosphorylated: Attached to a phosphate group. [NIH]

Photoreceptor: Receptor capable of being activated by light stimuli, as a rod or cone cell of the eye. [NIH]

Physiology: The science that deals with the life processes and functions of organismus, their cells, tissues, and organs. [NIH]

Plasmid: An autonomously replicating, extra-chromosomal DNA molecule found in many bacteria. Plasmids are widely used as carriers of cloned genes. [NIH]

Polymerase: An enzyme which catalyses the synthesis of DNA using a single DNA strand as a template. The polymerase copies the template in the 5'-3'direction provided that sufficient quantities of free nucleotides, dATP and dTTP are present. [NIH]

Polymorphism: The occurrence together of two or more distinct forms in the same population. [NIH]

Postsynaptic: Nerve potential generated by an inhibitory hyperpolarizing stimulation. [NIH]

Potassium: It is essential to the ability of muscle cells to contract. [NIH]

Prion: Small proteinaceous infectious particles that resist inactivation by procedures modifying nucleic acids and contain an abnormal isoform of a cellular protein which is a major and necessary component. [NIH]

Probe: An instrument used in exploring cavities, or in the detection and dilatation of strictures, or in demonstrating the potency of channels; an elongated instrument for exploring or sounding body cavities. [NIH]

Promoter: A chemical substance that increases the activity of a carcinogenic process. [NIH]

Promotor: In an operon, a nucleotide sequence located at the operator end which contains all the signals for the correct initiation of genetic transcription by the RNA polymerase holoenzyme and determines the maximal rate of RNA synthesis. [NIH]

Prone: Having the front portion of the body downwards. [NIH]

Protease: Any enzyme that catalyzes hydrolysis of a protein. [NIH]

Protocol: The detailed plan for a clinical trial that states the trial's rationale, purpose, drug or vaccine dosages, length of study, routes of administration, who may participate, and other aspects of trial design. [NIH]

Purifying: Respiratory equipment whose function is to remove contaminants from otherwise wholesome air. [NIH]

Recombination: The formation of new combinations of genes as a result of segregation in crosses between genetically different parents; also the rearrangement of linked genes due to crossing-over. [NIH]

Reentry: Reexcitation caused by continuous propagation of the same impulse for one or more cycles. [NIH]

Refer: To send or direct for treatment, aid, information, de decision. [NIH]

Repressor: Any of the specific allosteric protein molecules, products of regulator genes, which bind to the operator of operons and prevent RNA polymerase from proceeding into the operon to transcribe messenger RNA. [NIH]

Rett Syndrome: A neurological disorder seen almost exclusively in females, and found in a variety of racial and ethnic groups worldwide. [NIH]

Reversion: A return to the original condition, e. g. the reappearance of the normal or wild type in previously mutated cells, tissues, or organisms. [NIH]

Sarcomere: The repeating structural unit of a striated muscle fiber. [NIH]

Satellite: Applied to a vein which closely accompanies an artery for some distance; in cytogenetics, a chromosomal agent separated by a secondary constriction from the main body of the chromosome. [NIH]

Schizophrenia: A mental disorder characterized by a special type of disintegration of the personality. [NIH]

Schwann: A neurilemmal cell from the sheath of a peripheral nerve fiber. [NIH]

Scoliosis: A lateral curvature of the spine. [NIH]

Secretory: Secreting; relating to or influencing secretion or the secretions. [NIH]

Sendai: A virus that causes an important and widespread infection of laboratory mice; it belongs to the parainfluenza group of mixoviruses. The virus is widely used in cell fusion studies. [NIH]

Senescence: The bodily and mental state associated with advancing age. [NIH]

Senile: Relating or belonging to old age; characteristic of old age; resulting from infirmity of old age. [NIH]

Sequencing: The determination of the order of nucleotides in a DNA or RNA chain. [NIH]

Sequester: A portion of dead bone which has become detached from the healthy bone tissue, as occurs in necrosis. [NIH]

Specialist: In medicine, one who concentrates on 1 special branch of medical science. [NIH]

Specificity: Degree of selectivity shown by an antibody with respect to the number and types of antigens with which the antibody combines, as well as with respect to the rates and the extents of these reactions. [NIH]

Spectrometer: An apparatus for determining spectra; measures quantities such as wavelengths and relative amplitudes of components. [NIH]

Spectroscopic: The recognition of elements through their emission spectra. [NIH]

Stomatology: The branch of medical science concerned with the mouth and its diseases. [NIH]

Suppression: A conscious exclusion of disapproved desire contrary with repression, in which the process of exclusion is not conscious. [NIH]

Synapse: The region where the processes of two neurons come into close contiguity, and the nervous impulse passes from one to the other; the fibers of the two are intermeshed, but, according to the general view, there is no direct contiguity. [NIH]

Temporal: One of the two irregular bones forming part of the lateral surfaces and base of the skull, and containing the organs of hearing. [NIH]

Therapeutics: The branch of medicine which is concerned with the treatment of diseases, palliative or curative. [NIH]

Tonus: A state of slight tension usually present in muscles even when they are not undergoing active contraction. [NIH]

Transduction: The transfer of genes from one cell to another by means of a viral (in the case of bacteria, a bacteriophage) vector or a vector which is similar to a virus particle (pseudovirion). [NIH]

Translational: The cleavage of signal sequence that directs the passage of the protein through a cell or organelle membrane. [NIH]

Translocation: The movement of material in solution inside the body of the plant. [NIH]

Transmitter: A chemical substance which effects the passage of nerve impulses from one cell to the other at the synapse. [NIH]

Ubiquitin: A highly conserved 76 amino acid-protein found in all eukaryotic cells. [NIH]

Ulcer: A localized necrotic lesion of the skin or a mucous surface. [NIH]

Vacuole: A fluid-filled cavity within the cytoplasm of a cell. [NIH]

Vector: Plasmid or other self-replicating DNA molecule that transfers DNA between cells in nature or in recombinant DNA technology. [NIH]

Venom: That produced by the poison glands of the mouth and injected by the fangs of poisonous snakes. [NIH]

Villus: Cell found in the lining of the small intestine. [NIH]

Virion: A complete, mature, infectious virus particle. [NIH]

Vitro: Descriptive of an event or enzyme reaction under experimental investigation occurring outside a living organism. Parts of an organism or microorganism are used together with artificial substrates and/or conditions. [NIH]

General Dictionaries and Glossaries

While the above glossary is essentially complete, the dictionaries listed here cover virtually all aspects of medicine, from basic words and phrases to more advanced terms (sorted alphabetically by title; hyperlinks provide rankings, information and reviews at Amazon.com):

- **Dictionary of Medical Acronymns & Abbreviations** by Stanley Jablonski (Editor), Paperback, 4th edition (2001), Lippincott Williams & Wilkins Publishers, ISBN: 1560534605,
  http://www.amazon.com/exec/obidos/ASIN/1560534605/icongroupinter na

- **Dictionary of Medical Terms: For the Nonmedical Person (Dictionary of Medical Terms for the Nonmedical Person, Ed 4)** by Mikel A. Rothenberg, M.D, et al, Paperback - 544 pages, 4th edition (2000), Barrons Educational Series, ISBN: 0764112015,
  http://www.amazon.com/exec/obidos/ASIN/0764112015/icongroupinter na

- **A Dictionary of the History of Medicine** by A. Sebastian, CD-Rom edition (2001), CRC Press-Parthenon Publishers, ISBN: 185070368X,
  http://www.amazon.com/exec/obidos/ASIN/185070368X/icongroupinter na

- **Dorland's Illustrated Medical Dictionary (Standard Version)** by Dorland, et al, Hardcover - 2088 pages, 29th edition (2000), W B Saunders Co, ISBN: 0721662544,
  http://www.amazon.com/exec/obidos/ASIN/0721662544/icongroupinter na

- **Dorland's Electronic Medical Dictionary** by Dorland, et al, Software, 29th Book & CD-Rom edition (2000), Harcourt Health Sciences, ISBN: 0721694934,
  http://www.amazon.com/exec/obidos/ASIN/0721694934/icongroupinter na

- **Dorland's Pocket Medical Dictionary (Dorland's Pocket Medical Dictionary, 26th Ed)** Hardcover - 912 pages, 26th edition (2001), W B Saunders Co, ISBN: 0721682812,
  http://www.amazon.com/exec/obidos/ASIN/0721682812/icongroupinter na/103-4193558-7304618

- **Melloni's Illustrated Medical Dictionary (Melloni's Illustrated Medical Dictionary, 4th Ed)** by Melloni, Hardcover, 4th edition (2001), CRC Press-Parthenon Publishers, ISBN: 85070094X,

http://www.amazon.com/exec/obidos/ASIN/85070094X/icongroupintern
a

- **Stedman's Electronic Medical Dictionary Version 5.0 (CD-ROM for Windows and Macintosh, Individual)** by Stedmans, CD-ROM edition (2000), Lippincott Williams & Wilkins Publishers, ISBN: 0781726328, http://www.amazon.com/exec/obidos/ASIN/0781726328/icongroupinter na

- **Stedman's Medical Dictionary** by Thomas Lathrop Stedman, Hardcover - 2098 pages, 27th edition (2000), Lippincott, Williams & Wilkins, ISBN: 068340007X, http://www.amazon.com/exec/obidos/ASIN/068340007X/icongroupinter na

- **Tabers Cyclopedic Medical Dictionary (Thumb Index)** by Donald Venes (Editor), et al, Hardcover - 2439 pages, 19th edition (2001), F A Davis Co, ISBN: 0803606540, http://www.amazon.com/exec/obidos/ASIN/0803606540/icongroupinter na

INDEX